# Manual of Gynecologic Oncology

# Manual of Gynecologic Oncology

Editors

Christina S. Chu
Stephen C. Rubin
*University of Pennsylvania, USA*

World Scientific

NEW JERSEY • LONDON • SINGAPORE • BEIJING • SHANGHAI • HONG KONG • TAIPEI • CHENNAI

*Published by*

World Scientific Publishing Co. Pte. Ltd.
5 Toh Tuck Link, Singapore 596224
*USA office:* 27 Warren Street, Suite 401-402, Hackensack, NJ 07601
*UK office:* 57 Shelton Street, Covent Garden, London WC2H 9HE

**British Library Cataloguing-in-Publication Data**
A catalogue record for this book is available from the British Library.

**MANUAL OF GYNECOLOGIC ONCOLOGY**



ISBN-13 978-981-4343-69-5
ISBN-10 981-4343-69-2

Typeset by Stallion Press
Email: enquiries@stallionpress.com

Printed by FuIsland Offset Printing (S) Pte Ltd Singapore

*To our families*

# CONTENTS

# CONTRIBUTORS

**Sarah Adams, MD**
Assistant Professor
Division of Gynecologic Oncology
Pennsylvania Hospital
Ovarian Cancer Research Center
The University of Pennsylvania
1307 BRB II/III, 421 Curie Boulevard
Philadelphia, PA 19104, USA

**Peter A. Argenta, MD**
Associate Professor
Division of Gynecologic Oncology
Department of Obstetrics
Gynecology and Women's Health
University of Minnesota Medical School
MMC 395
420 Delaware St. SE
Minneapolis, MN 55455, USA

**Stephanie V. Blank, MD**
Director, Gynecologic Oncology Fellowship
Chief of Gynecologic Oncology at Bellevue Hospital
Assistant Professor

Department of Obstetrics and Gynecology
Division of Gynecologic Oncology
New York University School of Medicine
160 East 34th Street
New York, NY 10016, USA

**Raffi Chalian, MD**
Fellow
Division of Gynecologic Oncology
University of Pennsylvania Health System
Jordan Center for Gynecologic Cancer
3 West Pavilion
Perelman Center for Advanced Medicine at Penn
3400 Civic Center Boulevard
Philadelphia, PA 19104, USA

**Christina S. Chu, MD**
Associate Professor
Division of Gynecologic Oncology
University of Pennsylvania School of Medicine
Jordan Center for Gynecologic Cancer
3 West Pavilion
Perelman Center for Advanced Medicine at Penn
3400 Civic Center Boulevard
Philadelphia, PA 19104, USA

**Sarah Czok, MD**
Department of Obstetrics and Gynecology
Division of Gynecologic Oncology
New York University School of Medicine
160 East 34th Street
New York, NY 10016, USA

**Heidi J. Gray, MD**
Assistant Professor
Division of Gynecologic Oncology
Department of Obstetrics and Gynecology

University of Washington
Box 356460
Seattle, WA 98195, USA

**Andrea R. Hagemann, MD**
Assistant Professor, Department of Obstetrics and Gynecology
Division of Gynecologic Oncology
Washington University School of Medicine in St. Louis
4911 Barnes Hospital Plaza, Box 8064
St Louis, MO 63110, USA
3400 Spruce Street
Philadelphia, PA 19104, USA

**Yevgeniya J. Ioffe, MD**
Fellow in Gynecologic Oncology
Department of Obstetrics and Gynecology
Division of Gynecologic Oncology
Washington University School of Medicine in St. Louis
4911 Barnes Hospital Plaza, Box 8064
St Louis, MO 63110, USA

**Sarah H. Kim, MD, MSCE**
Assistant Professor
Division of Gynecologic Oncology
Department of Surgical Oncology
Fox Chase Cancer Center
333 Cottman Avenue
Philadelphia, PA 19111-2497, USA

**Rajul Kothari, MD**
Gynecologic Oncology Fellow
Department of Obstetrics
Gynecology and Women's Health
University of Minnesota Medical School
MMC 395
420 Delaware St. SE
Minneapolis, MN 55455, USA

**John B. Liao, MD, PhD**
Division of Gynecologic Oncology
Department of Obstetrics and Gynecology
University of Washington
Box 356460
1959 NE Pacific Street
Seattle, WA 98195, USA

**Lilie L. Lin, MD**
Assistant Professor
Department of Radiation Oncology
University of Pennsylvania
3400 Spruce Street
2 Donner Building
Philadelphia, PA 19104, USA

**Evelyn B. Marsh, MD**
Clinical Assistant Professor
Department of Obstetrics and Gynecology
Hospital of the University of Pennsylvania
3400 Spruce Street
5 Dulles
Philadelphia, PA 19104, USA

**Lara Bonner Millar, MD**
Resident
Department of Radiation Oncology
University of Pennsylvania
3400 Spruce Street
2 Donner Building
Philadelphia, PA 19104, USA

**Waleed S.W. Shalaby, MD, PhD**
Chief Science Officer
Poly-Med, Inc.
51 Technology Drive
Anderson, SC 29625, USA

**Janos L. Tanyi, MD, PhD, FACOG**
Assistant Professor of Gynecologic Oncology
Division of Gynecologic Oncology
University of Pennsylvania
Abramson Cancer Center
Perelman Center for Advanced Medicine
West Pavilion, 3rd Floor
3400 Civic Center Boulevard
Philadelphia, PA 19104, USA

**Premal H. Thaker, MD, MS, FACOG**
Assistant Professor
Department of Obstetrics and Gynecology
Division of Gynecologic Oncology
Washington University School of Medicine in St. Louis
4911 Barnes Hospital Plaza, Box 8064
St Louis, MO 63110, USA

# PREFACE

Since the recognition of Gynecologic Oncology as an official subspecialty in the United States in 1973, an increasing number of physicians have devoted themselves to the treatment of patients with gynecologic malignancies. This *Manual of Gynecologic Oncology* is designed to be a practical reference, appropriate for residents in Obstetrics and Gynecology, and fellows receiving training in Gynecologic Oncology. As the field is inherently collaborative, the text should also be of interest to those practicing and training in allied fields such as Medical Oncology and Radiation Oncology.

A wide range of topics are covered, with chapters addressing each major malignancy, as well as sections reviewing the basics of chemotherapy and radiation, and the management of common problems encountered in the daily practice of the specialty. The text was not designed as an exhaustive review and makes no effort to cover basic research, but it is intended to be highly readable and concise.

We are grateful to the contributing authors for their time and effort, as well as to Carmen Lord for her assistance in preparation of the manuscript.

We hope that this book will be a valuable tool for those aspiring to improve the lives of women with gynecologic cancer.

**Christina S. Chu, MD**
**Stephen C. Rubin, MD**

# 1

# CHEMOTHERAPY IN GYNECOLOGIC MALIGNANCIES

*Waleed S.W. Shalaby*

## INTRODUCTION

The modern era of cancer chemotherapy began in the 1940s with the use of nitrogen mustard as chemical warfare in World War II. It was observed that exposed victims had profound lymphoid and myeloid suppression. This observation in rapidly dividing cells led Louis Goodman and Alfred Gilman to investigate the potential therapeutic application of chemical warfare agents in cancer therapy.[1] Over the next 20 years, a number of agents were developed and found to have antitumor activity in clinical trials.

Despite many decades of basic and clinical research, cancer remains a major cause of morbidity and mortality. The basis of current cancer treatment, while still grounded in traditional cytotoxic agents, is rapidly evolving to incorporate targeted agents developed from advances in molecular pharmacology. The future emphasis of cancer therapy will undoubtedly rely on identifying new classes of molecules to optimize therapy. This chapter will address the basic concepts of cancer pharmacology and pharmacokinetics, their application in clinical trial design, drug delivery scheduling, mechanisms of existing cytotoxic agents, and new biological response modifiers. We conclude with an overview of current agents used in the treatment of gynecologic malignancies.

# GENERAL CHEMOTHERAPY PRINCIPLES AND TERMINOLOGY

Our understanding of cancer in the basic research, pre-clinical, and clinical settings have led to a number of principles that not only reflect the complexity of cancer research, but also the multi-disciplinary efforts required. The following terms are intended to provide a basic framework for conceptualizing the issues encountered with the use of cytotoxic agents as well as biologic response modifiers.

## General Characteristics of Cancer Cells

Several general properties displayed by cancer cells include unregulated proliferation, invasion of surrounding tissues, metastasis to secondary sites, failure of normal differentiation, and alteration of cellular components such as antigens, enzymes, and oncogenes. Cancers growing in the body also occupy space and crowd out normal cells. They produce nutritional deficits and weight loss due to their high metabolic rate. Cancer cells also decrease host defense mechanisms against infection.

## Tumor Factors that May Influence Drug Response

*Cell cycle* factors determine the percentage of cells in a sensitive phase during the time of exposure to pharmacologically effective concentrations of drug. In general, for cycle phase-specific agents, drug administration should allow for a duration of drug exposure of at least two cell cycles. Most drugs have their greatest activity during the S phase when cells are undergoing DNA synthesis. Cells in the G0 phase are, for the most part, refractory to chemotherapy. These cells may later re-enter the cell cycle and result in disease recurrence. Most anticancer drugs are effective against cells in one particular phase of the cycle (e.g., vincristine during M; cytarabine during S, etc.).

*Growth fraction* is the proportion of cells that are actively dividing with respect to the entire population of viable cells in any given tissue. High growth fraction tumors are more susceptible to the cytotoxic effects of anticancer drugs than those with a high percentage of dormant cells.

*Normal tissues* with high growth fractions (bone marrow, oral and intestinal mucosa, hair follicles) are also damaged by anticancer drugs, and treatment may produce predictable toxicity such as bone marrow depression (leukocytopenia and infection, thrombocytopenia and bleeding), stomatitis, GI tract ulceration, nausea/vomiting, and alopecia.

*Tumor burden* may limit successful chemotherapy. Drugs may be unable to penetrate tumor nodules in sufficient concentration to achieve cell killing. Also, most cells in a bulky tumor may be in a nonproliferative stage at the time of treatment and thus survive to re-establish the tumor mass.

*Tumor cell kill* follows first-order kinetics, i.e., each treatment results in killing a constant proportion, rather than a constant number of tumor cells, with deviation from first-order kinetics at the two ends of the response curve. After initial treatment, the rate of cell kill may change because the growth fraction and mass doubling time change as the tumor mass decreases. The slope of the response curve is also different for the residual cells because they are likely to be less sensitive to the drug or present in sites where the drug does not penetrate as well.

*Tumor doubling time* is the time it takes for the tumor to double in size.

*Tumor heterogeneity* leads to sub-populations of cells in different phases of the cell cycle, i.e., proliferative (G1S, G2M0), resting (G0), or apoptosis. The fact that tumors are not uniform must be considered.

## Mechanisms of Drug Resistance

Several mechanisms exist which afford tumor cells the opportunity to mitigate the effects of chemotherapy (see Table 1). Multidrug resistance (MDR) is a phenomenon whereby tumors become resistant to several, often unrelated drugs, simultaneously. The multidrug resistance (MDR1) gene encodes an ATP-dependent efflux pump, called P-glycoprotein, that may become amplified through stepwise selection in drug-resistant tumors. The degree of P-glycoprotein overproduction correlates well with the degree of drug resistance. MDR activity may be reversed by drugs such as calcium channel blockers (e.g., verapamil), cyclosporin, or tamoxifen.

Table 1. Mechanisms of drug resistance.

| Mechanism of resistance | Example |
|---|---|
| Altered amount of target enzyme or receptor (gene amplification) | Methotrexate resistance — tumor cells amplify the target enzyme dihydrofolate reductase |
| Decreased activity of an enzyme required for killing effect | Doxorubicin resistance — decreased activity of topoisomerase II |
| Decreased affinity of target enzyme or receptor for drug | Antimetabolite and hydroxyurea resistance |
| Decreased intracellular drug levels | Anthracyclines, dactinomycin, vinca alkaloids, epipodophyllotoxins |
| Enhanced repair of the drug-induced defect | Alkylating agents |
| Multidrug resistance (MDR) | Vinca alkaloids, etoposide, paclitaxel |

## Host Factors that Influence Response

Several host-related factors dictate effectiveness of therapy. The location of the neoplasm and available blood supply are crucial. If any drug is to be effective, it must be present in sufficient concentrations at the site of its action. In cancer chemotherapy, this means that tumor cells, even if very sensitive to the administered drug, cannot be destroyed unless they have reasonable access to blood supply. Failure of drug therapy may occur when tumors metastasize into the pleural space or the CNS. Host tolerance of toxicity governs the ability to administer therapy. Combination chemotherapy may decrease the overall toxicity to any one organ system by utilizing agents with differing toxicity profiles, allowing drugs to achieve a synergistic effect, resulting in decreased resistance. Immune status and more specifically cell-mediated immunity (i.e., the effects initiated by activated macrophages, cytotoxic T-lymphocytes, and natural killer cells) are also important in the response of malignant cells to therapy, especially given that some tumors such as ovarian cancer have been shown to be immune-mediated. Lastly, performance status is a useful index to assess patient tolerance of disease and therapy. The most commonly used scales are the Karnofsky score and the Zubrod score (see Table 2). In general, if the patient's Karnofsky

Table 2. Performance status.

| ECOG/WHO/Zubrod | Karnofsky |
|---|---|
| 0: Asymptomatic | 100%: Normal |
| 1: Symptomatic but completely ambulatory | 90%: Normal activity with few symptoms or signs |
| | 80%: Normal activity with some symptoms or signs of disease |
| 2: Symptomatic, <50% in bed during the day, ambulatory and capable of all self-care | 70%: Caring for self, not capable of work |
| | 60%: Requiring some help |
| 3: Symptomatic, >50% in bed, but not bedbound, capable of limited self-care | 50%: Often requires help, frequent medical care |
| | 40%: Disabled |
| 4: Bedbound, completely disabled | 30%: Seriously disabled, hospital admission indicated |
| | 20%: Very ill, urgently requiring admission |
| 5: Death | 10%: Moribund |
| | 0%: Death |

performance status is below 40%, it is less likely that his or her clinical condition can be markedly improved with chemotherapy.

## Timing of Chemotherapy

*Neoadjuvant chemotherapy* is also called primary or induction therapy. Chemotherapy is given prior to surgery and may confer several advantages, including the ability to monitor drug sensitivity in the intact primary tumor and decrease tumor burden, thereby minimizing the morbidity of any planned surgical resection.

*Adjuvant chemotherapy* is administered following initial surgery. This has the theoretical advantage of debulking tumor mass to minimize the burden of disease prior to chemotherapy, potentially improving survival.

*Salvage therapy* is given after the cancer has recurred or progressed after prior treatment.

*Consolidation therapy* is therapy prescribed after achieving clinical remission, with the intent of destroying all remaining occult cancer cells.

## Monitoring Tumor Response

The Response Evaluation Criteria in Solid Tumors (RECIST) has been adopted and updated to facilitate treatment decisions and comparisons among different chemotherapeutic regimens.[2] It is based on the prospective designation of at least one "target lesion" that measures at least 2 cm in one dimension, as well as "non-target lesions" that are used to corroborate response. Radiographic imaging by helical computed tomography (CT) or magnetic resonance imaging (MRI) is preferred for monitoring tumor response (see Table 3). The criteria were subsequently modified by the Gynecologic Oncology Group (GOG) to include pelvic lesions measurable by physical examination.

## Clinical Trial Design

The drug development process will normally proceed through several phases over many years. If the drug successfully passes through phase I, II, and III clinical trials, it will usually be approved by the FDA for use in the general population.

Table 3. RECIST.

| | |
|---|---|
| Complete Response (CR) | Disappearance of all target lesions. Any pathological lymph nodes (whether target or non-target) must have reduction in short axis to <10 mm |
| Partial Response (PR) | At least a 30% decrease in the sum of diameters of target lesions, taking as reference the baseline sum diameters |
| Progressive Disease (PD) | At least a 20% increase in the sum of diameters of target lesions, taking as reference the smallest sum on study (this includes the baseline sum if that is the smallest on study). In addition to the relative increase of 20%, the sum must also demonstrate an absolute increase of at least 5 mm. (Note: the appearance of one or more new lesions is also considered progression) |
| Stable Disease (SD) | Neither sufficient shrinkage to qualify for PR nor sufficient increase to qualify for PD, taking as reference the smallest sum diameters while on study |

*Pre-clinical studies* involve *in vitro* and *in vivo* experiments using wide-ranging doses of the study drug to obtain preliminary efficacy, toxicity, and pharmacokinetic information. Such tests assist researchers in deciding whether a drug candidate has scientific merit for further development as an investigational new drug.

*Phase 0* is for exploratory, first-in-human trials designed to speed up the development of promising drugs. A distinctive feature of phase 0 trials is micro-dosing, the administration of single sub-therapeutic doses of the study drug to a small number of subjects to gather preliminary data on the agent's pharmacokinetics and pharmacodynamics.

*Phase I trials* are usually the first stage of testing in a small group (20–100) of human subjects. This phase includes trials designed to assess the safety, tolerability, pharmacokinetics, and pharmacodynamics of a drug. Phase I trials also normally include dose escalation so that the maximum tolerated dose (MTD) for therapeutic use can be found.

*Phase II trials* are performed on larger groups (20–300) and are designed to assess efficacy, as well as to continue safety assessments. Phase II studies are sometimes divided into phase IIA and phase IIB, which are designed to assess dosing requirements and efficacy, respectively.

*Phase III studies* are randomized, controlled, multicenter trials on large patient groups aimed at comparing promising new therapy with the current "gold standard".

*Phase IV studies* are also known as post-marketing surveillance trials. Phase IV trials involve safety surveillance designed to detect any rare or long-term adverse effects over a much larger patient population after a drug receives permission to be sold by the FDA.

## Drug Toxicity

Each agent will have respective categories of toxicity that may be graded for the purpose of dose modification, addition of other agents to minimize specific side effects, determination of eligibility to continue with therapy, or reporting adverse drug reactions to the FDA. Table 4 illustrates the definition and grading of general toxicities commonly encountered with chemotherapy given in gynecologic malignancies.

Table 4. Common toxicity grading in gynecologic oncology.

| Adverse drug event | Grade 1 | Grade 2 | Grade 3 | Grade 4 | Grade 5 |
|---|---|---|---|---|---|
| **Allergy/Immunology** | | | | | |
| • Allergic reaction/ hypersensitivity (including drug fever) | Transient rash, drug fever <38°C (<100.4°F) | Urticaria, drug fever ≥38°C (≥100.4°F) | Symptomatic bronchospasm, with or without urticaria; parenteral medication(s) indicated; allergy-related edema/angioedema; hypotension | Anaphylaxis | Death |
| **Blood/Bone marrow** | | | | | |
| • Hemoglobin (Hgb) | <LLN to 10.0 g/dL | <10.0 to 8.0 g/dL | <8.0 to 6.5 g/dL | <6.5 g/dL | Death |
| • Neutrophils/ granulocytes (ANC/AGC) | <LLN to 1500/mm$^3$ | <1500 to 1000/mm$^3$ | <1000 to 500/mm$^3$ | <500/mm$^3$ | |
| • Platelets | <LLN to 75000/mm$^3$ | <75000 to 50000/mm$^3$ | <50000 to 25000/mm$^3$ | <25000/mm$^3$ | |
| **Constitutional symptoms** | | | | | |
| • Fatigue | Mild fatigue over baseline | Moderate or causing difficulty performing some ADL | Severe fatigue interfering with ADL | Disabling | — |
| • Weight loss | 5 to <10% of baseline | 10 to <20% of baseline | ≥20% of baseline | — | — |

(*Continued*)

Table 4. (*Continued*)

| Adverse drug event | Grade 1 | Grade 2 | Grade 3 | Grade 4 | Grade 5 |
|---|---|---|---|---|---|
| **Dematology/Skin** | | | | | |
| • Alopecia | Thinning or patchy | Complete | — | — | — |
| • Rash: hand-foot reaction | Minimal skin changes or dermatitis | Skin changes or pain not interefering with function | Ulcerative dermatitis or skin change with pain interfering with function | — | — |
| **Gastrointestinal** | | | | | |
| • Anorexia | Loss of appetite | Oral intake altered without significant weight loss | Significant weight loss | Life-threatening consequences | Death |
| • Diarrhea | Increase of <4 stools/day over baseline | Increase of 4–6 stools/day | Increase of ≥7 stools/day or incontinence; hospitalization | Life-threatening consequences or hemodynamic collapse | Death |
| • Nausea | Loss of appetite | Oral intake decreased without weight loss; IV fluids indicated <24 hours | Inadequate oral caloric or fluid intake requiring IV fluids, tube feeds or TPN >24 hours | Life-threatening consequences | Death |
| • Vomiting | 1 episode in 24 hours | 2–5 episodes in 24 hours; IV fluids indicated <24 hours | ≥6 episodes in 24 hours; IV fluids or TPN >24 hours | Life-threatening; disabling | Death |

(*Continued*)

Table 4. (*Continued*)

| Adverse drug event | Grade 1 | Grade 2 | Grade 3 | Grade 4 | Grade 5 |
|---|---|---|---|---|---|
| **Infection/Febrile Neutropenia** | | | | | |
| • Febrile neutropenia (fever of unknown origin without clinically or microbiologically documented infection) (ANC <1.0 × 109/L, fever ≥38.5°C) | — | — | Present | Life-threatening sepsis (e.g., septic shock) | Death |
| **Metabolic/Laboratory** | | | | | |
| • ALT | >ULN to 2.5 × ULN | >2.5 to 5.0 × ULN | >5.0 to 20.0 × ULN | >20.0 × ULN | — |
| • Amylase | >ULN to 1.5 × ULN | >1.5 to 2.0 × ULN | >2.0 to 5.0 × ULN | >5.0 × ULN | |
| • AST | | | | | |
| • Bilirubin | >ULN to 2.5 × ULN | >2.5 to 5.0 × ULN | >5.0 to 20.0 × ULN | >20.0 × ULN | |
| • Creatinine | >ULN to 1.5 × ULN | >1.5 to 3.0 × ULN | >3.0 to 10.0 × ULN | >10.0 × ULN | |
| • GGT | >ULN to 1.5 × ULN | >1.5 to 3.0 × ULN | >3.0 to 6.0 × ULN | >6.0 × ULN | |
| • Lipase | >ULN to 2.5 × ULN | >2.5 to 5.0 × ULN | >5.0 to 20.0 × ULN | >20.0 × ULN | |
| | >ULN to 1.5 × ULN | >1.5 to 2.0 × ULN | >2.0 to 5.0 × ULN | >5.0 × ULN | |

(*Continued*)

Table 4. (*Continued*)

| Adverse drug event | Grade 1 | Grade 2 | Grade 3 | Grade 4 | Grade 5 |
|---|---|---|---|---|---|
| **Neurology** | | | | | |
| • Neuropathy-sensory | Loss of deep tendon reflexes or paresthesia (including tingling) but not interfering with function | Sensory loss or paresthesia (including tingling), interfering with function, but not interfering with activities of daily living | Sensory loss or paresthesia interfering with activities of daily living | Disabling | Death |
| **Pain** | | | | | |
| | Mild pain not interfering with function | Moderate pain: pain or analgesics interfering with function, but not interfering with activities of daily living | Severe pain: pain or analgesics severely interfering with activities of daily living | Disabling | — |

(*Continued*)

Table 4. (*Continued*)

| Adverse drug event | Grade 1 | Grade 2 | Grade 3 | Grade 4 | Grade 5 |
|---|---|---|---|---|---|
| **Pulmonary** | | | | | |
| • Pulmonary fibrosis | Minimal radiographic findings, total lung volume that is fibrotic: <25% | Patchy or bi-basilar changes, total lung volume that is fibrotic: 25% to <50% | Dense or widespread infiltrates, total lung volume that is fibrotic: 50% to <75% | Total lung volume that is fibrotic: ≥75%; honeycombing | Death |
| **Renal/Genitourinary** | | | | | |
| • Cystitis | Asymptomatic | Frequency w/dysuria; macroscopic hematuria | Transfusion; IV pain medications; bladder irrigation indicated | Catastrophic bleeding; major non-elective intervention indicated | Death |
| • Renal failure | — | — | Chronic dialysis not indicated | Chronic dialysis or renal transplant indicated | Death |

*Source*: Adapted from the Cancer Therapy Evaluation Program (CTEP), Common Toxicity Criteria for Adverse Events (CTCAE), Version 3.0, DCTD, NCI, NIH, DHHS, March 31, 2003 (http://ctep.cancer.gov); published August 9, 2006.

# EMERGING CONCEPTS IN CANCER CHEMOTHERAPY

## Tumor Growth Theory

The complexity of *in vivo* cancer growth is influenced by a continuum of interrelated processes involving cell-cell, tumor-microenvironment, and tumor-host interactions. Gompertzian kinetics predict an initial period of increasing growth rate followed by a period of decreasing growth (Fig. 1). The point of inflection on the curve represents the maximum rate of tumor growth. Because of its wide applicability, the Gompertz model is felt to represent empiric properties inherent to the biology of tumor growth. Unfortunately, a clear understanding of these biological properties has yet to be achieved.

## Pharmacokinetic and Tumor Heterogeneity

Pharmacokinetic heterogeneity can be related to drug disposition as a function of drug delivery route, tumor perfusion, and elimination kinetics. Drug

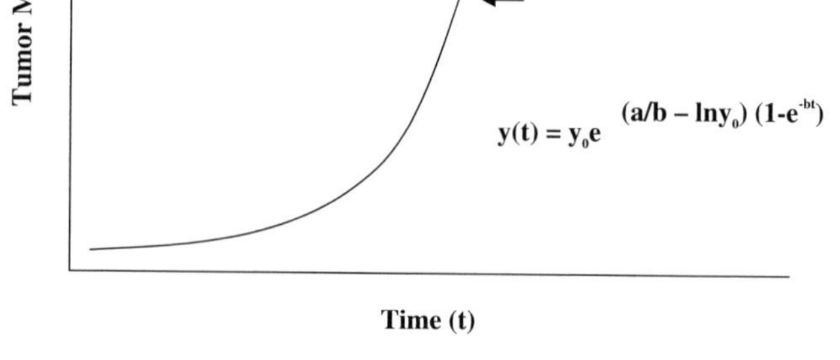


Figure 1. Theoretical tumor growth curve as predicted by Gompertzian kinetics. The model predicts an initial period of increasing growth rate followed by a period of decreasing growth. The inflection point (arrow) on the curve represents the maximum rate of tumor growth.

disposition is often a perfusion-dependent process whereby solid, necrotic, or ischemic tumors will receive only a fraction of the intended dose (see Fig. 2). Based on Table 5, it is observed that the majority of agents possess half-lives of 12 hours or less. Parenteral administration of most agents will result in large serum peaks and relatively rapid troughs, which marginalize drug distribution to solid tumors while the majority of the administered dose is seen by well-perfused tumor and normal tissue. Elimination

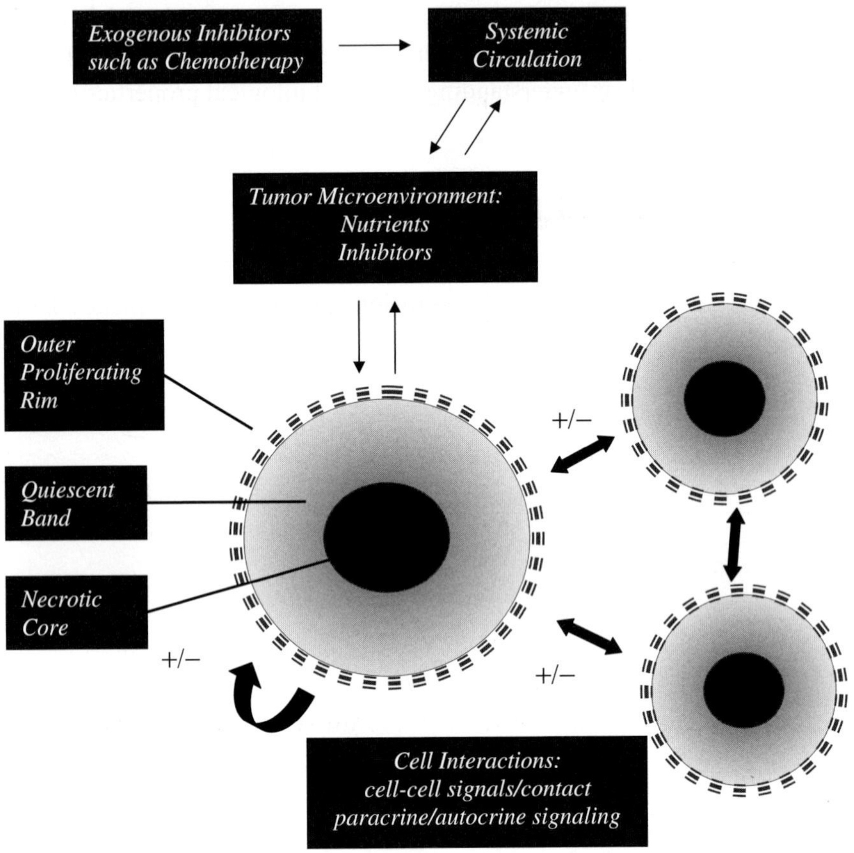


Figure 2. Conceptual description of an avascular tumor growth model. Tumor growth is represented as a layered structure consisting of an outer proliferating rim, quiescent band, and necrotic core. The model treats the proliferating, quiescent, and necrotic cells as a continuum under the influence of environmental factors such as nutrient/growth factors from underlying tissues, and cell movement in terms of migration and contact inhibition.

Table 5. Standard chemotherapy agents and associated plasma half-lives.

| Agent | Trade name | Plasma half-life (h) |
|---|---|---|
| Altretamine | Hexalen | 4.7–10.2 |
| Bleomycin | Blenoxane | 2–5 |
| Capecitabine | Xeloda | 0.7–10.6 |
| Carboplatin | Paraplatin | 2.6–5.9 |
| Cisplatin | Platinol | 0.4–0.8 |
| Cyclophosphamide | Cytoxan | 3–12 |
| Dacarbazine | DTIC-Dome | 5 |
| Docetaxel | Taxotere | 11.4–18.5 |
| Doxorubicin | Adriamycin | 20–48 |
| Epirubicin | Ellence | 11–25 |
| Etoposide, VP-16 | Vepesid | 3–11 |
| Fluorouracil, 5-FU | Adrucil | 0.1–0.33 |
| Gemcitabine | Gemzar | 0.7–1.6 |
| Ifosfamide | IFEX | 15 |
| Irinotecan | Camptosar | 11.7 |
| Methotrexate | Methotrexate | 8–15 |
| Mitomycin C | Mitozytrex | 0.28 |
| Paclitaxel | Taxol | 3–52.7 |
| Topotecan | Hycamtin | 2–3 |
| Vinblastine | Velban | 24 |
| Vincristine | Oncovin | 1 |
| Vinorelbine | Navelbine | 27.7–43.6 |

kinetics will also vary from patient to patient depending on how renal excretion and hepatic metabolism are biased by genetic predisposition, co-morbidities, and organ toxicities from prior chemotherapy. As a result, individual differences will unknowingly influence drug clearance, which could lead to significant underdosing as described by Gurney.[3]

Tumor heterogeneity represents a continuum of variation in terms of cell cycle kinetics and chemosensitivity. Cells within the same tumor can vary in terms of the cell cycle time or phase. Based on Gompertzian growth kinetics, as a solid tumor increases in size, the rate of cell proliferation decreases. Furthermore, such growth kinetics do not take into consideration the expansion of tumor sub-clones that develop from sporadic mutations or by selective pressure from chemotherapy. Thus, chemo-resistance can be related to the resting cell (G0 phase) fraction as well as the ability of sub-clones to inactivate the drug, alter its cell targets, amplify repair mechanisms, or decrease drug accumulation.

## Dose-Dense Scheduling

In the adjuvant setting, Gompertzian kinetics would predict that the probability of achieving log kill is greatest for small-volume tumors since they are likely to display the most rapid rate of proliferation. Thus, late intervention and delays in treatment due to toxicity or scheduling may actually work against the efficacy of the agent.[4,5] The concept of dose scheduling of chemotherapy described by Norton and Simon provides an alternative mode, which is to compress the conventional schedule by decreasing treatment intervals and using lower doses. In simulations, this simple manipulation achieves a considerably greater efficacy by minimizing the re-growth of cells between cycles of treatment (Fig. 3).[4,5]

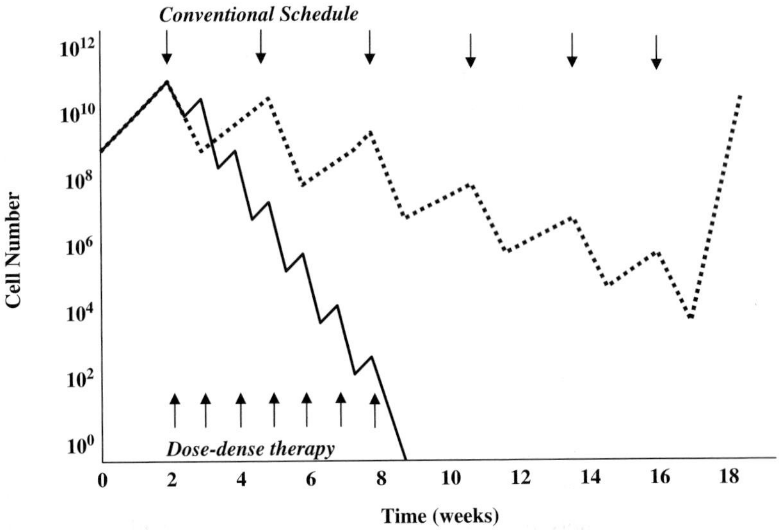


Figure 3. Simulated effect of dose-dense therapy versus conventional scheduling on log cell kill in Gompertzian growth (adapted from ref 5). The initial time zero may represent the time of initial diagnosis at the time of surgery with subsequent treatment.

## Intraperitoneal (IP) Drug Administration

In theory, the advantage of site-specific drug delivery is to produce high local drug concentrations at the tumor with limited systemic exposure. The intraperitoneal (IP) route of drug delivery has been extensively studied for ovarian cancer[6–8] and been recently shown to improve survival in patients with optimally resected ovarian cancer.[9] Certain drugs derive a "pharmacokinetic advantage" when administered into the peritoneal compartment: higher-molecular-weight agents such as paclitaxel would preferentially remain in the IP compartment with slow systemic absorption. Efforts to achieve optimal surgical cytoreduction through peritoneal stripping and tumor debulking, as well as post-operative adhesion formation, may compromise the peritoneum. The extent to which these factors influence the distribution of drug after IP administration adds another layer of complexity that is difficult to quantify when considering local drug penetration into tumors.

# CHEMOTHERAPEUTIC AGENTS (CYTOTOXIC)

The following chemotherapy agents described below have been used in the area of gynecologic malignancies. Currently used regimens will be discussed below. The goal of this section is to describe the basic classifications, mechanisms of action (MOA), dose-limiting toxicities, and clinical uses. Table 6 provides an overview for general reference.

## Alkylating Agents (Covalent Binding to DNA)

*Cyclophosphamide* was originally designed to be preferentially activated in tumor tissue. It was erroneously believed that tumor cells would contain higher levels of enzymes necessary to convert it into an active form. The drug undergoes metabolic activation in the liver, catalyzed by the cytochrome P-450 microsomal enzymes. One of the metabolites formed is believed to be active as a cytotoxic agent while another metabolite, acrolein, is believed to be responsible for the cystitis produced by cyclophosphamide. Prior to the taxanes, cyclophosphamide was used in the primary treatment of epithelial ovarian cancers.

Table 6. Overview of common chemotherapy agents used in the treatment of gynecologic malignancies.

| Agent | Mechanism of action | Dose-limiting toxicities or common side effects | Primary or adjuvant therapy | Recurrent, advanced, or metastatic therapy |
|---|---|---|---|---|
| Actinomycin-D | DNA intercalation (non-covalent binding) | Myelosuppression<br>Mucositis<br>Vomiting<br>Radiation recall | GTD | GTD*<br>O-GCT*<br>O-SCST* |
| Adriamycin (Doxorubicin) | DNA intercalation (non-covalent binding) | Myelosuppression<br>Dose-related cardiomyopathy<br>Stomatitis<br>Vesicant | — | UC-E, UC-S |
| Altretamine (Hexalen) | — | Nausea/vomiting<br>Neurotoxicity | — | EOC (PO) |
| Anastrozole (Arimidex) | Aromatase inhibitor | Diarrhea | — | UC-E<br>UC-ESS<br>EOC |
| Bevacizumab (Avastin) | Antiangiogenesis (binds to VEGF receptor) | Hypertension<br>GI bleeding, hematemesis<br>Delayed wound healing<br>GI perforation<br>Proteinuria | | EOC<br>CC |

(*Continued*)

Table 6. (*Continued*)

| Agent | Mechanism of action | Dose-limiting toxicities or common side effects | Primary or adjuvant therapy | Recurrent, advanced, or metastatic therapy |
|---|---|---|---|---|
| Bleomycin | DNA intercalation (forms ferrous chelation complex to cause DNA strand breaks) | Pulmonary toxicity | O-GCT* | |
| Carboplatin | DNA cross-linking | Myelosuppression<br>Hypersensitivity reaction | EOC (IV)*<br>O-GCT* | EOC, EOC*<br>UC-E<br>CC, CC*<br>O-GCT*, |
| Cisplatin | DNA cross-linking | Nephrotoxicity<br>Nausea/vomiting<br>Neurotoxicity | EOC (IV, IP)*<br>CC-r<br>O-GCT* | EOC, EOC*<br>UC-E<br>CC, CC*<br>O-GCT* |
| Cyclophosphamide | Alklyating agent (DNA covalent binding) | Myelosuppression<br>Hemorrhagic cystitis<br>SIADH | — | EOC<br>GTD*<br>O-SCST* |
| Etoposide (VP-16) | Topoisomerase inhibitor (type II) | Myelosuppression | O-GCT* | EOC (oral)<br>O-GCT* |
| Doxil (Liposomal doxorubicin) | DNA intercalation (non-covalent binding) | Palmar-plantar erythrodysesthesia (PPE)<br>Stomatitis | — | EOC, EOC* |

(*Continued*)

Table 6. (*Continued*)

| Agent | Mechanism of action | Dose-limiting toxicities or common side effects | Primary or adjuvant therapy | Recurrent, advanced, or metastatic therapy |
|---|---|---|---|---|
| 5-Fluorouracil | Antimetabolite (pyrimidine antimetabolite, TS inhibitor) | Myelosuppression<br>Nausea/vomiting | CC-r* | CC |
| Gemcitabine | Antimetabolite (pyrimidine antimetabolite)<br>RNR inhibitor | Myelosuppression | — | EOC, EOC*<br>UC-S*<br>CC, CC*<br>O-GCT* |
| Ifosfamide | Alkylating agent (DNA covalent binding) | Hemorrhagic cystitis<br>Nausea/vomiting<br>Lethargy/confusion | — | EOC<br>UC-S, UC-S*<br>O-GCT*<br>O-SCST* |
| Irinotecan (CPT-11, Camptosar) | Topoisomerase inhibitor (type I) | Myelosuppression<br>Diarrhea | — | EOC<br>CC |
| Letrozole (Femara) | Aromatase inhibitor | Bone pain, hot flushes, back pain, nausea | | UC-E<br>UC-ESS<br>EOC |
| Medroxyprogesterone (Provera) | ER/PR modulation | Nausea | UC-E† | UC-E, UC-E*<br>UC-ESS |
| Megestrol (Megace) | ER/PR modulation | Thrombophlebitis<br>Pulmonary embolism | UC-E† | UC-E<br>UC-ESS<br>EOC |

(*Continued*)

Table 6. (*Continued*)

| Agent | Mechanism of action | Dose-limiting toxicities or common side effects | Primary or adjuvant therapy | Recurrent, advanced, or metastatic therapy |
|---|---|---|---|---|
| Methotrexate | Antimetabolite (DHFR inhibitor) | Myelosuppression<br>Nausea/vomiting/ stomatitis/ulceration<br>Hepatoxicity | GTD | GTD* |
| Oxaliplatin | DNA cross-linking | Myelosuppression<br>Nausea/vomiting<br>Peripheral neuropathy | — | EOC |
| Pemetrexed (Alimta) | Antimetabolite (DHFR, TS, GARFT inhibitor) | Myelosuppression, stomatitis, pharyngitis, and rash | — | EOC<br>CC |
| Tamoxifen (Nolvadex) | SERM | Stroke, deep vein thrombosis, pulmonary embolism | — | EOC |
| Taxol (Paclitaxel) | Microtubule inhibitor | Myelosuppression<br>Hypersensitivity reaction<br>Neurotoxicity | EOC (IV, IP)* | EOC, EOC*<br>UC-E, UC-E*<br>UC-S<br>CC, CC*<br>O-GCT, O-GCT*<br>O-SCST, O-SCST* |

(*Continued*)

develop individual dosing algorithms.[13] This approach is supported by the clinical relationship between toxicity and efficacy as a function of the area under the concentration-time curve (AUC).[14] Calvert and colleagues showed that it was possible to predict clearance by measuring the glomerular filtration rate (GFR) using the [51Cr]-ethylenediamine tetraacetic acid (EDTA) method according to the equation[12,15]

$$\text{Cl (ml/min)} = \text{GFR (ml/min)} + 25$$

where the carboplatin dose given by

$$\text{Carboplatin dose (mg)} = \text{AUC (CrCl} + 25)$$

is calculated based on a target AUC and by substituting the creatinine clearance (CrCl) for GFR.[16] Several formulas exist for the calculation of CrCl, but the most commonly used in gynecologic oncology is the method of Jelliffe:

$$\text{CrCl} = 0.9 \times \{98 \times [0.8 \times (\text{age} - 20)]\} \,/\, \text{serum Cr.}$$

*Oxaliplatin* is a third-generation platinum agent. It is occasionally used in the salvage setting for ovarian cancer. Dose-limiting toxicities include peripheral neuropathy, myelosuppression, and nausea/vomiting.

## *Antitumor Antibiotics (Non-covalent DNA Binding)*

Most of these compounds have been isolated from natural sources and antibiotics; however, they lack the specificity of the antimicrobial antibiotics and thus produce significant toxicity. These drugs interact with DNA in a variety of ways including intercalation, DNA strand breakage, and inhibition of the enzyme topoisomerase II. Resistance to the anthracyclines is due to increased drug efflux due to amplification of the gene for P-glycoprotein, the multi-drug transporter.

Toxicity of doxorubicin (Adriamycin) includes nausea and vomiting; patients may experience anorexia and diarrhea. The drug and its metabolites may color the urine red for one or two days after administration. Bone marrow depression is dose-limiting and occurs in 60–80% of patients. Stomatitis is dose-related and may be severe. Alopecia also occurs in most patients. Doxorubicin is notorious for producing local skin and deep tissue damage with inadvertent extravasation. Cardiac toxicity is a peculiar adverse effect observed with the doxorubicin in both adults and children. The total cumulative dose should not exceed 550 mg/m$^2$ as the risk of progressive dose-dependent cardiomyopathy increases markedly at that level. Acute changes in the electrocardiogram, including tachycardia, extrasystolic contractions, and ST-T wave alterations, may occur in the week following drug administration. Due to liposomal encapsulation, *liposomal doxorubicin* (*Doxil*) has neither dose-related cardiac toxicity nor vesicant properties with inadvertent extravasation to the extent of its parent compound. Gastrointestinal and hematologic toxicities are less common, and alopecia is rare. A common side effect of liposomal doxorubicin is palmar-plantar erythrodysesthesia (PPE).

*Actinomycin-D* characteristically interacts with radiation therapy, producing delayed "radiation recall" skin damage. Previously irradiated or even irritated skin may become reddened and inflamed after drug administration. These reactions may occur months after radiation therapy.

*Bleomycin* is a glycopeptide antibiotic produced by the bacterium *Streptomyces verticillus*. Bleomycin acts by induction of DNA strand breaks through iron chelation, which acts to oxidize oxygen into superoxide and hydroxide free radicals. Bleomycin's dose-limiting side effect is pulmonary toxicity, which occurs in approximately 10% of treated patients. Bleomycin-induced lung damage can present as pneumonitis with dry cough, dyspnea, and rales, and may progress within weeks to pulmonary fibrosis.

## Antimetabolites

Antimetabolites are structural analogs of naturally occurring compounds. Antimetabolites interfere with the production of nucleic acids. They work through a variety of mechanisms, including competition for binding sites on enzymes and incorporation into nucleic acids.

*Methotrexate* is an antifolate that has been the agent of choice in the treatment of gestational trophoblastic disease and choriocarcinoma. It is often used in sequential therapy with actinomycin-D[17] or in combination for high-risk gestational trophoblastic disease.[18] The enzyme dihydrofolate reductase (DHFR) is the primary site of action of most folate analogs such as methotrexate. Inhibition of this DHFR leads to toxicity through partial depletion of cofactors required for the synthesis of purines and thymidylate, leading to the inhibition of DNA synthesis. Resistance to methotrexate may develop as a result of elevated dihydrofolate reductase activity or defective transport of methotrexate into malignant cells. Hematologic effects of methotrexate include leukopenia, thrombocytopenia, and anemia. Gastrointestinal side effects include nausea, vomiting, pharyngitis, stomatitis, and ulcerations. Hepatoxicity may also occur with high-dose regimens. Patients should also be counseled regarding photosensitivity and other dermatologic effects such as erythematous rashes, pruritus, depigmentation, or hyperpigmentation.

*5-Fluorouracil (5-FU)* is a pyrimidine antimetabolite that directly inhibits thymidylate synthetase (TS). It has radio-sensitizing properties and can be utilized with external beam radiation in combination with cisplatin for adjuvant treatment for patients with high-risk[19,20] or advanced[21] cervix cancer.

*Gemcitabine* (*Gemzar*) is a synthetic pyrimidine analog which competes with cytidine during DNA replication. Following insertion of gemcitabine, DNA replication is terminated. The diphosphate analog binds to the active site of ribonucleotide reductase (RNR) to irreversibly inactivate the enzyme. Gemcitabine has demonstrated significant activity in recurrent or refractory ovarian and cervical cancer. It also has known activity in less common gynecologic malignancies such as uterine leiomyosarcoma in combination with docetaxel.[22]

*Pemetrexed* (*Alimta*) is an antifolate antineoplastic agent which inhibits folate-dependent enzymes thymidylate synthetase (TS), dihydrofolate reductase (DHFR), as well as glycinamide ribonucleotide formyltransferase (GARFT). It can be used in the salvage setting for ovarian and cervix cancers. Dose-limiting toxicities are similar to methotrexate and include myelosuppression, stomatitis, pharyngitis, and rash.

## Microtubule Inhibitors

Microtubules are protein polymers that are responsible for various aspects of cellular shape and movement. The major component of microtubules is the polymer tubulin, a protein containing two non-identical sub-units (alpha and beta).

*Vinca alkaloids* (vincristine, vinblastine) are large, complex molecules produced by the leaves of the periwinkle plant. The mechanism of action involves specific binding to tubulin, preventing tubulin dimer aggregation and polymerization into microtubules. This effectively decreases the pool of free tubulin dimers available for microtubule assembly, resulting in a shift of the equilibrium toward disassembly. They block mitosis with metaphase arrest. Resistance is due primarily to decreased drug accumulation from overexpression of the P-glycoprotein (MDR). In gynecologic oncology, vincristine has been used in the treatment of high-risk gestational trophoblastic disease.[18] Dose-limiting toxicity consists mainly of peripheral sensory neuropathy. Autonomic neuropathy may result in abdominal pain, constipation, paralytic ileus, urinary retention, and orthostatic hypotension. Unlike most antineoplastic agents, vincristine usually does not cause significant bone marrow suppression and is therefore often combined with other drugs that are myelosuppressive. Gastrointestinal symptoms also are common.

*Paclitaxel* (*Taxol*) and *docetaxel* (*Taxotere*) are widely used in the treatment of many solid tumors including breast, lung, and head and neck carcinomas, in addition to gynecologic malignancies. Paclitaxel was first isolated from the bark of the Pacific yew (*Taxus brevifolia*). Docetaxel is a semisynthetic analog. Treatment causes both the stabilization of microtubules and the formation of abnormal bundles of microtubules. Resistance to these drugs arises through mechanisms similar to that of the vinca alkaloids. Toxicity includes bone marrow suppression with neutropenia. Of the two, paclitaxel has more neurotoxicity and docetaxel has more myelotoxicity. Hypersensitivity reactions are also common, characterized by dyspnea, urticaria and hypotension; hypersensitivity to docetaxel may include edema. Avoidance of bolus injections and short infusions can minimize this toxicity, as can pretreatment with steroids or antihistamines. Reactions appear to be related to the additive (Cremophor) required for paclitaxel preparation, though patients also experience hypersensitivity to docetaxel which is formulated in Tween. Mucositis is also common.

## Topoisomerase Inhibitors

This class of drugs causes disruption of chromosomal dynamics, in particular, the topoisomerase enzymes which unwind DNA to facilitate DNA replication.

*Etoposide* (*VP-16*) is a semisynthetic glycoside derivative of podophyllotoxin, a natural compound produced in the roots of the American mayapple plant. It is a type II topoisomerase inhibitor that has been used in recurrent epithelial ovarian cancer and in the treatment of germ cell malignancies in combination with bleomycin and cisplatin.[23] Myelosuppression is dose-limiting for both oral and intravenous administration.

*Topotecan* (*Hycamtin*) is a water-soluble semisynthetic analog of camptothecin. It acts by forming a stable covalent complex with type I topoisomerase, leading to breaks in double-stranded DNA resulting in apoptosis. It is widely used in the setting of recurrent/refractory ovarian cancer[24] as well as advanced cervix cancer in combination with cisplatin.[25] The dose-limiting toxicity is myelosuppression.

*Irinotecan* (*CPT-11, Camptosar*) is another water-soluble semisynthetic analog of camptothecin that forms a stable covalent complex with type I topoisomerase. It has been used in the salvage setting for ovarian and cervix cancers. Diarrhea and neutropenia are the major dose-limiting toxicities.

## Cytotoxic Agents with Unclear Mechanisms of Action

*Altretamine* (*Hexalen*) is a synthetic cytotoxic antineoplastic s-triazine derivative. The mechanism of action is not completely understood; however, it structurally resembles the alkylating agent triethylenemelamine. The drug is administered orally in refractory ovarian cancer patients. Nausea and vomiting of gradual onset occur frequently and are the dose-limiting toxicities. Neurotoxicity in terms of peripheral neuropathy and CNS symptoms (mood disorders, disorders of consciousness, ataxia, dizziness, vertigo) have also been reported in the continuous high-dose daily regimen.

# CHEMOTHERAPEUTIC AGENTS (TARGETED THERAPY)

In this section we will review targeted therapies that do not meet the historical definition of cytotoxic agents. Estrogen/progesterone receptor-modulating agents were the first targeted therapies used; however, in recent years, bevacizumab has been one of the more successful translation drugs used in recurrent ovarian cancer.

## Estrogen/Progesterone Receptor Modulation

*Medroxyprogesterone* (*Provera*) therapy is indicated for therapeutic use in women to treat atypical endometrial hyperplasia or in grade 1 endometrial cancer as a fertility-sparing measure.[26,27] Medroxyprogesterone has been found to have activity against advanced or recurrent endometrial cancer[28] and low-grade endometrial stromal sarcomas. *Megestrol* (*Megace*) is another agent that has been used with some success in similar settings. It may also have some activity in the treatment of recurrent ovarian cancer. *Tamoxifen* (*Nolvadex*) is a selective estrogen receptor modulator (SERM) widely used in the adjuvant treatment of node-positive breast cancer, which may also display some activity in recurrent ovarian cancer.

## Aromatase Inhibitors

The aromatase inhibitors anastrozole (Arimidex) and letrozole (Femara) have been used with limited success in advanced endometrial or ovarian cancers, as well as low-grade endometrial stromal sarcomas.

## Antiangiogenesis Agents

In tumors, vascular endothelial growth factor (VEGF) is considered to be the most potent and specific of the many angiogenic factors.[29] It is not only crucial for endothelial cell proliferation and blood vessel formation, but also induces significant vascular permeability and plays a key role in endothelial cell survival signaling in newly formed vessels.[29–31] VEGF is secreted by tumor cells and expression can be increased by environmental triggers such as hypoxia, loss of tumor suppressor gene function and oncogene activation.[32] Inhibition of VEGF functioning is therefore a key target in antiangiogenic approaches.

*Bevacizumab* (*Avastin*) is a chimeric murine/human monoclonal antibody, which specifically binds to the receptor of vascular endothelial cell growth factor (VEGFR). In gynecologic malignancies, bevacizumab has shown significant activity in recurrent ovarian cancer,[33,34] advanced cervical cancer,[35] and granulosa cell tumors of the ovary.[36] Bevacizumab toxicity is related to its mechanism of action. GI perforations are not uncommon and have been documented in approximately 11% of patients undergoing treatment for recurrent ovarian cancer. These events may be lethal. Bevacizumab can also induce hemorrhage or even intra-abdominal abscesses. Because of the drug's long 20-day half-life, surgery should be delayed at least 28 days after the last dose if possible. Other side effects include severe venous as well as arterial thromboembolism. Hypertension is relatively frequent and should be treated in order to avoid cerebral hemorrhage during hypertensive crisis. Far less common is congestive heart failure, which has been reported in 2% of patients. Renal effects have been observed such as proteinuria and nephrotic syndrome.

## Tyrosine Kinase Inhibitors

*Erlotinib* (*Tarceva*) is an orally administered selective epidermal growth factor receptor tyrosine kinase inhibitor. Activation of epidermal growth factor receptor (EGFR) results in a cascade of intracellular signaling events, leading to cell proliferation, differentiation, cell survival, angiogenesis, and invasion/metastasis. It is currently approved for treatment of non-small cell lung and pancreatic cancers. The most frequent adverse effects are acneiform-like skin rash, diarrhea, nausea, vomiting, cough, dyspnea, and fatigue. More severe reactions have included GI bleeding and interstitial lung disease. It is currently being studied in recurrent ovarian cancer and advanced endometrial and cervix cancers. It is too early to draw any convincing conclusions regarding efficacy.

*Lapatinib* (*Tykerb*) is an orally administered inhibitor of the intracellular tyrosine kinase domains of both epidermal growth factor receptor (EGFR [ErbB1]) and human epidermal receptor type 2 (HER2 [ErbB2]) receptors. It has been approved for hormone-positive and HER2-positive advanced breast cancer. It appears to be well tolerated with adverse reactions including diarrhea, rash, nausea, and fatigue. It is currently being studied in phase I trials involving ovarian cancer. It is too early to draw any convincing conclusions regarding efficacy.

*Sunitinib* (*Sutent*) is an orally administered agent that inhibits multiple receptor tyrosine kinases (RTKs), as well as platelet-derived growth factor receptors (PDGFR), vascular endothelial growth factor receptors (VEGFR), stem cell factor receptor (KIT), Fms-like tyrosine kinase-3 (FLT3), colony-stimulating factor receptor type 1 (CSF-1R), and the glial cell line-derived neurotrophic factor receptor (RET). It is approved for the treatment of advanced renal cell carcinoma and for gastrointestinal stromal tumor. GI adverse drug events include diarrhea, nausea, mucositis/stomatitis, vomiting, abdominal pain, and constipation. Cardiovascular effects include hypertension, left ventricular dysfunction, and QT interval prolongation. Hemorrhage can also be a severe adverse drug reaction with sunitinib. It is currently being studied in recurrent ovarian cancer and advanced endometrial and cervix cancers. It is too early to draw any convincing conclusions regarding efficacy.

*Pazopanib* (*Votrient*) is an orally administered, multi-targeted tyrosine kinase inhibitor that binds to VEGFR and PDGFR. It is approved for the treatment of advanced renal cell carcinoma. The most common adverse reactions are diarrhea, hypertension, hair color changes (depigmentation), nausea, anorexia, and vomiting. Increases in serum transaminase levels and bilirubin have been observed with severe and fatal hepatotoxicity in rare instances. Hypertension can be observed and usually easily controlled. However, prolonged QT intervals and torsades de pointes have been observed. In comparison to the preceding tyrosine kinase inhibitors, phase II activity has been more encouraging in recurrent ovarian[37] and cervical cancer.[38]

## Poly(Adenosine Diphosphate [ADP]-Ribose) Polymerase or PARP Inhibitors

One emerging area of targeted antitumor therapy is the concept of "synthetic lethality". In this case, an inhibitor of poly(adenosine diphosphate-ribose) polymerase (an enzyme that repairs DNA single-strand breaks through the repair of base excisions) that is tumoricidal in cancer cells deficient in BRCA1- or BRCA2-associated DNA repair mechanisms. By inhibiting the repair of DNA single-strand breaks, DNA single-strand breaks accumulate which can produce DNA double-strand breaks at replication forks. Under normal conditions, these breaks are repaired by homologous-recombination double-stranded DNA repair pathways, which are key components of the tumor-suppressor proteins BRCA1 and BRCA2.[39,40] It is well recognized that germ-line mutation in the BRCA1 or BRCA2 allele is associated with a high risk of developing breast, ovarian, and prostate cancers. Carcinogenesis can arise through genetic aberrations when cells carrying the heterozygous BRCA mutations lose the remaining wild-type allele. This loss of heterozygosity leads to the emergence of a tumor that carries a DNA-repair defect that is not shared by the normal tissues of the patient. Therefore, this tumor-specific defect can be exploited (i.e., synthetic lethality) using PARP inhibitors to induce selective tumor cytotoxicity while sparing normal cells. Olaparib (AZD2281), a novel, potent, orally active PARP inhibitor, has shown promising activity in phase I evaluation with carriers of BRCA1 or BRCA2 mutations,[41] including those with ovarian cancer.[42]

## REFERENCES

1. Goodman LS, Wintrobe MM, Dameshek W, Goodman MJ, Gilman A, McLennan MT. Nitrogen mustard therapy. Use of methyl-bis(beta-chloroethyl)amine hydrochloride and tris(beta-chloroethyl)amine hydrochloride for Hodgkin's disease, lymphosarcoma, leukemia, and certain allied and miscellaneous disorders. *J Am Med Assoc* 1946;105:475–476. Reprinted in *JAMA* 1984;251:2255–2261.
2. Eisenhauer EA, Therasse P, Bogaerts J, *et al.* New response evaluation criteria in solid tumours: revised RECIST guideline (version 1.1). *Eur J Cancer* 2009;45(2):228–247.
3. Gurney H. How to calculate the dose of chemotherapy. *Br J Cancer* 2002;86(8):1297–1302.
4. Norton L. Adjuvant breast cancer therapy: current status and future strategies — growth kinetics and the improved drug therapy of breast cancer. *Semin Oncol* 1999;26(3):1–4.
5. Norton L. Theoretical concepts and the emerging role of taxanes in adjuvant therapy. *Oncologist* 2001;6(3):30–35.
6. Howell SB, Zimm S, Markman M, *et al.* Long-term survival of advanced refractory ovarian carcinoma patients with small-volume disease treated with intraperitoneal chemotherapy. *J Clin Oncol* 1987;5(10):1607–1612.

7. Alberts DS, Liu PY, Hannigan EV, *et al.* Intraperitoneal cisplatin plus intravenous cyclophosphamide versus intravenous cisplatin plus intravenous cyclophosphamide for stage III ovarian cancer. *N Engl J Med* 1996; 335(26):1950–1955.
8. Markman M, Bundy BN, Alberts DS, *et al.* Phase III trial of standard-dose intravenous cisplatin plus paclitaxel versus moderately high-dose carboplatin followed by intravenous paclitaxel and intraperitoneal cisplatin in small-volume stage III ovarian carcinoma: an intergroup study of the Gynecologic Oncology Group, Southwestern Oncology Group, and Eastern Cooperative Oncology Group. *J Clin Oncol* 2001;19(4): 1001–1007.
9. Armstrong DK, Bundy B, Wenzel L, *et al.* Intraperitoneal cisplatin and paclitaxel in ovarian cancer. *N Engl J Med* 2006;354(1):34–43.
10. Markman M, Kennedy A, Webster K, *et al.* Clinical features of hypersensitivity reactions to carboplatin. *J Clin Oncol* 1999;17(4):1141.
11. Gurney H. Dose calculation of anticancer drugs: a review of the current practice and introduction of an alternative. *J Clin Oncol* 1996;14:2590–2611.
12. Gurney HP, Ackland S, Gebski V, Farrell G. Factors affecting epirubicin pharmacokinetics and toxicity: evidence against using body-surface area for dose calculation. *J Clin Oncol* 1998;16:2299–3004.
13. Chatelut E, Canal P, Brunner V, *et al.* Prediction of carboplatin clearance from standard morphological and biological patient characteristics. *J Natl Cancer Inst* 1995;87(8):573–580.
14. Duffull SB, Robinson BA. Clinical pharmacokinetics and dose optimisation of carboplatin. *Clin Pharmacokinet* 1997;33:161–183.
15. Calvert AH, Newell DR, Gumbrell LA, *et al.* Carboplatin dosage: prospective evaluation of a simple formula based on renal function. *J Clin Oncol* 1989;7(11):1748–1756.
16. Cockcroft DW, Gault MH. Prediction of creatinine clearance from serum creatinine. *Nephron* 1976;16(1):31–41.
17. Berkowitz RS, Goldstein DP, Bernstein MR. Ten years' experience with methotrexate and folinic acid as primary therapy for gestational trophoblastic disease. *Gynecol Oncol* 1986;23(1):111–118.
18. Escobar PF, Lurain JR, Singh DK, Bozorgi K, Fishman DA. Treatment of high-risk gestational trophoblastic neoplasia with etoposide, methotrexate, actinomycin D, cyclophosphamide, and vincristine chemotherapy. *Gynecol Oncol* 2003;91(3):552–557.

19. Morris M, Eifel PJ, Lu J, *et al.* Pelvic radiation with concurrent chemotherapy compared with pelvic and para-aortic radiation for high-risk cervical cancer. *N Engl J Med* 1999;340(15):1137–1143.
20. Peters WA 3rd, Liu PY, Barrett RJ 2nd, *et al.* Concurrent chemotherapy and pelvic radiation therapy compared with pelvic radiation therapy alone as adjuvant therapy after radical surgery in high-risk early-stage cancer of the cervix. *J Clin Oncol* 2000;18(8):1606–1613.
21. Whitney CW, Sause W, Bundy BN, *et al.* Randomized comparison of fluorouracil plus cisplatin versus hydroxyurea as an adjunct to radiation therapy in stage IIB-IVA carcinoma of the cervix with negative para-aortic lymph nodes: a Gynecologic Oncology Group and Southwest Oncology Group study. *J Clin Oncol* 1999;17(5):1339–1348.
22. Hensley ML, Blessing JA, Mannel R, Rose PG. Fixed-dose rate gemcitabine plus docetaxel as first-line therapy for metastatic uterine leiomyosarcoma: a Gynecologic Oncology Group phase II trial. *Gynecol Oncol* 2008; 109(3):329–334.
23. Williams S, Blessing JA, Liao SY, Ball H, Hanjani P. Adjuvant therapy of ovarian germ cell tumors with cisplatin, etoposide, and bleomycin: a trial of the Gynecologic Oncology Group. *J Clin Oncol* 1994;12(4): 701–706.
24. Clarke-Pearson DL, Van Le L, Iveson T, *et al.* Oral topotecan as single-agent second-line chemotherapy in patients with advanced ovarian cancer. *J Clin Oncol* 2001;19(19):3967–3975.
25. Long HJ 3rd, Bundy BN, Grendys EC Jr, *et al.* Gynecologic Oncology Group Study. Randomized phase III trial of cisplatin with or without topotecan in carcinoma of the uterine cervix: a Gynecologic Oncology Group Study. *J Clin Oncol* 2005;23(21):4626–4633.
26. Imai M, Jobo T, Sato R, *et al.* Medroxyprogesterone acetate therapy for patients with adenocarcinoma of the endometrium who wish to preserve the uterus — usefulness and limitations. *Eur J Gynaecol Oncol* 2001; 22(3):217–220.
27. Kobiashvili H, Charkviani L, Charkviani T. Organ preserving method in the management of atypical endometrial hyperplasia. *Eur J Gynaecol Oncol* 2001;22(4):297–299.
28. Thigpen JT, Brady MF, Alvarez RD, *et al.* Oral medroxyprogesterone acetate in the treatment of advanced or recurrent endometrial carcinoma: a

dose-response study by the Gynecologic Oncology Group. *J Clin Oncol* 1999;17(6):1736–1744.
29. Ferrara N, Gerber HP, LeCouter J. The biology of VEGF and its receptors. *Nat Med* 2003;9:669–676.
30. McMahon G. VEGF receptor signaling in tumor angiogenesis. *Oncologist* 2000;5 Suppl 1:3–10.
31. Dvorak HF, Brown LF, Detmar M, Dvorak AM. Vascular permeability factor/ vascular endothelial growth factor, microvascular hyperpermeability, and angiogenesis. *Am J Pathol* 1995;146:1029–1039.
32. Ferrara N. Role of vascular endothelial growth factor in physiologic and pathologic angiogenesis: therapeutic implications. *Semin Oncol* 2002;29: 10–14.
33. Burger RA, Sill MW, Monk BJ, Greer BE, Sorosky JI. Phase II trial of bevacizumab in persistent or recurrent epithelial ovarian cancer or primary peritoneal cancer: a Gynecologic Oncology Group Study. *J Clin Oncol* 2007; 25(33):5165–5171.
34. Cannistra SA, Matulonis UA, Penson RT, *et al.* Phase II study of bevacizumab in patients with platinum-resistant ovarian cancer or peritoneal serous cancer. *J Clin Oncol* 2007;25(33):5180–5186.
35. Monk BJ, Sill MW, Burger RA, Gray HJ, Buekers TE, Roman LD. Phase II trial of bevacizumab in the treatment of persistent or recurrent squamous cell carcinoma of the cervix: a gynecologic oncology group study. *J Clin Oncol* 2009;27(7):1069–1074.
36. Tao X, Sood AK, Deavers MT, *et al.* Anti-angiogenesis therapy with bevacizumab for patients with ovarian granulosa cell tumors. *Gynecol Oncol* 2009;114(3):431–436.
37. Friedlander M, Hancock KC, Rischin D, *et al.* A Phase II, open-label study evaluating pazopanib in patients with recurrent ovarian cancer. *Gynecol Oncol* 2010;119(1):32–37.
38. Monk BJ, Lopez LM, Zarba JJ, *et al.* Phase II, open-label study of pazopanib or lapatinib monotherapy compared with pazopanib plus lapatinib combination therapy in patients with advanced and recurrent cervical cancer. *J Clin Oncol* 2010;28(22):3562–3569.
39. McCabe N, Turner NC, Lord CJ. Deficiency in the repair of DNA damage by homologous recombination and sensitivity to poly(ADP-ribose) polymerase inhibition. *Cancer Res* 2006;66:8109–8115.

40. Gudmundsdottir K, Ashworth A. The roles of BRCA1 and BRCA2 and associated proteins in the maintenance of genomic stability. *Oncogene* 2006;25:5864–5874.
41. Fong PC, Boss DS, Yap TA, *et al.* Inhibition of poly(ADP-ribose) polymerase in tumors from BRCA mutation carriers. *N Engl J Med* 2009; 361(2):123–134.
42. Fong PC, Yap TA, Boss DS, *et al.* Poly(ADP)-ribose polymerase inhibition: frequent durable responses in BRCA carrier ovarian cancer correlating with platinum-free interval. *J Clin Oncol* 2010;28(15):2512–2519.

# 2

# RADIATION THERAPY FOR GYNECOLOGIC MALIGNANCIES

*Lara Bonner Millar and Lilie L. Lin*

## INTRODUCTION

Gynecologic cancers were among the first malignancies treated with ionizing radiation more than a century ago.[1] Today, radiation therapy remains an essential component of both the primary non-surgical management and the adjuvant postoperative treatment of malignancies arising in the female reproductive tract.

Current strategies for treating gynecologic cancers are tailored to the clinical and pathologic stage of disease. Early-stage lesions of the lower genitourinary tract can be treated surgically if resection can be accomplished without substantial tissue disruption. Postoperative radiotherapy is reserved for cases in which histopathologic analysis of the removed specimen reveals features suggesting a high risk for local recurrence.

Primary radiotherapy can be used for women with unresectable locally advanced disease, women with resectable disease in whom the risk of surgical morbidity is unacceptably high, or women with medical risk factors that contraindicate primary surgical therapy. For women with distant metastatic disease at presentation, palliative radiotherapy is used to relieve symptoms and improve quality of life.

## RADIATION PHYSICS

Radiation is grouped into two categories: non-ionizing radiation, which cannot ionize matter, and ionizing radiation. Ionization is a process whereby the radiation removes an outer-shell electron from an atom. There are two forms of ionizing radiation. Directly ionizing radiation comes from charged particles such as electrons, protons, alpha particles, and heavy ions. Indirectly ionizing radiation consists of neutral particles such as photons (X-rays and gamma rays) and neutrons.

X-rays and gamma rays are part of the high energy end of the electromagnetic radiation spectrum. X-ray radiation and gamma ray radiation have much shorter wavelengths than light, and hence have much higher energies than photons of light. The relationship between photon energy ($E$) and frequency ($v$) is given by $E = hv$ where $h$ is Planck's constant ($6.62 \times 10^{-34}$ J.s) and $v$ is the frequency. Frequency and wavelength are related by the expression $v = c/\lambda$ where $c$ is the speed of light in a vacuum. Therefore, $E = hc/\lambda$.[2]

The distinction between X-rays and gamma rays is based on the origin of the radiation, not on the frequency or wavelength of the electromagnetic waves. Gamma rays are produced by nuclear transitions, while X-rays are emitted during electron transitions between energy shells. Photons with energies between about 10 keV and a few hundred keV can be either X-rays or gamma rays.

## X-Ray Production

Diagnostic X-rays are generated by an X-ray tube, which is a vacuum tube that uses a high voltage to accelerate electrons released from the cathode (also called a filament) to a metal target, usually made of tungsten, embedded within the anode. The maximum energy of an X-ray is the energy of the incident electron, which is equal to the voltage on the tube. For example, a 90 kV tube cannot create X-rays with energy greater than 90 keV. When the electrons hit the target, X-rays are created by two different atomic processes. If the incident electrons have sufficient energy, they can knock an electron out of an inner shell of the target metal atoms. Then electrons from higher states drop down to fill the vacancy, emitting X-ray photons with precise energies determined by the electron energy levels. These X-rays are called *characteristic X-rays.* A second type of indirectly ionizing photon radiation is *bremsstrahlung* or "braking radiation", which is radiation given off by the electrons as they are scattered by

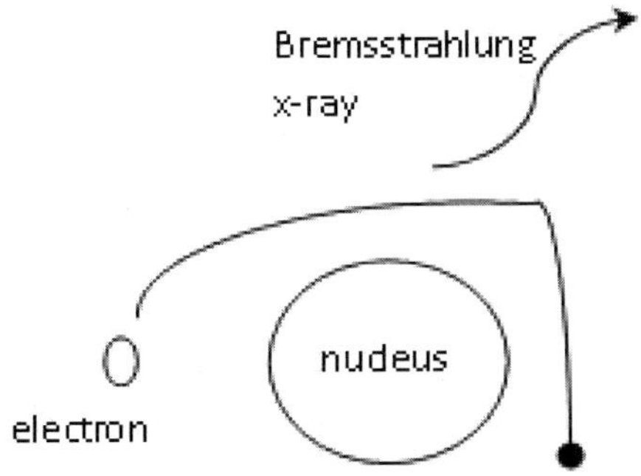


Figure 1. *Bremsstrahlung:* as the electron is deflected by the field of the atomic nucleus, radiation is produced.

the strong electric field near the positively charged nucleus (see Fig. 1). These X-rays have a continuous spectrum of energies.

## Photon Interactions with Matter

Photons interact *indirectly* with matter.[2] All ionization occurs after the photon has deposited its energy. Three major photon interactions with matter are:

- Photoelectric effect,
- Compton scattering,
- Pair production.

The *photoelectric effect* is an interaction between a photon and a tightly bound electron whose binding energy is equal to or less than the energy of the photon. The photon is absorbed by the electron and, as a result of the added energy, is ejected from the atoms with kinetic energy equal to the difference between the original gamma ray energy and the electron binding energy.

*Compton scattering* occurs when a photon interacts with a loosely bound outer-shell electron. The electron absorbs the photon, but will emit another photon at a lower energy. The incident photon energy is now shared between the scattered photon and electron.

*Pair production* occurs at photon energies greater than 1.02 MeV, which is equal to the rest mass of two electrons. As the photon approaches the nucleus of an atom, it completely disappears. The energy absorbed is then expressed by the emission of an electron-positron pair (which together has a mass of 1.02 MeV). Any remaining energy will be distributed between the two particles as kinetic energy.

The probability that a photon will undergo any one of the various interaction phenomena with an attenuator depends on the energy of the photon and on the atomic number $Z$ of the attenuating material. In general, the photoelectric effect predominates at low photon energies, the Compton effect at intermediate energies, and pair production at high photon energies.

## Radioactive Decay

The nucleus of each atom has a specific number of protons and neutrons and is either stable or unstable, depending on the relative number of each. Stable atoms have an equal number of protons and neutrons. Unstable atoms are radioactive, and are also known as radionuclides. Radionuclides undergo a process called radioactive decay to reach a more stable state. While a radionuclide is going through the process of decay, energy is released from the atom in one of the following modes: alpha, beta minus, beta plus, electron capture, or gamma radiation.[3] The particular mode of decay determines the type of radiation released from the atom.

Alpha decay is the emission of an alpha particle (two protons and two neutrons) from an unstable nucleus. The daughter nuclide has an atomic number two less than the parent nuclide and a mass number four less than the parent nuclide. The daughter nucleus commonly releases its excitation energy by gamma emission. Alpha decay occurs in nuclides where $Z > 83$.

$$^{238}_{92}\mathrm{U} \rightarrow {}^{234}_{90}\mathrm{Th} + {}^{4}_{2}\mathrm{He}$$

Beta-minus decay occurs in radionuclides with an excess of neutrons. This form of decay effectively converts a neutron into a proton and an electron, which is immediately ejected from the nucleus. The daughter nuclide has its atomic number increased by one and has the same mass number compared to the parent.

$$^{233}_{91}\text{Pa} \rightarrow {}^{233}_{92}\text{U} + \beta-$$

Beta-plus decay effectively converts a proton into a neutron and a positron, which is immediately ejected from the nucleus. The daughter nuclide has its atomic number decreased by one and has the same mass number compared to the parent.

$$^{11}_{5}\text{C} \rightarrow {}^{11}_{5}\text{B} + \beta+$$

Electron capture occurs when there are too many protons in the nucleus, and there isn't enough energy to emit a positron. One of the inner orbital electrons is captured by a proton in the nucleus, forming a neutron. Since the proton is essentially changed into a neutron, the number of neutrons increases by one, the number of protons decreases by one, and the atomic mass remains unchanged. By changing the number of protons, electron capture transforms the nuclide into a new element.

$$^{125}_{53}\text{I} + \text{e}^- \rightarrow {}^{125}_{52}\text{Te}*$$

The quantity of a radioactive substance is expressed as disintegrations per second, in units of curies (Ci), named for Marie Curie, or becquerels (Bq) in the SI system, named for Henri Becquerel. 1 Ci = $3.7 \times 10^{10}$ Bq. The rate at which a radionuclide decays depends on its half-life.

When a photon interacts with a material, it may be scattered, absorbed, or transmitted without interaction. Scattering involves a partial transfer of energy to tissue, with the resulting scattered X-ray having less energy and a different trajectory. A photon that is absorbed or scattered is described as being attenuated. The half-value layer (HVL or $x_{1/2}$) is the thickness in centimeters of the attenuator that reduces the photon beam intensity to 50% of its original value:

$$x_{1/2} = \text{HVL} = (\ln 2)/\mu$$

where $\mu$ is the linear attenuation coefficient. The value of $\mu$ depends on the photon energy and the atomic number of the attenuator.

Linear accelerators (linacs), which produce X-rays for therapeutic purposes, accelerate electrons to a target in a different way from a diagnostic machine. Linacs use microwave technology via a magnetron or klystron, which converts electrical power into microwaves. The microwaves accelerate electrons in a part of the accelerator called the "wave guide," and then the electrons collide with a heavy metal target. As a result of the collisions, high-energy X-rays are scattered from the target. The X-rays are collected and shaped by blocks or a collimator. The beam exits the part of the accelerator called the gantry, which rotates around the patient.

Historically, radiation was measured in rads. Today, radiation dose is measured using an SI term called gray (Gy), which is the energy absorbed per unit mass of the irradiated material; one Gy is one joule per kilogram. One Gy is equivalent to 100 centigray (cGy) or 100 rads. The roentgen is a unit of radiation exposure. The unit roentgen (R) is defined in terms of charge (coulombs) created by ionizing radiation per unit mass (kg) of air. $1\ R = 2.58 * 10^{-4}$ C/kg air. The unit roentgen is only defined for air and cannot be used to describe dose to tissue. Therefore patient exposures are described in gray.

Not all radiation has the same biological effect, even for the same amount of absorbed dose. For example, a photon has a different biologically effective dose than an alpha particle. The quantity of dose equivalent ($H$), measured in sieverts, was introduced to account for differences in biological effects. $H$ attempts to account for the different effects of different radiation types by using a dimensionless radiation "quality factor", $Q$. The quality factor is a unique value that relates the relative biological effectiveness to a value that is multiplied by the absorbed dose. Therefore, $H = Q \times$ absorbed dose. Per most government regulations, the $Q$ for electron and photon radiation is 1, for neutron radiation it is 10, and for alpha radiation it is 20.[4]

## RADIOBIOLOGY

Radiobiology is the study of the effect of radiation on tissues. Radiation imparts energy to tissues causing DNA damage with consequent loss of cellular reproductive ability. Some cells die through apoptosis, but most do not manifest evidence of damage until mitosis occurs, and several divisions may ensue before actual cell death, termed mitotic cell death. Radiation is known to damage a variety of cellular components. While the exact mechanism of cell death is still under investigation, evidence supports double-stranded breaks of nuclear DNA as the most important cellular effect of radiation.[5] This breakage leads to irreversible loss of the reproductive potential and eventual cell death. X-rays and gamma rays differ from other forms of EM radiation in that they are indirectly ionizing, meaning that they cannot eject electron from atoms; damage is most commonly via the formation of free-radical intermediaries such as $H_2O^+$ (water ion) and OH• (hydroxyl radical). The free radicals in turn can cause damage to the target within the cell.

## Cell Survival Curve

A logarithmic curve of survival versus dose characterizes cell survival after exposure (see Fig. 2). The curve forms an initial shoulder followed by a logarithmic decline in survival, which varies with the dose.[6] The linear (alpha) component is responsible for the initial shoulder on the cell survival curve and is caused by irreparable damage to the target. The quadratic (beta) component represents sub-lethal damage. The linear component is proportional to the dose, while the quadratic component is proportional to the dose squared. The equation for the survival curve is $S = e^{-(\alpha D+\beta D2)}$ where $D$ is the total dose in Gy, alpha ($\alpha$) is the cell kill per Gy of the initial linear component (on a log-linear plot) and beta ($\beta$) the cell kill per $Gy^2$ of the quadratic component of the survival curve.

Curves for the individual linear quadratic components $e^{-\alpha D}$ and $e^{-\beta D^2}$ intersect at the dose where the $\alpha D$ and $\beta D^2$ components of cell killing are equal. This intersection happens to occur at a dose equal to the ratio of $\alpha$ to $\beta$, and is referred to as $\alpha/\beta$. Alpha is measured in 1/Gy and beta in $1/(Gy)^2$ so $\alpha/\beta$ has the unit of dose (Gy). $\alpha$ defines the initial slope of the survival curve; larger values indicate a steeper slope. $\beta$ defines the bend of the curve and a larger $\beta$ indicates more curvature. Therefore, a large $\alpha/\beta$ means there is a steep, small shoulder with little curvature, and for a small $\alpha/\beta$, there is a large, shallow shoulder with a large curve. Since the size of the shoulder indicates the repair capacity, a small $\alpha/\beta$ tissue has

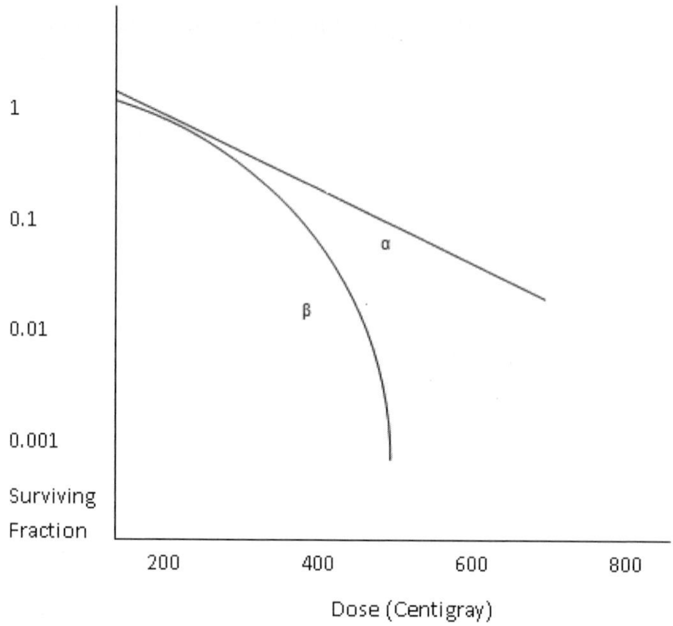


Figure 2. The cell survival curve depicts the relationship between the fraction of cells retaining their reproductive integrity with respect to absorbed dose. The linear quadratic or $\alpha/\beta$ model posits two components to cell killing, one that is linear ($\alpha$, proportional to dose) and one that is quadratic ($\beta$, proportional to dose squared). At low doses the linear portion predominates while at higher doses, it is the quadratic portion that predominates.

greater repair capacity than one with a large $\alpha/\beta$. Thus, for late effects, $\alpha/\beta$ is small, but for early responding tissue and tumors, which are mitotically active, $\alpha/\beta$ is large. The $\alpha$ and $\beta$ components of cell killing are equal at approximately $\alpha/\beta = 10$ Gy and $\alpha/\beta = 3$ Gy for early and late effects, respectively.

## Fractionation

This difference between tumors and late-responding tissues is useful in creating fractioned regimens, which have a larger sparing effect on late-responding tissues than on tumors and early-responding tissues. The rationale for fractionation, which refers to breaking up a total dose into smaller fractions, is based on the "four Rs" of radiobiology: redistribution, repair, repopulation, and re-oxygenation.[7] Conventional fractionation is a dose of 1.8 to 2.0 Gy given once per day until the specified total dose is delivered.

- Redistribution: Cells are more sensitive to radiation in certain phases of the cell cycle, particularly mitosis. By breaking up treatment into daily fractions, the chances of radiating cells in a radiation-sensitive portion of the cell cycle are increased. To review, mitosis (M) is the phase where division takes place. The S phase is a period of DNA synthesis. The S and M portions of the cell cycle are separated by two periods (gaps) called G1 and G2 when, respectively, DNA has not yet been synthesized or has been synthesized but other metabolic processes are taking place. In general, cells are most radiosensitive in the M and G2 phases, and most resistant in the late S phase.
- Repair: Fractionation also allows for repair of sub-lethal damage. As normal tissue requires time between doses to repair itself, this improves the therapeutic ratio.
- Repopulation: Accelerated repopulation can occur in tumors during a course of radiation. Accelerated repopulation of tumor cells is thought to influence local control of several malignancies, including cervical cancer, with a reduction in local control of 0.5% for each day of prolongation of time.[8] For a dose known to control a tumor according to a conventional fractionation schedule, the dose must be increased if the overall treatment time is prolonged. Overall treatment time is believed to be less critical in slower-growing tumors, such as prostate cancer. Ideally, a given fractionation schedule provides enough time for normal cells to repopulate, but limits time enough to prevent cancer cell repopulation.
- Reoxygenation: Tumor cell response to radiation is also influenced by hypoxia. Cancers often form tumors that outgrow their blood supply, resulting in hypoxia and radiation resistance, but over time, they may regain access to a blood supply and become re-oxygenated. The presence or absence of molecular oxygen within a cell influences the biological effect of ionizing radiation. The ratio of doses without and with oxygen to produce the same biological effect is called the oxygen enhancement ratio (OER). The OER for X-rays

and electrons is about three at high doses and falls to about two for doses of 1–2 Gy. The OER decreases as the linear energy transfer (LET) increases and approaches OER = 1 at about LET = 150 keV/m.

## TELETHERAPY

Teletherapy, from the Greek *tele* which means "at a distance," is given from a source outside the patient. Types of teletherapy can be thought of according to their energies:

- Superficial (10–80 kVp),
- Orthovoltage (100–500 kVp),
- Megavoltage (Co-60 to 35 MV).

The earliest teletherapy units were low-energy and were therefore limited to the treatment of superficial lesions.[2] Furthermore, the lack of a precise method of measuring dosage limited the early use of radiation therapy. An early prescription typically called for an erythema dose as the standard unit of radiation. One of the limiting factors in early treatment was skin tolerance. The use of fractionation helped to overcome this problem. Later, megavoltage radiotherapy units were introduced. External beam radiation therapy (EBRT) is delivered by photons, most commonly electrons or protons from a source outside the body. Less frequently, electrons, which have a sharp dose gradient, are also used, generally to treat superficial lesions. For example, in the treatment of vulvar cancer, electrons can supplement the dose to the inguinal lymph nodes or be used to deliver a boost to the primary tumor.

Conventional external beam radiation therapy, called 2D-XRT, is planned using two-dimensional, fluoroscopic radiographs. Beam arrangements are designed in reference to bony landmarks to encompass regions of interest to be treated. This technique has been used for many decades, but in contrast to newer techniques, does not allow visualization of soft tissue.

In the United States, three-dimensional conformal radiation therapy (3D-CRT) is the most widely used method of treatment planning and delivery. CT images are obtained with the patient in treatment position; this process is also known as "CT simulation." The CT images are then transferred to the treatment planning system. CT simulation allows for delineation of the tumor and normal structure in three-dimensions. The physician uses the clinical and radiographic findings to determine the gross tumor volume (GTV).[9] The clinical tumor volume (CTV) is defined to include microscopic extension of the disease. The planning treatment volume (PTV) adds an additional margin to account for day-to-day variations in patient setup as well as organ motion. Using beam's-eye-view technology, the field of radiation can be planned so that the physician is assured that the radiation field adequately covers the target and spares or minimizes the dose to the non-target healthy tissues known as organs at risk (OAR). For many gynecologic radiation plans, OARs would include the bowel, bladder, rectum, and bone marrow. In order to minimize any variation in patient positioning, precise immobilization is essential.

## Endometrial Carcinoma

The treatment of endometrial cancer is individualized depending on patient factors and disease stage. Although surgical therapy and surgicopathologic staging is the mainstay of therapy for most endometrial cancers and uterine sarcomas, radiation therapy may be used as primary therapy for early endometrial cancer and uterine sarcomas for patients who have unresectable disease. Primary radiotherapy (total dose to tumor of up to approximately 80 Gy) is the treatment of choice for those patients who are poor surgical candidates. Radiation therapy is more often employed in the adjuvant setting, particularly vaginal brachytherapy, as the sole adjuvant treatment for patients with high-intermediate-risk endometrial cancer (see *Brachytherapy*), and pelvic radiation for patients with high-risk endometrial cancer. When delivered in the adjuvant setting for high-risk disease, volume-directed radiotherapy is usually employed in addition to chemotherapy. Generally this includes pelvic radiotherapy with doses ranging from 45 to 50.4 Gy in 1.8 to 2 Gy daily fractions. If para-aortic lymph nodes are involved, the radiation field is extended to include this region.

Indications for adjuvant radiation after surgery for endometrial cancer are based on the stage and grade of disease. Whole-pelvis external beam

(see *Brachytherapy*). These implants are typically done after several weeks of external beam radiotherapy in order to allow for shrinkage of the tumor.

## Vulvar Carcinoma

For clinical stage I or II disease, postoperative radiotherapy is indicated when pathologic evidence suggests inguinal node metastasis or close (<8 mm) resection margins around the primary site.[14] A dose of 45–50 Gy is given in fractions of 1.8–2 Gy to regions at risk for residual microscopic disease, which includes the inguinal lymph nodes.

Using the proper technique to treat the inguinal nodes is important and excessive irradiation of the femoral neck should be avoided. Appropriate options include a wide AP photon field prescribed to the depth of the external iliac artery as it crosses the inguinal ligament, supplemented by a narrow PA field to ensure adequate coverage of the pelvic nodes. As an alternative, electrons may be used to cover some of the entire region of the inguinal nodes, but the energy must be carefully selected to achieve a sufficiently deep distribution of radiation dose to the full nodal area.[15]

Radical vulvectomy has historically been considered sufficient central treatment to the primary site, with postoperative irradiation directed only to the nodes. Thus, to protect the vulva, a midline block was often used. However, the use of a midline block is not recommended because of the high recurrence rate within the shielded area.[16]

## Vaginal Carcinoma

Definitive radiotherapy is the treatment of choice in most localized vaginal cancers as it tends to provide a better functional outcome than surgical treatment. Radiation consists of external beam radiotherapy with or without a brachytherapy boost. EBRT is typically 40–45 Gy in 1.8 Gy fractions, with a brachytherapy boost to 70–80 Gy. Inserting a radiopaque marker at the time of CT simulation allows one to determine the caudal extent of disease. When vaginal carcinoma occurs in the distal 1/3 of the vagina, the inguinal lymph nodes should be included in the radiation volume, following the drainage pattern of the distal vaginal to the inguinal and femoral vessels. External beam alone is generally not used except for palliation; however, brachytherapy alone may be used for small, well-differentiated lesions less than 0.5 cm thick.[17]

## INTENSITY-MODULATED RADIATION THERAPY

Conventional external beam radiotherapy, while highly effective, delivers ionizing radiation not only to the target tumor volume but also to the surrounding adjacent normal tissues, accounting for many of the observed acute (diarrhea, cystitis) and late (small bowel obstruction, urethral stricture) tissue toxicities.[18] These potential complications limit the total radiation dose that can be safely delivered by conventional radiotherapy techniques. In an attempt to increase the ratio of prescribed radiation dose given to the tumor as opposed to the surrounding normal tissues, a technique of intensity-modulated radiation therapy (IMRT) has recently been developed. IMRT differs from three-dimensional conformal radiotherapy (3D-CRT) by modifying the intensity of radiation within each of the radiation beams. Unlike conventional RT, IMRT uses an inverse planning process, whereby the planner first delineates the target and designated OARs and then uses a computerized algorithm to set priorities to areas that require treatment and limits (often referred to as constraints) to those that should be avoided. The computer then generates a plan that meets the specifications determined by the planner. This allows selective avoidance of critical normal tissues without compromising the tumor doses. IMRT utilizes variable, computer-controlled intensities within each radiation beam, in contrast to the uniform doses within each 3D-CRT beam. This is accomplished by dividing each beam into smaller "beamlets." Compared to most other treatment techniques, IMRT can achieve a higher degree of conformality to the target while sparing high dose to normal tissue, particularly when the target volumes have complex shapes or concave regions. IMRT, however, is not necessarily superior to 3D-CRT in all cases, and no randomized trials have been conducted to date. In patients who are treated with extended field radiation, where the volume of bowel treated is greater than in whole-pelvis treatment, IMRT has been used with favorable acute toxicity outcomes.[19] One intricacy of IMRT is the increased volume of normal tissue exposed to low-dose radiation, as compared to 3D-CRT, which, theoretically, could increase the incidence of secondary malignancies.[20]

Other potential uses for IMRT include the ability to administer higher doses to target tissues and lower doses to OARs with the goal of improving the therapeutic ratio.[21] Dosimetric studies have shown that IMRT is as good as or better than 3D-CRT at covering the target while reducing the volume of OARs receiving high dose.[22] For example, in patients with positive nodes or with gross residual disease post-surgery, one might use IMRT to boost the dose to the nodes to a higher dose than could safely be achieved with 3D-CRT while maintaining high local-regional control.[23] A dosimetric comparison of IMRT with traditional planning for treatment of pelvic and inguinal nodes demonstrated a reduced volume of the bladder, bowel, and rectum in the IMRT plans.[24] While it is still in relative infancy and although long-term patient follow-up is not yet available, the use of IMRT in the treatment of gynecologic cancer is increasing and, when properly utilized, has the potential not only to reduce normal tissue toxicity but also improve oncologic outcomes.

## PROTON THERAPY

The development of proton therapy, which uses protons (rather than X-rays) to irradiate tissues, began in the 1950s in accelerator laboratories, but in the last 20 years has expanded to hospital-based facilities. The chief advantage of proton therapy is the ability to reduce exit dose when compared with other types of external beam radiotherapy (see Fig. 4). The reason for this is a physical property unique to protons: the dose delivered to tissue is at a maximum just over the last few millimeters of the particle's range; this maximum is called the Bragg peak.[25] In contrast, X-rays penetrate completely through tissue while losing some energy along the way.

Consequently, the increased precision of proton therapy may be used to reduce unwanted side effects, by limiting the dose to normal tissue, as has been demonstrated in certain pediatric tumors.[26] Proton therapy has been studied retrospectively in cervical cancer. Patients who were unable to receive intracavitary brachytherapy treatment and were instead treated with a proton boost following external beam therapy had similar local control and overall survival as conventionally treated patients.[27]

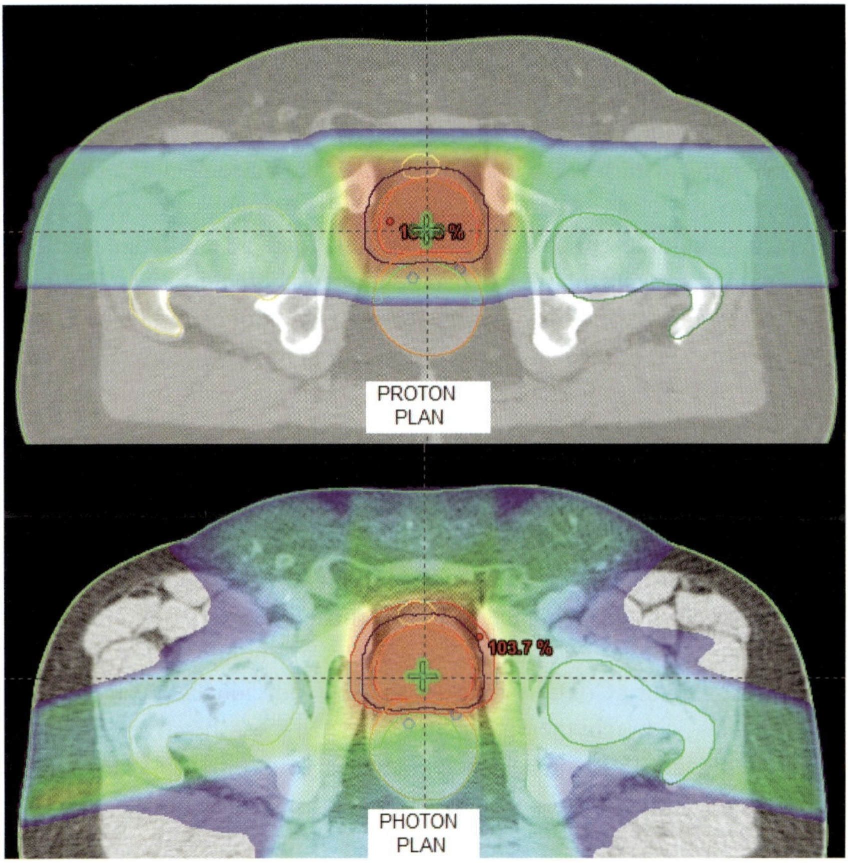


Figure 4. The photon plan depicts beam entering, passing through the target, and exiting normal tissue, while in the proton plan, two opposed lateral beams enter and converge in the target, with no exit through normal tissue.

## BRACHYTHERAPY

Brachytherapy (*brachy*, derived from Greek, meaning "short distance") places radioactive sources in direct contact with or adjacent to the tumor. An advantage of brachytherapy is the ability to treat the tumor with high doses locally, with rapid dose fall-off to surrounding tissues. Brachytherapy may be either intracavitary, interstitial, or intraluminal. The first two forms are used to treat gynecologic malignancies. Optimal treatment with brachytherapy requires that the tumor must be accessible, well-demarcated, and cannot be the only modality for tumors with high risk of regional lymph node metastasis. Intracavitary treatments are always temporary, while interstitial treatments may be temporary or permanent. Curative intracavitary brachytherapy involves the placement of a source in a body cavity. It is frequently used to treat malignancies of the vagina, cervix, and endometrium. While smaller tumors are generally amenable to intracavitary implants, more extensive tumors may require treatment with interstitial implants and may involve a combination of external beam radiation therapy and intracavitary and/or interstitial brachytherapy. Interstitial implants use radioactive needles, wires, or seeds, which are directly inserted into the tumor.

The methods of brachytherapy may be broadly described as manual, where the radioactive material is placed by hand, or remote, and source placement is at least partially automated. An automated machine used to place a radioactive material during a brachytherapy procedure is known as "a remote afterloader." The licensing of radioactive sources and the safety of the general public and healthcare workers are regulated by either the Nuclear Regulatory Commission (NRC) or by individual state agencies.[28]

The classic brachytherapy source, Ra-226, was discovered by the Curies in the late 1800s. It has an average energy of 0.83 MeV and a half-life of 1,600 years. Radium sources are manufactured as needles or tubes in a variety of lengths and activities. Unfortunately, radium-226 leaks radon gas, and was replaced by cesium-137, which has an energy of 0.662 MeV and a half-life of 30 years. Iridium-192 is also used and is available in the form of thin, flexible wires that can be cut to the desired length. It has an average energy of 0.38 MeV so it requires less shielding for personnel protection. The half-life of Ir-192 is 73.8 days (see Table 1).

Table 1. Commonly used brachytherapy sources.

| Radionuclide | Half-life | Energy |
|---|---|---|
| Cesium-137 | 30.17 years | 0.662 MeV |
| Iridium-192 | 74.0 days | 0.38 MeV (mean) |
| Iodine-125 | 59.6 days | 31.4 and 35.5 keV |
| Palladium-103 | 17.0 days | 21 keV (mean) |

Factors influencing the dose distribution of brachytherapy treatments include distance (inverse square law), attenuation from the source capsule, attenuation within the surrounding tissue, and build-up from scattered photons. The inverse square law indicates that doubling the distance from a radiation source decreases the radiation level by a factor of four. Conversely, decreasing the distance by half increases the radiation level by a factor of four.

Brachytherapy is described according to the length of time that a procedure is performed. For low-dose-rate (LDR) temporary implants, treatments take place over a few days. In some cases (i.e., prostate brachytherapy), permanent interstitial implants may be preferred; in such cases, the source should have a short half-life, so that the dose is delivered within a few weeks or months, as well as low energy, to reduce exposure to others. During most LDR brachytherapy procedures, a dose of radiation in the range of about 0.4–2 Gy/h is administered. High-dose-rate (HDR) brachytherapy typically uses high-specific-activity, gamma-emitting radionuclides to deliver a much greater dose rate (>12 Gy/h) of radiation. A typical HDR source is Ir-192. Because of the higher dose rate, HDR brachytherapy procedures are shorter in duration as compared to LDR. The short treatment times, the ability to perform HDR procedures on an outpatient basis, and improved patient comfort are all advantages of HDR brachytherapy.

## Tandem and Ovoid Brachytherapy

Tandem and ovoid brachytherapy is most commonly used for the treatment of intact uterine cervical cancer. The treatment consists of the temporary placement of an intrauterine tandem and intravaginal ovoids to deliver treatment via HDR or LDR. A tandem and ovoid applicator consists of a pencil-thin, hollow, metal tube (the tandem) that is inserted through the cervix into the uterus. The ovoids are hollow, metal capsules that are small enough to fit in the vaginal fornices. The radionuclides are loaded into the hollow spaces within the tandem and ovoids. In place of the tandem and ovoid applicator, some facilities will use a tandem and ring applicator. Prior to the first treatment, a Smit sleeve is placed in the uterus and its base is sutured to the cervix to secure it. The Smit sleeve is a hollow, plastic tube wide enough to accommodate the flange of the tandem, which is designed to keep the os open, allowing for comfortable and reproducible positioning of the tandem. Because it is close-ended, the Smit sleeve also protects against uterine perforation. After the tandem and ovoids are placed, radiopaque vaginal gauze is applied to secure the devices in place and fix their position relative to the bladder and rectum. Intraoperative radiographs or digital fluoroscopic images document appropriate device positioning. Contrast material in a Foley catheter and a rectal tube can be used to identify the International Commission on Radiological Units and Measurements (ICRU) reference points of interest. A CT or MRI is recommended after placement of the applicators for treatment planning. Figure 5 shows a CT-based tandem and ovoid plan; note the typical pear-shaped dose distribution.[29]

The standard prescription for treatment for decades has been based on point A in the following list of ICRU reference points for gynecologic brachytherapy doses.

- Point A = 2 cm cephalic to the external os along the tandem and 2 cm perpendicular to the plane of the tandem.
- Point B = 2 cm cephalic to the os and 5 cm lateral to the patient's midline.

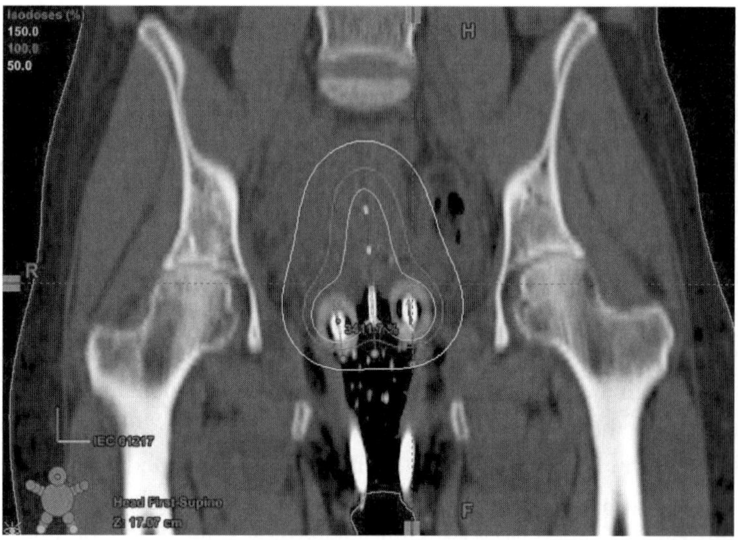


Figure 5. The HDR tandem and ovoid treatment reflects the standard pear-shaped dose distribution.

- Bladder point = Most posterior point in the bulb of the Foley catheter along a direct AP line through the center of the bulb.
- Rectal point = 0.5 cm posterior to the vaginal mucosa in the patient's midline at the level of the posterior aspect of the ovoid.

Doses are prescribed to ICRU points A and B. The reference point of origin for points A and B is the cervical os, which is identified by its relationship to the flange of the tandem. Placing a non-radioactive gold seed marker near the os also helps to corroborate localization of the cervical os on radiography.

HDR brachytherapy typically involves 5–7 weekly outpatient procedures using an Ir-192 source. Point A is given a dose of 5–7 Gy during each treatment, which typically is delivered over 10–15 minutes depending on the activity of the source. LDR brachytherapy usually involves 1 or 2 placement procedures in which the radioactive source is Cs-137. Each time, the sources are left in place for approximately two days, during which a dose of 20–40 Gy is administered to point A.

The timing of brachytherapy is important. For women receiving both external beam radiation and brachytherapy, high-dose-rate brachytherapy may begin during the conclusion of external beam radiation and it may start as early as after 20 Gy of an external beam course. Pelvic examination of patients undergoing external beam radiation helps the physician determine if brachytherapy at that time point would provide adequate tumor coverage. When brachytherapy procedures are performed along with adjuvant external beam therapy, some physicians use custom blocking called a "midline block" when administering EBRT, in order to shield areas of the bladder and rectum that have received a high dose from brachytherapy.

The most frequent clinical complications of intracavitary radiation treatments of cervical cancer result from a high dose delivered to the portions of the rectum and bladder that are in close proximity to the sources. Applicator placement is important in order to keep the dose to these critical structures as low as possible. Packing with gauze helps to displace the OARs away from the applicators.

The cumulative dose from external beam radiation and HDR brachytherapy to point A usually is 75–80 Gy, somewhat lower than the total dose of LDR brachytherapy. A typical dose would be 50 Gy via external beam and then five HDR treatments of 5.5 Gy each for a total of 77.5 Gy. For LDR, the biologically equivalent total dose to point A is 85–90 Gy. The reason for this difference is related to the anticipated intracellular radiation repair mechanisms active during the prolonged LDR application.

The basic approach for treating medically inoperable uterine cancer involves brachytherapy treatment with disposable afterloading Heyman capsules or tandems with colpostats (ovoids). Heyman capsules are well suited to a large uterus, and the current practice is to load as many capsules into the uterus as possible, to stretch the uterus and obtain the best isodose distribution. Typically, at least four Heyman capsules are inserted through the dilated cervix, but as many as ten may be necessary. A problem encountered with Heyman capsules is that they have relatively thick stems and the dilation of the cervix from multiple Heyman capsule stems may cause patients discomfort. Heyman capsules are numbered and should always be removed in the reverse order in which they were inserted to avoid jamming.

For patients with small uteri, it may be preferable to administer intrauterine brachytherapy with tandem and ovoids. Other afterloading systems used to administer brachytherapy for cervical cancer include the Henschke and Fletcher-Suit systems. The procedure may either take place in the operating room under anesthesia, or in the clinic using a patient-controlled anesthesia pump. The procedure may take as long as 30 minutes. Brachytherapy with tandem and ovoids may be performed with LDR or HDR applications.

## Interstitial Brachytherapy

Intracavitary brachytherapy devices are sometimes difficult to position because of anatomic distortion due to tumoral infiltration into the surrounding structures. In high-stage vaginal disease, the vaginal fornices are commonly effaced because the tumor erodes the cervix. The lateral distribution of the radiation dose to the parametrium is compromised when ovoids cannot be placed at a level near the cervical os. This may result in undesirably high doses to the bladder and rectal reference points.

In such circumstances, an alternative is to use interstitial brachytherapy, where blind-ended catheters are placed through the perineum into areas of tumor infiltration in the lower pelvis lateral to the cervix. Thin, plastic threads studded with Ir-192 sources are loaded into the catheters placed at the desired positions within a plastic Syed template (see Fig. 6) to provide the necessary lateral dose distribution. In many institutions, when interstitial brachytherapy is indicated, patients undergo CT-based treatment planning prior to implantation to determine the amount of Ir-192 needed and the optimal spatial arrangement of catheters. Other indications for interstitial brachytherapy include treatment of cervical cancer where the extent of parametrial disease precludes adequate coverage when intracavitary technique is used, treatment of vaginal cancer when paravaginal extension is not encompassed with standard intracavitary brachytherapy, and treatment of vaginal recurrence of endometrial cancer.[30–33] It is important to note that there are no randomized trials assessing the role of interstitial brachytherapy versus endocavitary brachytherapy in cervical cancer.

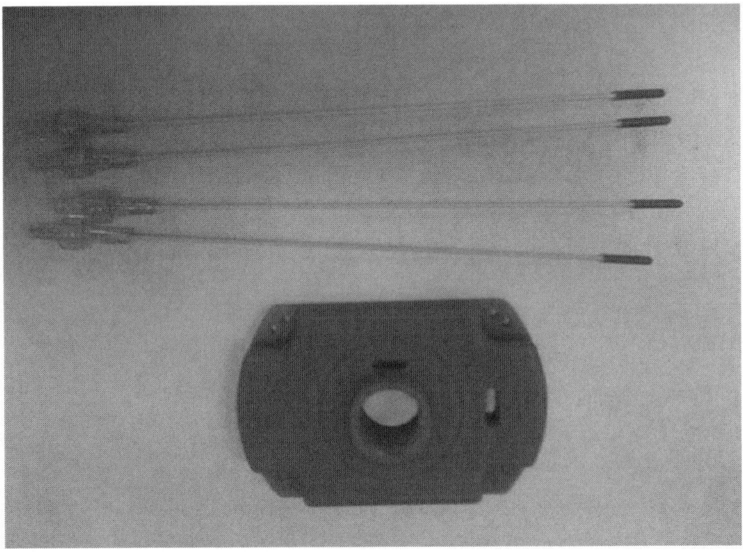

Figure 6. Interstitial brachytherapy is delivered through thin plastic catheters which are placed at pre-determined points within the grid of the Syed template.

## Vaginal Intracavitary Treatment

For adjuvant treatment of intermediate-risk endometrial cancer, the use of a vaginal cylinder in conjunction with a HDR source has become popular because of its convenience as a well-tolerated outpatient regimen.[34] When intravaginal brachytherapy is given, either after monotherapy or after pelvic EBRT, the goal is to treat the proximal 3–5 cm of vagina, given that the vagina has been identified as the region of highest risk for local failure after surgery.[35] Figure 7 shows vaginal cylinders, which are sized according to diameter.

When HDR intravaginal brachytherapy is administered without pelvic EBRT, a dose of 21 Gy to a depth of 0.5 cm given in three fractions is commonly prescribed. Lower doses of vaginal cuff brachytherapy can also be delivered after EBRT for high-risk factors including high-grade disease, papillary serous histology, or cervical involvement. A typical dosage schedule for HDR intravaginal brachytherapy after EBRT is 15 Gy prescribed to a depth of 0.5 cm over 3–5 cm of the upper vagina given in three weekly fractions of 5 Gy each.[10] When HDR intravaginal brachytherapy is administered without pelvic EBRT, a dose of 21 Gy to a depth of 0.5 cm given in three fractions is commonly prescribed. The dose

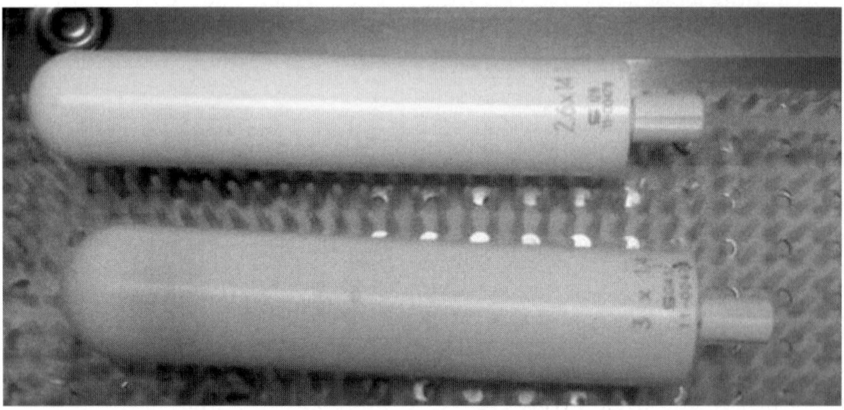

Figure 7. The vaginal cylinders are available in various sizes, according to diameter. The largest size a patient can comfortably tolerate is chosen to ensure contact between vaginal mucosa and the cylinder for a more homogeneous dose delivery.

may either be prescribed to the surface or to a depth of 0.5 cm with appropriate adjustments in the dose. Vaginal intracavitary brachytherapy may also be done with an LDR technique. When LDR is delivered without external beam, the dose prescription should be 50–60 Gy at 0.5 cm depth over 72 h (70–80 cGy/h). When used in conjunction with external beam radiation, the LDR dose is 30 Gy.

## Low-Dose Rate or High-Dose Rate

While many institutions have adopted HDR brachytherapy for vaginal intracavitary treatments, the choice of LDR versus HDR brachytherapy has been a source of controversy for the treatment of locally advanced cervical cancer. LDR brachytherapy has a much longer history, having been used over many decades. Advantages of LDR brachytherapy include a requirement for just two cesium insertions. Disadvantages of LDR include the need for inpatient treatment with prolonged bedrest (with a concomitant risk of venous thromboembolism), radiation exposure to staff, and limitations of source strengths. Disadvantages of HDR, on the other hand, include a higher risk of amplifying dosimetry errors, expense, the need to replace iridium sources frequently (due to the short half-life), and the need for multiple applications.[36] Practically speaking, not all institutions are able to offer both LDR and HDR treatments, which requires a significant commitment of resources in terms of both equipment and personnel.

## Clinical Outcomes

Although there are no randomized studies conducted in the United States, several randomized studies have been performed in Asia with results demonstrating no difference in long-term outcomes with HDR versus LDR brachytherapy; Osaka University Hospital[37] reported no significant differences in five-year cause-specific survival for HDR versus LDR. Moderate to severe complications, however, were higher in the HDR than LDR group (10% vs 4%). Patel *et al.*[38] reported no significant differences in five-year survival or pelvic control for HDR versus LDR brachytherapy, but they noted a statistically significant higher rate of rectal complications for patients in the LDR group (19.9% vs 6.4%).

Hareyama *et al.*[39] randomized 132 patients with stage II or stage IIIB cervical cancer to LDR versus HDR; no statistically significant differences were noted in survival or complication rates. Finally, Lertsanguansinchai *et al.*[40] randomized 237 patients between HDR and LDR brachytherapy and reported comparable outcome.

Within the United States, Petereit *et al.*[41] reviewed outcomes in patients treated with LDR versus HDR brachytherapy. The authors reported no statistically significant difference in pelvic control or other outcomes in stages IB or II, but outcomes in some patients with stage IIIB disease were inferior, which has not been demonstrated in other studies.

## TOXICITY

Radiation effects on the normal tissues are divided into acute and late effects. Acute effects occur during the course of therapy and during the post-therapy period, usually within three months of the start of radiation. The tissues that divide rapidly (e.g., mucous membranes) respond acutely to radiation and are responsible for much of the acute morbidity of the treatment. While patients are usually most bothered by the acute effects, physicians are at least equally concerned about the chronic effects. The acute effects can be quite uncomfortable but generally resolve, and include fatigue, urinary frequency, dysuria, diarrhea, fecal urgency, and hair loss within the radiation field. Late effects can manifest anytime thereafter, from weeks to years after the treatment. Late tissue responses occur in organs whose cells do not divide frequently and they also occur in tissues that manifest early reactions, though the nature of these reactions is different from that of early reactions. Late responses determine the maximum dose that can be safely delivered. One rare late effect is radiation-induced fibrosis. In patients who receive pelvic radiation, GI tract fibrosis may contribute to stricture formation and in severe cases, small bowel obstruction; the incidence of small bowel obstruction is less than 5% and is related to the dose of radiation delivered.[42] Other possible late side effects of pelvic EBRT and/or brachytherapy include urine leakage, pain or bleeding with bowel movements, fistula formation, and narrowing or scarring of the vagina,[43] which can cause pain with sexual intercourse. With regard to vaginal stenosis, patients who complete radiation treatment should be instructed on the use of vaginal dilators, plastic rods of varying widths, which are effective in preventing stenosis when used on a regular basis.

The late effects of radiation can be a source of ongoing morbidity from a course of radiation therapy. Other treatment modalities, such as surgery and chemotherapy, can increase the probability and severity of radiation-related morbidity. Just as with the acute effects, the chronic effects are related to site, dose, volume, and time. Much of the effort that goes into treatment planning goes towards minimizing the effects of treatment on normal tissue while ensuring adequate treatment of the tumor and areas at risk.

## REFERENCES

1. Cleaves M. Radium: with a preliminary note on radium rays in the treatment of cancer. *Med Rec* 1903;64:1719–1723.
2. Khan F. *The Physics of Radiation Therapy.* Baltimore: Lippincott Williams & Wilkins, 2010.
3. Stanton R, Stinson D. *Applied Physics for Radiation Oncology.* Madison: Medical Physics Publishing Corporation, 1996.
4. Wrixton D. New ICRP recommendations. *J Radiol Prot* 2008;28:161–168.
5. Nunez MI, McMillan TJ, Valenzuela MT, *et al.* Relationship between DNA damage and cell killing by radiation in mammalian cells. *Radiother Oncol* 1996;39:155–165.
6. Hall E, Giaccia A. *Radiobiology for the Radiologist.* Philadelphia: Lippincott Williams & Wilkins, 2006.
7. Withers R. The four Rs of radiotherapy. *Adv Radiat Biol* 1975;5:241–271.
8. Fyles A, Keane TJ, Barton M, *et al.* The effect of treatment duration in the local control of cervix cancer. *Radiother Oncol* 1992;25(4):273–279.
9. International Commission on Radiation Units and Measurements. ICRU Report 62. Prescribing, recording, and reporting photon beam therapy, Supplement to ICRU Report No. 50. Bethesda, 1999.
10. Nag S, Erickson B, Parikh S, *et al.* The American Brachytherapy Society recommendations for high-dose-rate brachytherapy for carcinoma of the endometrium. *Int J Radiat Oncol Biol Phys* 2000;48(3):779–790.
11. Landoni F, Maneo A, Colombo A, *et al.* Randomized study of radical surgery versus radiotherapy for stage Ib-IIa cervical cancer. *Lancet* 1997;350: 535–540.

12. Peters WA III, Liu PY, Barrett RJ II, *et al.* Concurrent chemotherapy and pelvic radiation therapy compared with pelvic radiation therapy alone as adjuvant therapy after radical surgery in high-risk early-stage cancer of the cervix. *J Clin Oncol* 2000;18:1606–1613.
13. Rotman M, Sedlis A, Piedmonte MR, *et al.* A phase III randomized trial of postoperative pelvic irradiation in Stage IB cervical carcinoma with poor prognostic features: follow-up of a Gynecologic Oncology Group study. *Int J Radiat Oncol Biol Phys* 2006;65(1):169–176.
14. Faul CM, Mirmow D, Huang Q, *et al.* Adjuvant radiation for vulvar carcinoma: improved local control. *Int J Radiat Oncol Biol Phys* 1997;38(2): 381–389.
15. Koh WJ, Chiu M, Stelzer KJ, *et al.* Femoral vessel depth and the implications for groin node irradiation. *Int J Radiat Oncol Biol Phys* 1993;27(4): 969–974.
16. Dusenbery KE, Carlson JW, LaPorte RM, *et al.* Radical vulvectomy with postoperative irradiation for vulvar cancer: therapeutic implications of a central block. *Int J Radiat Oncol Biol Phys* 1994;25(9):989–998.
17. Mock U, Kucera H, Fellner C, *et al.* High-dose-rate (HDR) brachytherapy with or without external beam radiotherapy in the treatment of primary vaginal carcinoma: long-term results and side effects. *Int J Radiat Oncol Biol Phys* 2003;56(4):950–957.
18. Perez CA, Breaux S, Bedwinek JM, *et al.* Radiation therapy alone in the treatment of carcinoma of the uterine cervix. II. Analysis of complications. *Cancer* 1984;54:235–246.
19. Salama JK, Mundt AJ, Roeske J, *et al.* Preliminary outcome and toxicity report of extended-field intensity-modulated radiation therapy for gynecologic malignancies. *Int J Radiat Oncol Biol Phys* 2006;65:1170–1176.
20. Kry SF, Salehpour M, Followill DS, *et al.* The calculated risk of fatal secondary malignancies from intensity-modulated radiation therapy. *Int J Radiat Oncol Biol Phys* 2005;62(4):1195–1203.
21. D'Souza WD, Ahamad AA, Iyer RB, *et al.* Feasibility of dose escalation using intensity-modulated radiotherapy in post-hysterectomy cervical carcinoma. *Int J Radiat Oncol Biol Phys* 2005;61:1062–1070.
22. Roeske JC, Lujan A, Rotsmensch J, *et al.* Intensity-modulated whole pelvic radiation therapy in patients with gynecologic malignancies. *Int J Radiation Oncol Biol Phys* 2000;28:1613–1621.

23. Grigsby PW, Singh AK, Siegel BA, *et al.* Lymph node control in cervical cancer. *Int J Radiat Oncol Biol Phys* 2004;59:706–712.
24. Beriwal S, Heron D, Kim H, *et al.* Intensity-modulated radiotherapy for the treatment of vulvar carcinoma: a comparative dosimetric study with early clinical outcome. *Int J Radiat Oncol Biol* 2006;64(5):1395–1400.
25. DeLaney T, Kooy H. *Proton and Charged Particle Radiotherapy.* Philadelphia: Lippincott Williams & Wilkins, 2008.
26. St. Clair *W*, Adams J, Bues M, *et al.* Advantage of protons compared to conventional X-ray or IMRT in the treatment of a pediatric patient with medulloblastoma. *Int J Radiat Oncol Biol Phys* 2004;58:727–734.
27. Kagei K, Tokuuye K, Okumura T, *et al.* Long-term results of proton beam therapy for carcinoma of the uterine cervix. *Int J Radiat Oncol Biol Phys* 2003;55(5):1265–1271.
28. NRC. Uses of Radiation. http://www.nrc.gov/about-nrc/radiation/around-us/uses-radiation.html#medical.
29. Haie-Meder C, Pötter R, Van Limbergen E, *et al.* Recommendations from gynaecological (GYN) GEC-ESTRO Working Group (I): concepts and terms in 3D image-based 3D treatment planning in cervix cancer brachytherapy with emphasis on MRI assessment of GTV and CTV. *Radiother Oncol* 2005;74(3):235–245.
30. Eifel PJ, Moughan J, Owen J. Patterns of radiotherapy practice for patients with squamous carcinoma of the uterine cervix: patterns of care study. *Int J Radiat Oncol Biol Phys* 1999;43:351–358.
31. Haie-Meder C, Breton C, de Crevoisier R, *et al.* Therapeutic orientations in brachytherapy in uterine cervix carcinoma. *Cancer Radiother* 2000;4: 133–139.
32. Charra C, Roy P, Coquard R. Outcome of treatment of upper third vaginal recurrences of cervical and endometrial carcinomas with interstitial brachytherapy. *Int J Radiat Oncol Biol Phys* 1998;40:421–426.
33. Lin LL, Grigsby PW, Powell MA, *et al.* Definitive radiotherapy in the management of isolated vaginal recurrences of endometrial cancer. *Int J Radiat Oncol Biol Phys* 2005;63(2):500–504.
34. Nout RA, Smit VT, Putter H, *et al.* Vaginal brachytherapy versus pelvic external beam radiotherapy for patients with endometrial cancer of high-intermediate risk (PORTEC-2): an open-label, non-inferiority, randomised trial. *Lancet* 2010;375:816–823.

35. Keys HM, Roberts JA, Brunetto VL, *et al.* A phase III trial of surgery with or without adjunctive external pelvic radiation therapy in intermediate risk endometrial adenocarcinoma: a Gynecologic Oncology Group study. *Gynecol Oncol* 2004;92(3):744–751.
36. Stewart AJ, Viswanathan AN. Current controversies in high-dose-rate versus low-dose-rate brachytherapy for cervical cancer. *Cancer* 2006; 107(5):908–915.
37. Teshima T, Inoue T, Ikeda H, *et al.* High-dose rate and low-dose rate intracavitary therapy for carcinoma of the uterine cervix. Final results of Osaka University Hospital. *Cancer* 1993;72:2409–2414.
38. Patel FD, Sharma SC, Negi PS, *et al.* Low dose rate vs. high dose rate brachytherapy in the treatment of carcinoma of the uterine cervix: a clinical trial. *Int J Radiat Oncol Biol Phys* 1994;28(2):335–341.
39. Hareyama M, Sakata K, Oouchi A, *et al.* High-dose-rate versus low-dose-rate intracavitary therapy for carcinoma of the uterine cervix: a randomized trial. *Cancer* 2002;94(1):117–124.
40. Lertsanguansinchai P, Lertbutsayanukul C, Shotelersuk K, *et al.* Phase III randomized trial comparing LDR and HDR brachytherapy in treatment of cervical carcinoma. *Int J Radiat Oncol Biol Phys* 2005;59(5):1424–1431.
41. Petereit D, Sarkaria J, Potter D. High-dose-rate versus low-dose-rate brachytherapy in the treatment of cervical cancer: analysis of tumor recurrence — the University of Wisconsin experience. *Int J Radiat Oncol Biol Phys* 1999;45(5):1267–1274.
42. Perez CA, Grigsby PW, Lockett MA, *et al.* Radiation therapy morbidity in carcinoma of the uterine cervix: dosimetric and clinical correlation. *Int J Radiat Oncol Biol Phys* 1999;44(4):855–866.
43. Brand A, Bull C, Cakir B. Vaginal stenosis in patients treated with radiotherapy for carcinoma of the cervix. *Int J Gynecol Cancer* 2006; 16(1):288–293.

# 3

# PREINVASIVE DISEASE OF THE LOWER GENITAL TRACT

*Sarah H. Kim*

## INTRODUCTION

The widespread use of screening with cervical cytology has led to a significant decline in the incidence of cervical cancer in the United States in the past 30 years. The American Cancer Society estimated 11,270 new cases and 4,070 deaths from cervical cancer in the United States in 2009. However, cervical cancer remains the second most common cancer among women worldwide, accounting for approximately 20% to 30% of all female cancers with almost 500,000 new cases and 240,000 deaths per year. The cancer incidence and mortality is disproportionately high in the developing countries, which largely reflects the impact of cervical cytology screening.[1]

There has been a marked increase in human papillomavirus-(HPV) associated disease in North America and Western Europe. HPV is the most commonly diagnosed sexually transmitted disease in the United States. More than half of sexually active women and men will be infected with HPV within their lives. This increase in the incidence of HPV-associated disease is in part due to increased prevalence of infection, but also secondary to heightened public awareness of HPV infection given the recent introduction of HPV vaccines against high-risk subtypes of HPV, and utilization of highly sensitive tests to detect high-risk HPV infections. The purpose of this chapter is to provide an overview in diagnosis, management, and treatment of preinvasive disease of the cervix, vagina, and vulva.

## HUMAN PAPILLOMAVIRUS

HPVs are small double-stranded DNA viruses with a genome of approximately 8,000 base pairs that belong to their own family, the papillomaviridae. The HPV genome encodes eight genes including two encapsulating structural proteins L1 and L2, which encode for major and minor capsid proteins, respectively. The L1 protein self-assembles in the absence of the viral genome to form a virus-like particle (VLP). The L1 VLP is the immunogen used in HPV vaccines.[2] The upstream regulatory region (URR) contains about 400 base pairs that code for binding sites of transcriptional activators and repressors; this region regulates the production of viral proteins and infectious particles.[3] Located downstream from the URR is the early region, which encodes for six proteins E1, E2, E4, E5, E6, and E7. The E6 and E7 proteins are involved in the transforming and immortalizing functions of HPV. The E2 protein is involved in the regulation of transcription of the viral genome, and both E1 and E2 proteins are required for replication and infection of HPV. The E4 protein is produced late in the viral life cycle and facilitates the release of assembled virus particles from infected epithelial cells. E5 is involved in stimulation of cell growth through the interaction with the epidermal growth factor receptor, platelet-derived growth factor receptor, and colony-stimulating factor-1 receptor.

There are more than 100 types of HPV and over 40 mucosal HPV serotypes can infect the lower female genital tract. Of these, approximately 20 types can cause anogenital cancers. These high-risk subtypes include 16, 18, 26, 31, 33, 35, 39, 45, 51, 52, 56, 58, 59, 66, 68, 73, and 82. Each varies in its carcinogenic potential.[4] HPV targets the basal cells in stratified squamous epithelium and the metaplastic cells at the cervical squamocolumnar junction. HPV can also infect the glandular epithelium of the endocervix, resulting in adenocarcinoma *in situ* (AIS) or invasive endocervical adenocarcinoma. HPV infects basal cells following microabrasion of cervical epithelium. Infected basal cells undergo proliferation and expansion. As HPV-infected cells progress through the more differentiated layers of the epithelium, viral replication is enhanced and large numbers of HPV DNA copies are produced. Late genes, including the viral capsid proteins, are produced and HPV virons are assembled.

Table 1. Classification of human papillomavirus types by risk of neoplasia and cancer.[5]

| High risk | Intermediate risk | Low risk |
|---|---|---|
| 16, 18, 45, 56 | 31, 33, 35, 39, 51, 52, 55, 58, 59, 66, 68 | 6, 11, 26, 42, 44, 54, 70, 73 |

This produces koilocytosis, the characteristic cytopathic effect of HPV infection.[3]

HPV 16 and 18 represent approximately 70% of all cervical cancers worldwide. Table 1 classifies the HPV subtypes by their oncogenic potential.[5] The E6 and E7 genes of high-risk HPV types, particularly HPV 16 and 18, are directly involved in cellular transformation. The E6 protein of high-risk HPV binds the tumor suppressor protein p53[5] and induces degradation of p53. As a result, the p53-dependent repair mechanism is lost and an increase in cellular proliferation is observed. The E7 protein is a nuclear phosphoprotein that transforms infected epithelium by binding and inactivation of the retinoblastoma gene (Rb), resulting in impeded function of endogenous tumor suppression.[3] The disruption of normal cell cycle control and abrogation of cellular apoptosis leads to chromosomal destabilization and inhibits cyclin-dependent kinase inhibitors and host interferons.[6] Telomerase is also activated, further augmenting oncogenic changes.

# CERVIX

## Epidemiology

Virtually all cases of cervical cancer can be attributed to persistent infection with carcinogenic genotypes of HPV. HPV 16 is the most carcinogenic subtype, accounting for approximately 50% of all cervical cancers. High-risk, oncogenic HPV types (HPV 16 and 18) are associated with 99.7% of all cervical cancers, as well as low-grade squamous intraepithelial lesions (LSIL), high-grade squamous intraepithelial lesions (HSIL), and abnormal Papanicolaou (Pap) test results. Low-risk HPV types (HPV 6 and 11) are also associated with abnormal Pap tests as well as almost all cases of genital warts. The degree of expression of HPV E6 and E7 is highly correlated with the severity of the cervical lesion. In low-grade lesions, these levels are expressed at low levels in the basal cells and at higher levels in the upper layers of the cervical epithelium. In high-grade lesions, E6 and E7 are expressed at high levels throughout the epithelium.[7] In low-grade lesions, HPV is in episomal form, whereas in higher-grade lesions and cervical cancer, the HPV DNA is more often integrated into host DNA.[7] This integration is a critical precursor for enhanced cellular proliferation and carcinogenesis.

Although the majority of sexually active adults will be infected with HPV at least once in their lives, sexually active women less than 25 years of age consistently have the highest rates of infection. Besides youth and gender, common risk factors for HPV infection and clinical sequelae of infection (including dysplasia and cancer) include high number of sexual partners, early age at first pregnancy and first intercourse, and coinfection with *Chlamydia trachomatis* or herpes simplex virus. In addition, lower socioeconomic class, cigarette smoking, oral contraceptive use, specific HLA-DR haplotypes, and immunosuppression are associated with both cervical cancer and its precursors (see Table 2). Most HPV infections are cleared by the immune system and do not result in clinical complications.[3]

## Natural History of Cervical Neoplasia

Infection with the HPV virus is a prerequisite for developing squamous cervical neoplasia. Fortunately, most HPV-infected women will not

Table 2. Risk factors for cervical intraepithelial neoplasia and cervical cancer.

| |
|---|
| Early sexual activity (before age 17) |
| Multiple sexual partners |
| HPV infection |
| Smoking |
| Human immunodeficiency virus |
| Parity |
| History of sexually transmitted diseases (herpes simplex, Chlamydia, and bacterial vaginosis) |
| Oral contraceptive use |
| Low socioeconomic status |

develop significant cervical abnormalities.[8] HPV infection is easily transmitted during sexual intercourse and is spread by skin-to-skin sexual contact. Non-penetrative sexual contact can also transmit HPV. Viral infection is cleared on average by eight months. This clearance is the consequence of host immunity, which leads to spontaneous regression of infection. More than 80% of low-grade squamous intraepithelial lesion regress within a period of two years. The major factor which permits the progression to high-grade squamous intraepithelial lesions is the persistence of HPV infection.[9] Studies show that the longer an infection persists, the more likely the patient is to develop CIN 2, 3.[3]

The National Health and Nutrition Examination Survey (NHANES) collected vaginal swabs for HPV DNA in 1,921 women to determine the prevalence of HPV infection in the United States.[10] The prevalence of HPV infection in young females aged 20 to 24 years was 45%. The prevalence of the specific serotypes of HPV 6, 11, 16, and 18 were 17%, 7%, 16%, and 7%, respectively. The overall prevalence of HPV infection in this study was 27%. A follow-up study prospectively examined 553 college-aged women every four months for up to five years with HPV DNA testing and cervical cytology.[11] The mean age of study participants was 19 and mean follow-up was 41.2 months. Over two years, 39% of HPV-negative women became HPV-positive with high-risk HPV types (HPV 16, 18, 51, 56, 33, 35, 39). The authors reported the cumulative incidence of HPV infection to be 38.9% at 24 months. HPV 16 was the most common type, with a cumulative infection rate of 10.4% at 24 months. For HPV 18 infection, the cumulative infection rate was 4.1% for the same time period. The median time to detection of severe dysplasia (CIN 2, 3) was 14 months after HPV detection. Brown *et al.* studied a smaller cohort of adolescent females for two years and found that 82% were infected with HPV during the study period.[12] High-risk HPV infection was detected in 77% of adolescents in a two-year period. In addition, cytological abnormalities were commonly found in adolescent females with atypical squamous cells of undetermined significance (ASCUS), LSIL, and HSIL occurring in 17%, 19%, and 2%, respectively. Therefore, adolescent and young women can present with high rates of cytological abnormalities and CIN 2, 3 can develop quickly after initial HPV exposure. In contrast, there is a very low rate of invasive cervical cancer in this group of women.

receiving placebo. The primary efficacy endpoint examined was reduction in the incidence of anogenital warts, vulvar intraepithelial neoplasia (VIN) and vaginal intraepithelial neoplasia (VAIN) grades 1 to 3, or invasive cancer associated with HPV 6, 11, 16, or 18. Secondary endpoints assessed included reduction in CIN 1 or higher abnormalities. At mean follow-up of three years, the vaccine was 100% effective at preventing anogenital disease in HPV-naïve women. In addition, vaccine efficacy was 100% at preventing CIN 1 or higher abnormalities in HPV-naïve women. The vaccine was well tolerated.[15] In both FUTURE II and I trials, there was no evidence that vaccination altered the course of disease infection in women who had evidence of incident HPV infection at the time of first vaccine dose. These data stress the importance of utilizing HPV vaccine as primary prevention, rather than as treatment of pre-existing HPV-related infections.

Cervarix is a bivalent recombinant vaccine that also targets high-risk types 16 and 18. It is a recombinant subunit vaccine produced with a baculovirus system in insect cells. Each dose is composed of 20 ug of L1 particles of each type absorbed into 500 ug of a novel adjuvant called AS04, composed of 500 ug of aluminum hydroxide and 50 ug of 3-O-deacetyl monophosphoryl lipid A, derived from liopolysaccharide of *Salmonella typhimurium*.[13] Cervarix is administered in three doses at time zero, and at one and six months of follow-up.

Cervarix has been evaluated by one large, randomized clinical trial, PATRICIA (PApilloma TRIal against Cancer In young Adults), an autonomous US National Cancer Institute (NCI)-sponsored trial in Costa Rica.[16,17] This study included more than 18,000 women aged 15 to 25 years (mean age of 20 years) who were randomly assigned to receive bivalent HPV vaccine or a control hepatitis A vaccine. Similar to previous FUTURE trials, approximately 26% of women demonstrated past or current infections with HPV 16 and 18. The primary vaccine efficacy was determined for HPV-naïve women who received all three doses of vaccine (ATP[16] analysis) in preventing CIN 2 or higher lesions. At mean follow-up of three years, vaccine efficacy for prevention of CIN 2, CIN 3, AIS, or cancer was 93%. The prevention of persistent six- and twelve-month HPV 16 and 18 infections were 94% and 91%, respectively.[16]

In summary, Gardasil and Cervarix have been shown to be highly immunogenic in clinical trials, resulting in essentially 100% seroconversion. The antibody titers generated by vaccine are about 50- to 100-fold higher than those obtained from natural infection; titers generally peak at seven months, decline over the next year, and then remain relatively stable for 7.3 to 9.5 years. Both vaccines also have been shown to induce production of memory B cells. The key differences between the two vaccines are 1) inclusion of HPV 6 and 11 in the Gardasil vaccine, and 2) higher antibody production by the Cervarix vaccine, though impact of the higher titers is not yet known. Several large clinical trials including over 40,000 individuals have been conducted to determine the efficacy of both vaccines. Table 3 summarizes the current recommendation for prophylactic HPV vaccination. Widespread immunization of children and adolescents may result in a substantial decline in HPV 16- and HPV 18-related cervical disease.

Table 3. Recommendation for prophylactic HPV vaccination in females.

| **Organization** | **Recommendation for HPV vaccine** |
|---|---|
| Advisory Committee on Immunization Practices (ACIP) | Routinely offered to females between the ages of 11 and 12 (may begin at 9 years of age)<br>Sexually active women through age 26 years should receive "catch-up" vaccination<br>Do not recommend pre-vaccination screening with HPV high-risk testing or HPV 16/18 genotyping<br>No exclusion if prior abnormal cervical cytology/CIN, history of genital warts, or prior HPV DNA testing<br>No preference between bivalent versus quadrivalent vaccines |
| American Congress of Obstetricians and Gynecologists (ACOG) | Same as ACIP guidelines |
| American Cancer Society (ACS) | Routinely offered to females between ages 11 and 18 (may begin at 9 years of age)<br>Do not recommend "catch-up" vaccination in women aged 19 to 26 years |

## Recommendations for Cervical Cytologic Screening

Cervical cancer screening should begin at age 21 years regardless of the age of onset of sexual intercourse and HPV vaccination status.[18] Squamous metaplasia at the transformation zone is active during adolescence and early adulthood. HPV infections are commonly acquired by young women shortly after initiation of sexual intercourse, but most infections and low-grade dysplasia are cleared spontaneously by the immune system within 1–2 years without producing clinical sequelae. Screening before age 21 should be avoided because it may lead to unnecessary and harmful evaluation and treatment in young women who have a very low risk of cancer. In 2006, the American Society for Colposcopy and Cervical Pathology-sponsored consensus conference set conservative guidelines for managing ASC-US or LSIL cytology for adolescent and young women.[19]

Cervical cancer screening with Pap testing is now recommended every two years for women aged 21–29 years. Women aged 30 years or older who have had three negative consecutive cervical cytology results may be screened every three years. The rate of dysplasia decreases as the number of sequential Pap tests increases.[20] In a recent study of 31,728 women 30–64 years of age, the prevalence of CIN 2 and CIN 3 in those women with three or more consecutive Pap results was 0.028% and 0.019%, respectively.[21] Most importantly, no invasive cervical cancer was detected in this cohort of women.

Women with HIV infection should have cervical Pap screening twice in the first year after initial diagnosis and annually thereafter. Women with a previous history of CIN 2, CIN 3, or cervical cancer remain at risk for persistent or recurrent disease even after treatment, and therefore should have screening annually for at least 20 years.[19]

There is no consensus as to when to discontinue cervical screening. The American Cancer Society recommends that screening may be discontinued at age 70 in low-risk women after three consecutive negative cervical cytologic screens in the prior 10 years. The US Preventive Services Task Force has set age 65 years as an appropriate age to discontinue screening.[19] Because cervical cancer develops slowly and risk factors decrease with age, it is reasonable to discontinue cervical cancer screening between age 65 and 70 years when women have three consecutive negative Pap results and no abnormal Pap results in the past 10 years. However, it is important to assess risk factors during annual gynecological exams to determine if reinitiating screening is appropriate.

Because of very low rates of vaginal cancers, women who underwent hysterectomy for benign indications and without prior history of high-grade CIN may have their cervical screening discontinued. However, women who have had total hysterectomy with history of prior treatment for high-grade CIN (CIN 2 or 3) or in whom negative cervical history cannot be confirmed should continue to be screened. There are no good data to support or refute discontinuing screening in this group.[19]

## CYTOLOGIC NOMENCLATURE AND INTERPRETATION OF CERVICAL CYTOLOGY

The terminology used in the description of preinvasive epithelial lesions of the cervix has undergone substantial revision in the last few decades. The term *dysplasia* refers to a spectrum of changes in the surface epithelium that ranges from minor changes in squamous metaplastic epithelium to near complete replacement of the epithelial layer by immature neoplastic cells. Cervical intraepithelial neoplasia (CIN) describes abnormal proliferation or overgrowth of the undifferentiated basal cell layer. Mild dysplasia (or CIN 1) describes the condition in which undifferentiated cells occupy approximately the lower one-third of the epithelium. Moderate dysplasia (or CIN 2) represents replacement of two-thirds of the thickness of the normal epithelium, and severe dysplasia (or CIN 3) denotes full-thickness replacement of epithelial cell layers with undifferentiated, hyperchromatic cells.[5]

The Bethesda System of reporting is the most widely used system in the United States (Table 4).[22] The Bethesda System nomenclature abolished the three-tiered CIN classification and replaced it with a two-tiered classification of high-grade squamous intraepithelial lesion (HSIL) and low-grade squamous intraepithelial lesion (LSIL). In this system, lesions previously classified as mild dysplasia, koilocytic atypia, koilocytosis, flat condylomata, and CIN 1 are grouped under LSIL, and those previously classified as moderate dysplasia (CIN 2), severe dysplasia (CIN 3), and

Table 4. The 2001 Bethesda classification of cervical cytology.[22]

**Specimen type:**

Conventional smear, liquid-based, or other techniques

**Specimen adequacy:**

Satisfactory for evaluation: description includes quality indicators, endocervical/ transformation zone component and obscuring blood or inflammation

Unsatisfactory for evaluation: reason specified

**Interpretation/Results:**

***Negative for intraepithelial lesion or malignancy***

Infections: *Trichomonas vaginalis*, *Candida* spp, bacterial vaginosis, *Actinomyces* spp, cellular changes

Other non-neoplastic findings: Reactive cellular changes associated with inflammation/cellular repair, radiation, or IUD

- Glandular cells post-hysterectomy
- Atrophy

Endometrial cells in woman ≥ age 40 years

***Epithelial cell abnormality: specify squamous or glandular***

*Squamous cell*

Atypical squamous cells (ASC)

- Of undetermined significance (ASC-US)
- Cannot exclude HSIL (ASC-H)

Low-grade squamous intraepithelial lesion (LSIL): cellular changes consistent with HPV, mild dysplasia, CIN 1

High-grade squamous intraepithelial lesion (HSIL): moderate and severe dysplasia, CIN 2, CIN 3, CIS

Squamous cell carcinoma

*Glandular cell*

Atypical

- Endocervical cells (not otherwise specified or specify in comment)
- Endometrial cells (not otherwise specified or specify in comment)
- Glandular cells (not otherwise specified or specify in comment)

Atypical

- Endocervical cells, favor neoplastic
- Glandular cells, favor neoplastic

Endocervical adenocarcinoma *in situ* (AIS)

Adenocarcinoma (endocervical, endometrial, extrauterine, not otherwise specified)

Modified from Soloman D, Davey D, Kurman R, *et al.* The 2001 Bethesda System: terminology for reporting results of cervical cytology. Forum Group members; Bethesda 2001 Workshop. *JAMA* 2002;287:2114–2119.

carcinoma *in situ* (CIS) are grouped together under HSIL.[3] The shift to two-tier terminology was made in recognition of the differing clinical course of these two levels of cellular change. Histological high-grade lesions almost uniformly represent lesions with high-risk oncogenic HPV types, but low-grade lesions represent a clinically more heterogeneous group. LSIL, especially in young women, is generally a sign of transient HPV infection, whereas HSIL is more likely to be associated with persistent HPV infection and a higher risk of progression to cervical cancer. Regardless of the system used, communication between pathologist and clinician is imperative when any diagnosis is not clear.[3]

The results of cervical cytology should not be used to make definite diagnosis or initiate treatment. Cytology serves as a screen for cellular abnormalities that are associated with the development of cervical cancer. Approximately 7–10% women require additional evaluation following Pap screening.[23] Cytologic abnormalities must be further evaluated with colposcopy and biopsy to determine histologic diagnosis and treatment options.

## Cervical Transformation Zone

The cervix and vagina are embryologically derived from the müllerian ducts. Prior to 18 to 20 weeks of gestation, the ducts are lined by a single layer of columnar epithelium, which is then replaced by squamous epithelium derived from cloacal endoderm.[5] The junction of the squamous epithelium of the exocervix and vagina and the columnar epithelium originating in the endocervix forms the squamocolumnar junction. During adolescence and first pregnancy, metaplastic squamous epithelium replaces the columnar epithelium to form a new squamocolumnar junction that is progressively closer to the external os of the cervix. The area between the original and new columnar squamocolumnar junction is referred to as the transformation zone. The position of the original squamocolumnar junction varies greatly, lying on the ectocervix in 66%, within the endocervical canal in 30%, and on the vaginal fornices in 4% of female infants.[5] The transformation zone is the region that undergoes squamous metaplasia and is the pivot site where cervical carcinogenesis and neoplastic cervical lesions originate.

## Techniques of Cervical Cytology

Cervical cytology is prepared by collecting exfoliated cells from the transformation zone of the cervix and then transferring the cells to a glass slide, in the case of a conventional Pap smear, or into a liquid-based, thin-layer preparation (e.g. ThinPrep, SurePath). In the United States, liquid-based methods are the predominant method of cervical cytology screening. Liquid-based preparation filters out most contaminating blood, lubricant, debris, and inflammatory cells. Immediate suspension of exfoliated cells decreases drying of cells and prevents formation of artifacts that may interfere with interpretation. Specimen adequacy is reported as "satisfactory" or "unsatisfactory" for interpretation. The presence or absence of an endocervical component or transformation zone is described in the narrative portion of the report. If a specimen is classified as "unsatisfactory", a reason must be specified in the report.

The major advantage of ThinPrep is the ability to use a single specimen for cytology, HPV, gonorrhea, and Chlamydia testing.[19] The rate of specimen adequacy is also improved with liquid-based techniques;[24] however, a recent systematic review failed to demonstrate a clinical benefit achieved from improved specimen adequacy.[25] The rate of false negatives is the same for liquid-based and traditional Pap tests, and disadvantages of liquid-based methods include higher cost and decreased specificity. In a systematic review of five high-quality studies, there was no evidence that liquid-based cytology significantly improved detection of HSIL compared with conventional smears.[25] In addition, meta-analysis of eight studies found no significant differences in sensitivity or specificity between the two methods of cytology in their ability to diagnose CIN 2 or higher using LSIL or HSIL cytology. If the threshold for colposcopy was lowered to ASC-US, liquid-based cytology had significantly lower specificity.[26] The systematic review and two randomized trials found that liquid-based techniques detected ASC-US and LSIL better than conventional smears,[19,24,25] however, one randomized trial found no difference.[27] Therefore, choosing an appropriate cervical cytological screening method depends upon a variety of factors including specimen adequacy, preference by the pathology laboratory, ability to perform concurrent testing, and cost.

## HPV Testing

Currently, HPV DNA testing is used as a method to triage patients to colposcopic exam for women with a cytology result of ASC-US, or postmenopausal women with LSIL.[19] HPV testing is reported as either positive or negative for oncogenic HPV types (HPV 16, 18, 31, 33, 35, 39, 45, 51, 52, 52, 56, 58, 59, 68, 69, 82). Negative test results may indicate no detection of oncogenic HPV types or presence of only low-risk HPV types. The method of HPV DNA testing is performed by the Hybrid Capture 2 HPV assay. A type-specific test for HPV 16 and 18 (Cervista HPV 16/18) was approved by the FDA in 2009. PCR-based assays are expected in 2010. There is limited data to suggest that stratifying high-risk HPV women by specific genotype will improve management. In a population-based randomized Finnish study, HPV DNA testing with cytology triage was both more sensitive and more specific than conventional cytology in women 35 years and older. HPV-based screening caught 44% more cases of severe dysplasia and cervical cancer overall than did conventional cytological screening (95% CI 1% to 205%).[28] An Italian study concluded that for women 35–60 years of age, HPV testing alone with a cutoff of 2 pg/ml achieved a substantial gain in sensitivity with only a minor reduction in positive predictive value compared to cytology.[29]

## Recommendations for Colposcopy

For patients who have an abnormal screening Pap test, colposcopy is the examination of cervical, vaginal, vulvar, and anogenital epithelium using magnified illumination, which facilitates the identification of abnormal cellular changes that suggest neoplasia. The colposcope allows biopsies to target areas of greatest cellular abnormality. Low power (2× to 6×) is often used to obtain an overall impression of the surface epithelium. Medium (8× to 15×) and high (15× to 25×) powers are used for close inspection of vascular patterns, which can signify high-grade or invasive lesions. Table 5 illustrates indications for colposcopic examination. Initial clinical workup should include a complete medical history, explanation of the indication for colposcopy, and a thorough description of the procedure to the patient. Pertinent history includes pregnancy history, last menstrual period,

Table 5. Indications for colposcopy.

| |
|---|
| **Specific cytological abnormalities:** |
| Persistent ASC-US or ASC-US with positive high-risk HPV |
| ASC-H |
| AGC |
| LSIL |
| HSIL |
| Suspicious for invasive cancer |
| Malignant cells present |
| **Other indications:** |
| Women exposed to diethylstilbestrol (DES) exposure *in utero* |
| Evaluation of grossly visible or palpable abnormality in cervix, vagina, or vulva |
| Used during treatment of lower genital neoplasia |

use of hormones or oral contraceptive pills, history of abnormal cervical cytologies and prior cervical procedures, allergies, medication, HIV status, immunosuppressive conditions, and iodine allergy. A pregnancy test is generally recommended prior to the procedure in order to avoid endocervical curettage (ECC) which may cause rupture of the gestational sac and miscarriage. Informed consent should be obtained prior to the procedure. Colposcopy is satisfactory if the transformation zone and entire extent of any lesions are fully visualized and if the ECC is without dysplasia.[5]

A thorough examination of the cervix, vagina, vulva, and perineum should accompany colposcopic examination. Squamous neoplasia may be multicentric and involve more than one genital tract region. The colposcopic examination involves speculum examination of the cervix. Normal saline is initially applied to remove obscuring mucus and debris, to moisten the cervix, and to visualize the cervix. Hyperkeratosis is a finding where a white, thickened cervical epithelial area is seen prior to application of acetic acid solution. Three- to five-percent acetic acid solution is then used to improve visualization of abnormal areas and the squamocolumnar junction. After application, the acetic acid solution dehydrates squamous cells that have relatively large or dense nuclei (including metaplastic cells, dysplastic cells, and HPV-infected cells), producing acetowhite changes. Atypical vascular patterns are characterized as mosaicism, punctuation, or simply abnormal-appearing vessels. As the acetic acid effect fades, mosaicism and punctuation become more pronounced. Green-filter examination enhances the abnormal vasculature. Use of a green or blue filter darkens blood vessels and sharpens the contrast between vessels and the surrounding epithelium. Ulceration and erosive changes are also seen and may be secondary to microtrauma, infection, or neoplasm. Heaped-up epithelium may represent mitotically active tissue such as in neoplasm or condyloma. Colposcopic examination should also include the upper one-third of the vagina, particularly the lateral vaginal fornices. Although visual changes are helpful for directing biopsies, an accurate diagnosis can only be established definitively by pathologic examination of the biopsied tissue. Tissue biopsy is indicated to exclude an underlying neoplastic process. If no lesions are seen, a quarter-strength Lugol's iodine solution may be applied to the cervix and vagina to aid in identification (Schiller's test). Normal ectocervical and vaginal squamous epithelium contains glycogen, which stains dark brown after application of iodine solution. Normal columnar epithelium and immature squamous metaplastic or neoplastic epithelium do not contain glycogen, and so are not stained by iodine solution and appear mustard-yellow. ECC is performed in patients with ASC-H, HSIL, AGC, AIS, LSIL without visible lesion, in patients anticipating ablative treatment, and for those with an unsatisfactory colposcopic examination.[5]

In 2006, the American Society for Colposcopy and Cervical Pathology created guidelines for management of women with abnormal cervical cancer screening tests and cervical intraepithelial neoplasia.[30,31] The ASCCP guidelines may be found on their website http://www.asccp.org/ConsensusGuidelines/ConsensusGuidelinesOverview/tabid/5956/Default.aspx

## Treatment for Cervical Intraepithelial Neoplasia

The methods of treatment for preinvasive cervical disease include ablative procedures, such as cryosurgery, electrocoagulation diathermy, and $CO_2$ laser, as well as excisional procedures, including loop electrosurgical excision procedure (LEEP), cervical conization, $CO_2$ laser excision, or hysterectomy. Ablative therapy is an effective treatment for women with high-grade and persistent low-grade CIN in whom there is no suspicion of glandular or invasive squamous disease and who are compliant with follow-up. Candidates for ablative therapy must have satisfactory colposcopy with biopsy confirming CIN. Cytology and histology findings must correlate and ECC must be negative for dysplasia. The most commonly used techniques for cervical ablation are cryotherapy and laser ablation. Cryotherapy can be performed in the office setting. Both $CO_2$ laser ablation and electrocoagulation diathermy may also be performed in the office, but cause more discomfort to the patient and general anesthesia may be indicated.

Cryotherapy causes destruction of lesions via cryonecrosis produced by the evaporation of liquid refrigerants (carbon dioxide or nitrous oxide). The ectocervix is cooled to –20ºC to cause crystallization of intracellular water, resulting in cell death. Cryoprobe tips are flat or cone-shaped, and 19 mm or 25 mm in diameter. A water-soluble gel is used to coat the cryoprobe tip before the procedure. To ensure a 5 mm depth of cryonecrosis, a total lateral freeze should be at least 7 mm and must cover the lesion and the entire transformation zone. A freeze-thaw-freeze technique is commonly used. This method reduced the failure rate from 29% to 7%.[32] A recent meta-analysis of randomized trials demonstrated a decline in residual disease at 27 months with the two freeze-thaw cycle method versus the single-freeze method (6% versus 16%).[33] Patients experience a watery, malodorous, blood-tinged vaginal discharge for several weeks and should be counseled to maintain pelvic rest for four weeks following cryotherapy.

Laser ablation techniques use a $CO_2$ laser directed at the lesion under colposcopic guidance. A typical setting uses a power density of 600–1200 watts/cm$^2$. A 2 mm laser spot size at 35 watts will produce a power density of 875 watts/cm$^2$. Intracellular water absorbs the laser energy and causes vaporization and destruction of tissue. Similar to cryotherapy, a depth of 5 mm is needed to ablate lesions on the ectocervix, with of depth of approximately 8–9 mm necessary around the endocervix. Protective eye gear and blackened instruments are used to avoid damage to other areas due to reflected beams. Wet towels are draped over the patient's perineum and thighs to avoid intraoperative fires.

Other infrequently used ablative techniques are cold coagulation and electrocoagulation diathermy. In cold coagulation, a thermosound probe is used to conduct heat to the cervix at lower temperatures (50–120°C). The diathermy technique uses electrically induced heat generated by a needle attached to a cautery device at 30–35 watts to destroy cervical lesions. The diathermy needle is passed into and out of the cervix multiple times to ablate the transformation zone. These methods are infrequently utilized in the treatment of CIN.

An excisional procedure should be performed in patients who are not appropriate candidates for ablative therapy. It provides both diagnostic information as well as therapeutic benefit. Excisional treatment can be performed by cold-knife conization, laser conization, or the loop electrosurgical excision procedure (LEEP). LEEP is an office procedure which uses a thin wire loop electrode, 1–2 cm in width and 0.7–1.5 cm in depth, connected to an electrosurgical generator delivering 35–55 watts to excise the entire transformation zone. Lugol's iodine solution helps to demarcate the outer margin of the excision during colposcopic exam. The cervix is infiltrated with 5–10 mL of local anesthetic (1% lidocaine with diluted epinephrine) at the 3, 6, 9, and 12 o'clock positions after a test dose. A grounding pad is attached to the patient. The cervical lesion is excised and the base of the crater is gently fulgurated with a 5 mm ball cautery using 40–60 watts of coagulation current. Significant postoperative bleeding occurs in approximately 2–5% of patients. Clinically significant cervical stenosis and cervical incompetence are rare complications.[5] Treatment effectiveness is greater than 95% and is comparable to that achieved with $CO_2$ laser or cold-knife conization.[33]

Excisional conization can be performed with a scalpel (also known as cold-knife conization) or using $CO_2$ laser. The following are indications for cervical conization: nonconcordance between cytology and histology, positive ECC for dysplasia, inadequate colposcopy, suspected microinvasion, and AIS. Conization is required for definite diagnosis of microinvasive carcinoma. In general, with suspected microinvasion or AIS, cold-knife conization is often recommended so that margins can be evaluated without cautery artifact. Cervical conization achieves cure rates for high-grade CIN greater than 96%. The risk of cervical stenosis and cervical incompetence is higher for cervical conization performed with a scalpel than for $CO_2$ laser and LEEP as demonstrated in a systematic review of 27 retrospective cohort studies.[34] Cold-knife conization and

LEEP were associated with a significantly increased risk of preterm delivery (14%, RR 2.59, 95% CI 1.80–3.72 for cold-knife; 11%, RR 1.70, 95% CI 1.24–2.35 for LEEP). Laser conization and laser ablation were not associated with significant increased risk of adverse pregnancy outcome. A deep excisional procedure with cone depth of greater than 1 cm appears to be an independent risk factor for preterm birth and preterm rupture of membranes in subsequent pregnancies.[35] Thus, excisional procedures in women planning future pregnancies should remove the minimum amount of tissue necessary for appropriate treatment.

In general, both ablative methods and excisional procedures are effective treatments for CIN.[36–38] A meta-analysis of randomized trials evaluated outcomes in women with any degree of CIN.[33] Laser ablation compared to LEEP or laser conization showed no significant difference in effectiveness of treatment defined as absence of persistent or recurrent disease, and laser ablation compared to cryotherapy also showed no significant difference in effectiveness of treatment.[33] There are no randomized studies to date comparing the effectiveness of cryotherapy or laser ablation to cold-knife conization. Overall, the rate of recurrent or persistent CIN is 5–17% following excisional or ablative therapy for CIN 2, 3.[33] Higher rates of persistent disease are associated with large lesion size,[38] endocervical gland involvement,[39] positive margin status,[40] and continuing HPV 16 DNA-positivity post-treatment.[41] However, as mentioned above, the risk of subsequent preterm delivery appears to be higher with excisional procedures rather than ablation. Selection of the most appropriate method of treatment depends on operator experience, equipment availability, lesion size, and other factors such as convenience and future reproductive plans. Ablative treatment should only be used after invasive cancer is excluded. Laser and LEEP minimize blood loss by thermal cautery during excision, but may impair the interpretability of the specimen secondary to cautery effect.

Lastly, hysterectomy should not be performed as an initial treatment of CIN 2, 3. The incidence of significant morbidity with hysterectomy is higher than with the less invasive modalities discussed above. The most common indication for hysterectomy in the management of CIN is the presence of other concurrent gynecologic conditions that warrant hysterectomy, such as dysfunctional uterine bleeding, symptomatic fibroids, uterovaginal prolapse, or undesired fertility. An excisional conization must be performed to exclude invasive cancer before hysterectomy is performed. In addition, 2–3% of patients with CIN 2, 3 have disease extending into the vaginal vault. High-grade vaginal intraepithelial neoplasia (VAIN) occurs in the vaginal vault in 0.9–6.8% of patients who have undergone hysterectomy to treat CIN.[42]

## VAGINA AND VULVA

### Epidemiology

Vulvar and vaginal cancers account for approximately 4–7% of gynecologic cancers.[43] Over the past few decades, the incidence of vulvar cancer and vulvar intraepithelial neoplasia (VIN) seems to be increasing, particularly among younger women. Topical treatment of vulvar precancerous lesions has been shown to be effective as an alternative to surgery. Comparatively, vaginal cancer is often found at relatively more advanced stages and has a lower overall five-year survival rate than vulvar cancer in the United States (39.8% compared with 79.3%.[44] HPV DNA has also been detected in notable proportions of invasive vulvar and vaginal cancers, VIN, and vaginal intraepithelial neoplasia (VAIN) cases.[45] A recent systematic review of HPV type distribution demonstrated that the HPV prevalence in vulvar cancer, VIN 2/3 and VIN 1 was 40.1%, 80.4%, and 77.5%, respectively.[46] HPV prevalence in vaginal cancer, VAIN 2/3, and VAIN 1 was relatively higher at 65.55%, 92.6%, and 98.5%, respectively. HPV 16 was the most common type in vulvar (29.3%) and vaginal (55.4%) cancers, VIN 2/3 (71.2%), and VAIN 2/3 (65.8%).[46] HPV-associated lesions in the lower genital tract are often multifocal. In addition to HPV infection, potential risk factors for vulvar and vaginal cancers include smoking, herpes simplex virus 2 infection, and a previous history of anogenital cancer.[47] Exposure to diethylstilbestrol and prior hysterectomy are also considered risk factors for vaginal cancer.[47]

### Classification

The vulvar and vaginal intraepithelial neoplasia terminology is consistent with the grade classification for CIN and is defined by the presence of squamous cell atypia without invasion. Although the progression to invasive

5-FU, $CO_2$ laser ablation, and surgical excision (local excision, partial or total vaginectomy). There are no randomized trials in the literature, making a direct comparison very difficult. Even though most lesions regress after initial treatment. Some may recur, sometimes repeatedly, and may progress to invasive cancer. Recurrence is more common for high-grade lesions, multifocal lesions, and VAIN associated with other anogenital neoplasia. The recurrence rates after partial vaginectomy, 5-fluorouracil (5-Fu), and $CO_2$ laser are approximately 0–20%, 7–20%, and 0–42%, respectively. Therefore, long-term follow-up is important to influence the success of treatment.

Surgical management of VAIN can be performed by local excision or upper vaginectomy. Small lesions can be removed entirely with a biopsy or simple excision. Local excision has a remission rate of approximately 65%.[49] Partial vaginectomy is the best treatment option for unifocal lesions or multifocal lesions with involvement limited to the upper third of the vagina. Most vaginectomies are performed trans-vaginally, though sometimes they may be approached trans-abdominally. Vaginectomy may be associated with complications such as bleeding, bladder or rectal injury, and shortening or stenosis of the vagina. A literature review of the surgical treatment of VAIN reported a recurrence rate of approximately 18%.[50]

$CO_2$ laser vaporization is the preferred option for lesion ablation. Because the vaginal mucosa contains no gland crypts or skin appendages, only superficial treatment is required to eradicate the lesion. Treatment complications include pain, bleeding, scarring, and delayed healing. Laser ablation should not be performed if the full extent of the abnormal vaginal epithelium cannot be visualized, if there is any suspicion of invasive cancer, or if there is gross scarring or distortion of the vaginal vault.

Topical application of chemotherapeutic agents, primarily 5-FU, is thought to be an ideal method for multifocal VAIN, for recurrent disease, and for primary treatment of poor surgical candidates. 5-FU can be applied to the entire vaginal mucosa and allows treatment of multifocal disease throughout the vault. In addition, this therapy is relatively inexpensive and can be applied in an outpatient setting. A series of 74 patients treated with excision with or without 5-FU showed 70.3% remission rates following initial biopsy or excision. Progression to invasive vaginal cancer was approximately 5.4% and duration to invasion was 14 months to 5 years.[49] As with ablation, it is prerequisite that invasion should be excluded prior to topical 5-FU treatment. Complications of topical 5-FU may include significant vaginal irritation, burning, and ulceration. Several dosing protocols have been suggested. One commonly used regimen prescribes one quarter of an applicator of 5-FU cream instilled per vagina every night for 5–8 nights followed by a 10–14 day rest. These cycles may be repeated. Another common regimen recommends one third of an applicator applied once a week at bedtime for 10 weeks. Patients may place a cotton ball in the introitus to help hold the medication in the vagina and to protect the perineum from leakage.

Treatment strategies for VIN are similar to those discussed above. For low-grade VIN, it is imperative that a thorough evaluation of entire vulva is performed to exclude the presence of high-grade VIN either in the same lesion or in other coexisting lesions. If true VIN 1 is confirmed, the treatment recommendation is observation. The goals of treatment for high-grade VIN are to control symptoms and prevent progression to invasive cancer. Management options include surgical excision (wide local excision or simple vulvectomy), $CO_2$ laser ablation, and topical treatment. Local excision with a 5–10 mm margin is performed with a scalpel or electrocautery. Removal of the epidermis provides sufficient depth for treatment of VIN as long as margins are negative. Skinning vulvectomy is performed for more extensive lesions that are multifocal, large, or confluent. The epidermis is removed and closed primarily, or via skin graft or flap. Wide local excision with negative margins achieves a cure rate of greater than 90%. If the margins are involved, the cure rate declines to approximately 50%.[5] Laser vaporization is used to treat multifocal, small lesions. The goal of laser ablation is to treat the entire area of intraepithelial abnormality with a 3 mm depth of destruction required in hairy areas of the vulva. Superficial laser vaporization may provide a better cosmetic result than skinning vulvectomy. Since tissue is ablated rather than excised, invasive cancer must be excluded. The depth of ablation should be 1–3 mm to avoid scar formation.[5]

Conservative therapy with preservation of vulvar anatomy may be indicated, particularly in younger women. Topical treatment with imiquimod, an immune response modifier, has been used to treat VIN. Imiquimod stimulates local cytokine production and improves cell-mediated immunity, which translates into its antiviral and antitumor effects. A randomized control trial examined the use of imiquimod for 16 weeks in women with biopsy-proven VIN 2, 3.[51] At 20 weeks for follow-up, 81% of women had a complete response and 10% had a partial response, compared to no responses in the placebo arm. Local side effects were common. In another randomized trial, at 20 weeks' of follow-up, 81% of women treated with imiquimod had at least a 25% reduction in size of their lesion as compared to controls, and 35% had complete clinical response and remained recurrence-free for 12 months.[52] Both of these studies were performed with small numbers of subjects and with short follow-ups. Mild to moderate erythema and erosions were the most common side effects, though approximately 20% of women had severe local inflammation. Typically, treatment was recommended three times a week for 16 weeks.

## REFERENCES

1. American Cancer Society. *Cancer Facts and Figures 2007*. Atlanta: American Cancer Society, 2007.
2. Lowy D, Schiller J. Prophylactic human papilloma vaccines. *J Clin Invest* 2006;116:1167.
3. Wright T. Pathogenesis and diagnosis of preinvasive lesions of the lower genital tract. Barakat R, Markman M, Randall M. eds., *Principles and Practice of Gynecologic Oncology*, 5th ed. Baltimore, MD: Lippincott Williams & Wilkins, 2009, pp. 523–552.
4. Bosch F, de Sanjose S. Human papillomavirus and cervical cancer burden and assessment of causality. *J Natl Cancer Inst Monogr* 2003;31:20–28.
5. Campion M. Preinvasive disease. Berek J, Hacker N. *Practical Gynecologic Oncology*, 4th ed. Philadelphia, PA: Lippincott Williams & Wilkins, 2005.
6. zur Hausen H. Papillomaviruses causing cancer: evasion from host-cell control in early events in carcinogenesis. *J Natl Cancer Inst* 2000;92(9): 690–698.
7. Scheurer M, Tortolero-Luna G, Adler-Strorthz K. Human papillomavirus infection: biology, epidemiology, and prevention. *Int J Gynecol Cancer* 2005;15(5):727–746.

8. Ho G, Bierman R, Beardsley L, Chang CJ, Burk RD. Natural history of cervicovaginal papillomavirus infection in young women. *N Engl J Med* 1998; 338:423–428.
9. Ault K. Epidemiology and natural history of human papillomavirus infections in the female genital tract. *Infect Dis Obstet Gynecol* 2005;2006:1–5.
10. Dunne E, Unger E, Sternber M, *et al.* Prevalence of HPV infection among females in the United States. *JAMA* 2007;297:813.
11. Winer R, Lee SK, Hughes JP, Adam DE, Kiviat NB, Koutsky LA. Genital human papillomavirus infection: incidence and risk factors in a cohort of female university students. *Am J Epidemiol* 2003;157(3):218–226.
12. Brown D, Shew M, Qadadri B, *et al.* A longitudinal study of genital human papillomavirus infection in a cohort of closely followed adolescent women. *J Infect Dis* 2005;191(2):182–192.
13. Madrid-Marina V, Torres-Poveda K, López-Toledo G, García-Carrancá A. Advantanges and disadvantages of current prophylactic vaccines against HPV. *Arch Med Res* 2009;40:471–477.
14. The FUTURE II Study Group. Quadrivalent vaccine against human papillomavirus to prevent high-grade cervical lesions. *N Engl J Med* 2007; 356(19):1915–1927.
15. Garland, S, Hernandez-Avila M, Wheeler C, *et al.* Quadrivalent vaccine against human papillomavirus to prevent anogenital diseases. *N Engl J Med* 2007; 356:1928–1943.
16. Paavonen J, Naud P, Salmeron J, *et al.* Efficacy of human papillomavirus (HPV)-16/18 AS04-adjuvanted vaccine against cervical infection and precancer caused by oncogenic HPV types (PATRICIA): final analysis of a double-blind, randomised study in young women. *Lancet* 2009;374:301–314.
17. Herrero R, Hildesheim A, Rodriguez A, *et al.* Rationale and design of a community-based double-blind randomized clinical trial of an HPV 16 and 18 vaccine in Guanacaste, Costa Rica. *Vaccine* 2008;26(4):4795.
18. Cervical Cytology Screening. *ACOG Practice Bulletin* 2009;109.
19. Beerman H, van Dorst EB, Kuenen-Boumeester V, Hogendoorn PC. Superior performance of liquid-based versus conventional cytology in a population-based cervical cancer screening program. *Gynecol Oncol* 2009; 112:572.
20. Cervical cytology screening: ACOG Practice Bulletin Number 109. *Obstet Gynecol* 2009;114:1409–1420.

46. Smith JS, Backes DM, Hoots BE, Kurman RJ, Pimenta JM. Human papillomavirus type-distribution in vulvar and vaginal cancers and their associated precursors. *Obstet Gynecol* 2009;113(4):917–924.
47. Daling J, Madeleine MM, Schwartz, *et al.* A population-based study of squamous cell vaginal cancer: HPV and cofactors. *Gynecol Oncol* 2002; 84:263–270.
48. Sideri M, Jones R, Wilkinson E, *et al.* Squamous vulvar intraepithelial neoplasia: 2004 modified terminology, ISSVD Vulvar Oncology Subcommittee. *J Reprod Med* 2005;50:807.
49. Sillman FH, Fruchter RG, Chen YS, Camilien L, Sedlis A, McTingue E. Vaginal intraepithelial neoplasia: risk factors for persistence, recurrence, and invasion and its management. *Am J Obstet Gynecol* 1997;176:93–99.
50. Dodge J, Eltabbakh G, Mount S, *et al.* Clinical features of risk and recurrence among patients with vaginal intraepithelial neoplasia. *Gynecol Oncol* 2001; 83:363–369.
51. Mathlesen O, Buus S, Cramers M. Topical imiquimod can reverse vulvar intraepithelial neoplasia: a randomized, double-blinded study. *Gynecol Oncol* 2007;107(2):219–222.
52. van Seters M, van Beurden M, ten Kate, *et al.* Treatment of vulvar intraepithelial neoplasia with topical imiquimod. *N Engl J Med* 2008;358:1465–1473.

# 4

# VULVAR CANCER

*Raffi Chalian and Christina S. Chu*

## INTRODUCTION

Vulvar cancer is an uncommon form of gynecological cancer with 3,580 new diagnoses in 2009 and 900 deaths.[1] It affects less than 5% of women afflicted with gynecological cancers. The incidence of vulvar cancer between 2000 and 2004 has been 2.2 per 100,000 women, with a mortality rate of 0.5 deaths per 100,000 women. Overall five-year survival is 77.8%.[2] Thirty percent of patients present at the age of 70 years or older, and the incidence rate increases with age, peaking at age 75 when it afflicts 20 per 100,000 women.[3]

## EPIDEMIOLOGY

Even though historically the disease burden of vulvar cancer has been relatively small when compared to other gynecological malignancies such as endometrial or ovarian cancer, the incidence of vulvar cancer has increased dramatically over the past 30 years. It is currently the fourth most common gynecological malignancy. The incidence of invasive and *in situ* vulvar carcinoma has been increasing at a rate of 2.4% per year. In the US population there has been an increase in the number of cases by 20% between the years 1973 and 2000. The National Cancer Institute has identified vulvar cancer as 1 of 12 cancers with rising incidence.[4] Even though there has been an increase in the number of cases in all age groups, there has been a dramatic increase in early-stage and *in situ* vulvar cancers particularly in the population under 50 years of age.[5–7] Hampl *et al.* reported a nearly four-fold increase in the number of younger patients with vulvar cancer presenting to one university hospital in Germany over three decades (+372%).[8] These tumors were associated with high-risk human papillomavirus (HPV) infection. Overall, 50% of all vulvar cancers are associated with HPV infection.[9] The risk factors for developing vulvar cancer in younger patients are dramatically different from those seen in the older patient population. Vulvar cancer in younger patients is associated with cervical neoplasia, presence of HPV virus, pre-existing vulvar intraepithelial neoplasia (VIN), strong association of sexually transmitted diseases, condyloma, and cigarette smoking.[3] Unlike cervical cancer, the time course between HPV infection and the development of vulvar cancer is not well described, though it is postulated to be shorter than the 10–12 year process seen between HPV infection and the development of cervical cancer.

In older patients, vulvar cancer is rarely associated with condyloma, sexually transmitted diseases, and cigarette smoking. The risk factors for vulvar cancer in this population are loosely identified and include hypertension, obesity, and diabetes mellitus. It is unclear whether these are co-morbid diseases or causative in nature. Cancers in the older population also have a high incidence of p53 tumor suppressor gene mutation. Lichen sclerosus is also associated with vulvar squamous cell cancer: approximately 4% of affected women will subsequently develop vulvar cancer.[10]

## PRESENTATION

Vulvar carcinoma is infrequently encountered in a general outpatient obstetrics and gynecology practice; in contrast, the symptoms of vulvar cancer, including pruritus and/or a mass lesion, are very common complaints. A considerable number of patients are asymptomatic and only present with a visible lesion. The lesion can be solitary or multifocal. Other less common symptoms include pain, ulceration, bleeding, discharge, dysuria, and occasionally a groin mass.

Traditionally, the labia majora and minora were the most frequently affected sites, with the left side being affected more frequently than the right. Labial lesions accounted for up to 60% of cases. The clitoris and posterior fourchette were involved less frequently. However, with the changing demographics of the disease has come a shift in location of the primary lesions. In the last decade, primary lesions have been noted to occur periclitorally in almost 40% of cases, in contrast to a labial location in only 27%.[8]

As symptoms of itching and palpable bumps are very non-specific, there can be a significant delay in the diagnosis of vulvar cancer. It is estimated that symptomatic patients delay presentation to a provider for approximately 2–16 months.[11] Self-medication with over-the-counter agents can be effective in controlling symptoms. Further adding to the delay in diagnosis is often the physician's empiric treatment of symptoms without biopsy. Fortunately, the non-aggressive nature of vulvar cancer usually results in a significant time interval between the development of a primary lesion and metastasis to the lymphatics. Thus, delay in diagnosis does not always reflect a decline in life expectancy in patients afflicted with vulvar cancer.

Both gynecologic oncologists and general obstetrician gynecologists should have a low threshold for biopsy of visible lesions on the vulva whether they are symptomatic or not. Cancer may be multifocal in 5% of cases; hence extensive evaluation of the vulvar and perianal skin must be performed. The examination must be extensive and all areas that are suspicious should be biopsied. Careful evaluation of the vagina and cervix must also be performed. A colposcopic examination of the cervix is also warranted as cervical neoplasia is found in 22% of patients with vulvar malignancy.[12]

## SQUAMOUS CELL CARCINOMA

### Pathology and Natural History

Squamous cell carcinoma of the vulva is the most common type of vulvar cancer, accounting for approximately 80–90% of cases (see Table 1). There are multiple subtypes of squamous cell carcinoma, the most common being the squamous keratinizing type. HPV-associated squamous cell carcinoma is more likely to be multi-centric and arise in a background of VIN. It is estimated that 80% of untreated women with warty VIN may develop invasive cancer.[13] Fortunately, these lesions have a more favorable prognosis. They are often associated with concomitant tumors of the cervix and vagina, and may present with varied appearances ranging from small nodules, to ulcerated lesions, or cauliflower-like exophytic growths.

Table 1. Histologies of vulvar cancer.

| |
|---|
| **Squamous cell carcinoma** |
| Keratinizing type |
| Nonkeratinizing type |
| Verrucous carcinoma |
| Basal cell carcinoma |
| **Melanoma** |
| **Sarcoma** |
| **Bartholin's gland carcinoma** |
| Squamous cell carcinoma |
| Adenocarcinoma |
| Adenoid cystic carcinoma |
| Transitional cell carcinoma |
| Adenosquamous carcinoma |
| **Basal cell carcinoma** |
| **Lymphoma** |
| **Endodermal sinus tumors** |
| **Merkel cell carcinoma** |
| **Dermatofibrosarcoma protuberans** |
| **Malignant schwannoma** |
| **Metastatic** |

Various grading schemes exist, but that proposed by the Gynecologic Oncology Group (GOG) utilizes four grades. Well-differentiated tumors that contain no poorly differentiated components are Grade 1 tumors and have the best prognosis. As the undifferentiated portion of the whole tumor increases, so does the grade. Grade 4 tumor is noted to have finger-like projections which aggressively invade the normal tissue. Grade 1 disease has the best prognosis and the lowest risk of lymph node metastasis. As the grade of tumor increases, so does the risk of lymph node metastasis.

The incidence of squamous carcinoma of the vulva peaks in the seventh decade of life, though with the increase in patients of younger ages, the mean age is falling.[8] The slow progression characteristic of vulvar cancer accounts for the majority of cases being diagnosed at an early stage, with over 65% being diagnosed as either *in situ*, International Federation

Table 2. Survival by FIGO stage for patients with vulvar cancer, 1999 to 2001; FIGO statistics.

| | | **Overall survival, percent** | | |
|---|---|---|---|---|
| **FIGO stage** | **Number of patients** | **1 year** | **2 years** | **5 years** |
| I | 286 | 96.4 | 90.4 | 78.5 |
| II | 266 | 87.6 | 73.2 | 58.8 |
| III | 216 | 74.7 | 53.8 | 43.2 |
| IV | 71 | 35.3 | 16.9 | 13.0 |

*Source*: Beller U, Quinn MA, Benedet JL, *et al.* Carcinoma of the vulva. *Int J Gynaecol Obstet* 2006;95:S7.

of Gynecology and Obstetrics (FIGO) stage I or II disease (see Table 2). Initial spread occurs predominately to local tissues via direct invasion which may result in the involvement of surrounding organs such as the urethra, vagina, and anus; metastasis to the draining lymphatics occurs later.

## Lymphatic Metastasis

Lymphatic drainage of the vulva commences with minute papillae which join to form a multilayer network of fine vessels extending over the entire region to the hymenal ring. This network of vessels consolidates to form 3–4 collecting trunks towards the anterior portion of the labium minus which then turn laterally (bypassing the clitoris) and drain into superficial inguinal lymph nodes. The superficial inguinal lymph nodes communicate with the deep inguinal nodes via multiple lymphatic channels. The deep inguinal (femoral) nodes lead to the external iliac pelvic nodes. Metastasis occurs predominantly via the lymphatic system in a predictable fashion, initially invading the superficial lymphatics surrounding the lesion, then subsequently the draining inguinal lymph nodes, finally progressing to the pelvic lymph nodes. The periclitoral tissues drain directly into the pelvic and obturator nodes, leading to potential extension of the disease to the pelvis, though this is not often seen in clinical practice[14] (see Fig. 1). Lesions which are more than 2 cm from the midline drain into ipsilateral nodes, while tumors within 2 cm of the

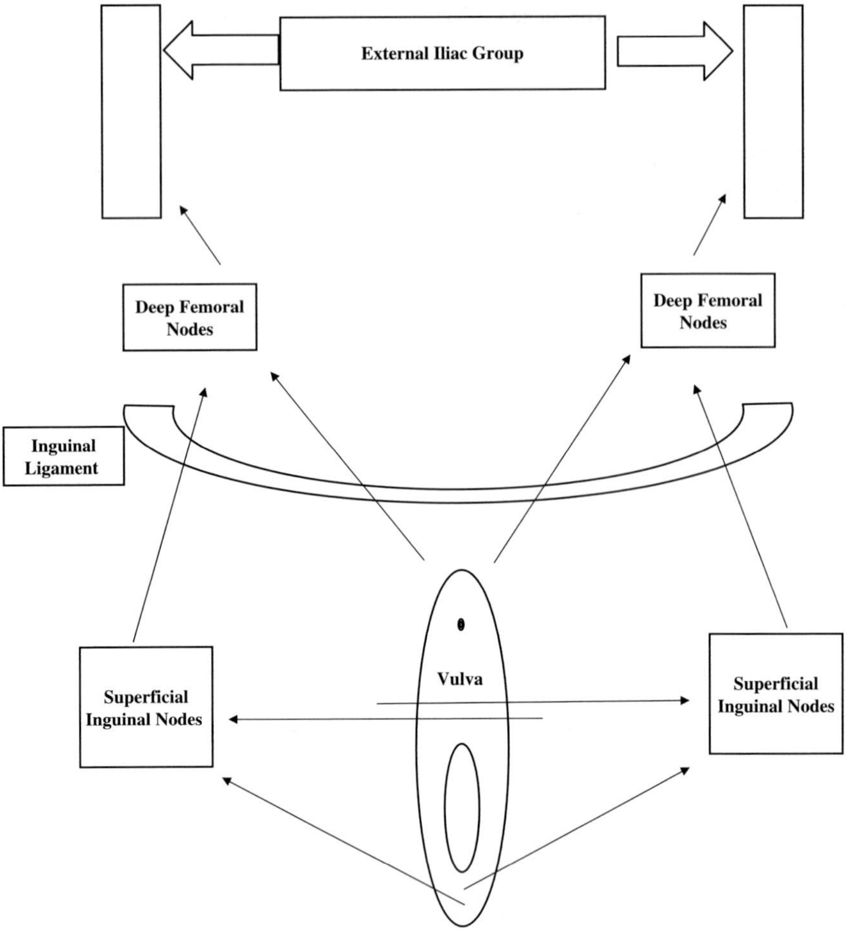


Figure 1. Schematic representation of lymphatic spread from vulvar cancer.

midline drain into both the right and left inguinal lymph nodes due to decussation of the lymphatics.

The risk of metastasis to the lymphatics increases as the size of the lesion increases. Patients whose tumors were found to be less than 1 cm in diameter had an 18% risk of spread to groin lymph nodes, while tumors greater than 5 cm had a 51.8% risk of having positive lymph nodes at the time of surgical resection[15] (see Table 3). There is a significant correlation between tumor thickness and incidence of positive groin nodes. This is

Table 3. Groin node metastasis in relation to tumor diameter.

| Tumor diameter (cm) | N | Groin nodes positive (%) |
|---|---|---|
| <1.0 cm | 61 | 18.0 |
| 1.1–2.0 cm | 129 | 19.4 |
| 2.1–3.0 cm | 175 | 31.4 |
| 3.1–4.0 cm | 81 | 54.3 |
| 4.1–5.0 cm | 48 | 39.6 |
| >5 cm | 85 | 51.8 |
| **Total** | **579** | **34.2** |

*Source*: Homesley HD, Bundy BN, Sedlis A, *et al.* Prognostic factors for groin node metastasis in squamous cell carcinoma of the vulva (a Gynecologic Oncology Group study). *Gynecol Oncol* 1993;49(3):279–283.

Table 4. Groin node metastasis in relation to tumor thickness (invasion).

| Tumor thickness (mm) | N | Groin nodes positive (%) |
|---|---|---|
| ≤1 mm | 38 | 2.6 |
| 2 mm | 56 | 8.9 |
| 3 mm | 59 | 18.6 |
| 4 mm | 68 | 30.9 |
| 5 mm | 57 | 33.3 |
| >5 mm | 286 | 47.9 |
| **Total** | **564** | **34.4** |

*Source*: Homesley HD, Bundy BN, Sedlis A, *et al.* Prognostic factors for groin node metastasis in squamous cell carcinoma of the vulva (a Gynecologic Oncology Group study). *Gynecol Oncol* 1993;49(3):279–283.

illustrated in Table 4 which shows a 2.6% chance of nodal disease in tumors less than 1 mm compared to a 47.9% chance of nodal disease in patients with lesions thicker than 5 mm.

## Staging

The initial staging of vulvar cancer was clinical. However, the inaccurate assessment of groin node involvement in 20–30 % of cases resulted in the

Table 5. FIGO staging.

| | |
|---|---|
| **Stage I** | Tumor confined to the vulva |
| IA | Lesions ≤2 cm in size, confined to the vulva or perineum and with stromal invasion ≤1.0 mm,* no nodal metastasis |
| IB | Lesions >2 cm in size or with stromal invasion >1.0 mm,* confined to the vulva or perineum, with negative nodes |
| **Stage II** | Tumor of any size with extension to adjacent perineal structures (1/3 lower urethra, 1/3 lower vagina, anus) with negative nodes |
| **Stage III** | Tumor of any size with or without extension to adjacent perineal structures (1/3 lower urethra, 1/3 lower vagina, anus) with positive inguino-femoral lymph nodes |
| IIIA | (i) With 1 lymph node metastasis (≥5 mm), or<br>(ii) 1–2 lymph node metastasis(es) (<5 mm) |
| IIIB | (i) With 2 or more lymph node metastasis (≥5 mm), or<br>(ii) 3 or more lymph node metastasis (<5 mm) |
| IIIC | With positive nodes with extracapsular spread |
| **Stage IV** | Tumor invades other regional (2/3 upper urethra, 2/3 upper vagina), or distant structures |
| IVA | Tumor invades any of the following:<br>(i) upper urethral and/or vaginal mucosa, bladder mucosa, rectal mucosa, or fixed to pelvic bone, or<br>(ii) fixed or ulcerated inguino-femoral lymph nodes |
| IVB | Any distant metastasis including pelvic lymph nodes |

*The depth of invasion is defined as the measurement of the tumor from the epithelial stromal junction of the adjacent most superficial dermal papilla to the deepest point of invasion.

Reprinted with permission granted by the International Federation of Gynecology and Obstetrics (FIGO) from: FIGO Committee on Gynecologic Oncology. Revised FIGO staging for carcinoma of the vulva, cervix, and endometrium. *Int J Gynaecol Obstet* 2009;105:103–104.

adoption of surgical staging by FIGO in 1989. FIGO staging was modified twice, in 1995 and 2009 (see Table 5). The American Joint Committee on Cancer (AJCC) has a tumor-node-metastasis (TNM) classification schema that is correlated to the FIGO staging schema (see Table 6). Any spread beyond the pelvic lymph nodes is considered distant metastasis and confers reduced survival. Distant metastases are hematogenously spread and can occur to a multitude of locations including bone, liver, and lung.

Table 6. American Joint Committee on cancer staging (1992).

**Primary Tumor (T)**

| | |
|---|---|
| TX | Primary tumor cannot be assessed |
| T0 | No evidence of primary tumor |
| Tis | Carcinoma *in situ* (preinvasive carcinoma) |
| T1 | Tumor confined to the vulva or to the vulva and perineum, 2 cm or less in greatest dimension |
| T2 | Tumor confined to the vulva or to the vulva and perineum, more than 2 cm in greatest dimension |
| T3 | Tumor invades any of the following: lower urethra, vagina, or anus |
| T4 | Tumor invades any of the following: bladder mucosa, upper urethral mucosa, or rectal mucosa, or is fixed to the bone |

**Regional Lymph Nodes (N)**

| | |
|---|---|
| NX | Regional lymph nodes cannot be assessed |
| N0 | No regional lymph node metastasis |
| N1 | Unilateral regional lymph node metastasis |
| N2 | Bilateral regional lymph node metastasis |

**Distant Metastasis (M)**

| | |
|---|---|
| MX | Presence of distant metastasis cannot be assessed |
| M0 | No distant metastasis |
| M1 | Distant metastasis (pelvic lymph node metastasis is M1) |

**Stage Groupings**

| | | | |
|---|---|---|---|
| Stage 0 | Tis | N0 | M0 |
| Stage I | T1 | N0 | M0 |
| Stage II | T2 | N0 | M0 |
| Stage III | T1 | N1 | M0 |
| | T2 | N1 | M0 |
| | T3 | N0 | M0 |
| | T3 | N1 | M0 |
| Stage IVA | T1 | N2 | M0 |
| | T2 | N2 | M0 |
| | T3 | N2 | M0 |
| | T4 | Any N | M0 |
| Stage IVB | Any T | Any N | M1 |

*Source*: Beahrs OH, Henson DE, Hutter RVP, *et al.*, eds. *Manual for Staging Cancer*, 4th ed. Philadelphia: JB Lippincott, 1992.

## Treatment

### *Vulvectomy*

Vulvar cancer is primarily treated with surgical resection of the primary tumor and excision of inguinal-femoral nodes. Over the decades, initial efforts at radical en bloc dissection have given way to more limited resections and even sentinel node biopsy in attempts to limit morbidity without compromising outcome. Traditionally, vulvar cancer has been treated with en bloc radical vulvectomy, groin and pelvic lymph node dissection based on work by Stoeckel, Taussig, and Way.[16] They showed that surgical resection and lymphadenectomy improved survival in patients with vulvar cancer. En bloc resection removes the vulvar skin and the underlying lymphatics which may harbor tumor via a "butterfly-shaped" incision. The superior margin of the skin incision extends from one anterior superior iliac spine to the other in a downward arc fashion. The lateral aspects of the incision follow the inguinal ligaments along the path of the lymphatic drainage toward the vulva. The vulvar component of the incision incorporates the whole vulva and the underlying subcutaneous tissue.

A less morbid, skin-sparing "longhorn" incision can also be utilized. The incision is smaller, extending superiorly from the anterior superior iliac spines to the mons pubis, incorporating the labia, and extending laterally to the labiocrural folds. The incisions are dissected down to the deep inguinal and perineal fascia thus ensuring the en bloc removal of the inguinal lymphatics. Even with this modified approach, there is considerable morbidity associated with the procedure. The most common complication is skin breakdown. This is in part due to the extensive resection of normal tissue surrounding the affected tissue, resulting in a large defect in an area of the body where tension is inevitably placed on the resection site. There is a 50% risk of some level of wound breakdown resulting in long-term morbidity.[17,18] Fortunately, in the majority of the cases, the wound site heals by primary intention resulting in an acceptable outcome. Lymphocysts can develop, presenting as a soft mass at the incision site. They may resolve spontaneously but persistence requires needle or catheter drainage and sclerosis.

Theoretically, removing the skin bridge between the vulva and groin ensures resection of any malignant cells that may be in transit, though this instance is rarely observed. The triple incision technique utilizes separate incisions for each groin and the vulva, preserving the intervening tissues. Sparing of the skin bridge dramatically decreases the incidence and severity of wound breakdown to approximately 15–20%.[19,20]

Currently, radical wide excision is the technique most commonly utilized for smaller tumors. This entails the resection of the tumor and a 1–2 cm gross margin of normal tissue, down to the level of the deep perineal fascia to allow preservation of more normal anatomy. Berek *et al.* examined the surgical samples of 135 patients, noting that even an 8 mm pathologic margin ensured a low risk of local recurrence. This 8 mm pathologic margin translates into a 1 cm gross surgical margin. Resection margins of less than 1 cm increased the risk of recurrence by up to 48%.[21]

Depending on the size of the primary lesion, the defect may still be substantial. In most circumstances primary closure is possible. In some cases, mobilization of normal tissue surrounding the resection site may facilitate closure. Some patients require rhomboid flaps or Z-plasty. The rhomboid flap (see Fig. 2) consists of a wide V-shaped incision placed at the lateral margin of the deficit. The subcutaneous tissue is undermined and the tissue flap is approximated to the medial edge of the deficit. In certain circumstances when the vulvar resection is extensive, reconstruction with a myocutaneous gracilis flap may be necessary. An area of skin, subcutaneous tissue, and underlying muscle are freed, preserving the

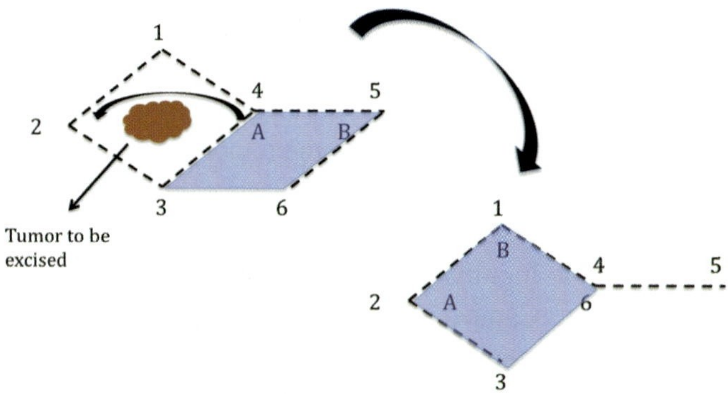


Figure 2. Diagrammatic representation of rhomboid flap repair.

underlying vascular pedicle. The flap is tunneled under the subcutaneous tissue of the medial thigh and secured over the site to ensure full-thickness coverage of the defect.

### *Lymphadenectomy*

Early vulvar cancers may be adequately treated with wide local excision, forgoing lymphadenectomy. Podratz *et al.* performed a retrospective review comparing 10 patients who underwent vulvar resection with groin lymphadenectomy and 30 patients who underwent vulvar resection without lymphadenectomy. In the 10 patients who underwent lymphadenectomy, vulvar recurrences developed in two patients (five-year recurrence rate, 5.9%). There were no groin recurrences in this group of patients. Of the 30 patients who underwent resection only, only one (ten-year rate, 6.7%) developed groin metastases at 7.5 years. The five- and ten-year cause-specific survivals were similar at 100% and 94.7%, respectively.[22] Berek *et al.* showed that the five-year survival was identical for those patients who had a wide local excision and lymphadenectomy versus wide local excision alone.[23] Thus lymph node dissection appears to be unnecessary after wide local excision of the primary lesion.

However, for larger lesions, particularly those with invasion greater than 1 mm, lymphadenectomy is indicated. The resection of both superficial and deep lymph nodes in the groin is called inguinofemoral lymphadenectomy. The superficial lymph node chain consists of 8–10 lymph nodes which are superficial to the cribriform plate and contained superiorly by the inguinal ligament, laterally by the sartorius muscle, medially by the adductor longus, and anteriorly by Camper's fascia. Deep inguinal lymph nodes consist of 3–5 nodes which lie medial to the femoral vein beneath the cribriform fascia.

Superficial lymphadenectomy is performed by first making a skin incision parallel to the inguinal ligament; the skin is elevated and the tissue is dissected along Camper's fascia to retain the blood supply to the overlying skin. The anatomical boundaries of the dissection are identified and the specimen is removed from the inguinal ligament and dissected along the sartorius and adductor longus muscles. When developing the plane, the saphenous vein in the lower medial aspect of the field may be ligated or preserved. To remove deep inguinal nodes, the cribriform fascia is penetrated, and the underlying tissue is removed medial to the femoral vein. Unilateral dissection can be utilized when the primary lesion is well lateralized (more than 2 cm from the midline).

Sentinel lymph node biopsy in vulvar cancer has been actively investigated as an alternative to full inguinal femoral lymphadenectomy. Sentinel lymph node biopsy in breast cancer patients has reduced the rate of lymphedema without compromising survival. Multiple observational studies using the technique in patients with vulvar cancer have shown promise as well. De Hullu *et al.* performed sentinel lymph node biopsy in 59 patients (107 groins) followed by full lymphadenectomy. The nodal specimens were evaluated separately. Negative sentinel lymph node biopsies were re-evaluated with ultrastaging. Routine evaluation showed positive nodes in 27 groins that were all identified by a positive sentinel lymph node. An additional four cases were identified as having metastatic disease in the sentinel node upon further ultrastaging. The authors concluded that the negative predictive value for sentinel lymph node evaluation was 100%.[24]

Sentinel lymph node biopsy identification occurs by using both radioactive $^{99m}$technetium and isosulfan blue. Dye alone results in unacceptably low sensitivity. The patient's primary tumor is preoperatively injected with both agents. The sentinel node is identified using a hand-held gamma probe. Once the high-intensity signal is identified in the groin, an incision is made on the overlying skin and the sentinel node is localized visually by the blue dye and with the assistance of the gamma probe. If the node is noted to be negative for metastases then full inguinal femoral dissection is unwarranted.

Patients who undergo sentinel lymph node biopsy alone versus lymphadenectomy have been shown to experience a shorter hospital stay, decreased risk of wound breakdown, infection, lymphedema, and recurrent erysipelas in the long-term.[25] Barriers to routine performance of the procedure include the ability to adequately learn the procedure given their relative rarity, concerns over groin failure with conservative surgery, and lack of long-term improvement in overall quality of life.[26,27]

## *Radiation*

Stage I and II disease is treated with surgical resection without the addition of radiotherapy. Primary radiotherapy in early-stage disease is only considered in patients who cannot tolerate surgery. The role for adjuvant radiotherapy to the primary tumor site in individuals with high-risk, node-negative primary tumors is not clear. A retrospective study performed by Jones *et al.* examined the use of adjuvant radiotherapy in patients with either positive margins or close margins (less than 8 mm), and showed an improvement in locoregional recurrence rate,[28] though in margin-positive tumors, re-excision is also an alternative.

GOG 88 randomized patients with stage I squamous cell vulvar cancer to bilateral/unilateral groin dissection or 5,000 cGy of groin radiation administered to 3 cm of depth. The study was stopped prematurely due to the high failure rate in the radiation arm.[29] GOG 88 has been criticized for failing to completely cover the inguinofemoral lymph nodes, the reliance on physical exam to detect nodal disease, failure to include distal pelvic lymph nodes in the radiation field, and significant underdosage (shallow depth) of radiation. Petereit *et al.*[30] and Levenback *et al.*[31] suggest that when clinically negative nodes are adequately radiated, an acceptable inguinal node recurrence rate of 11% or less may be achieved.

In the case of documented disease in the groin, adjuvant radiation is indicated when there are two or more microscopically positive groin nodes, one or more macroscopically involved lymph nodes, or evidence of extracapsular spread. GOG 37 demonstrated that when patients were noted to have positive inguinal lymph nodes, randomization to either radiation or pelvic lymph node dissection resulted in superior outcome for those treated with radiation in both the short two years[32] and long-term.[33]

Vulvar tissue does not tolerate radiotherapy very well. Other organs in the beam of radiation, including the bladder, rectum, and femoral head, also have a low tolerance for treatment. The morbidity of radiotherapy can be acute or late. In the acute phase, the skin displays inflammation, moist desquamation, and erythema. These symptoms improve with good perineal care over a 3–4-week period after radiotherapy is stopped. These symptoms may be severe enough to necessitate treatment delay between radiotherapy sessions. Late-phase complications include fibrosis, swelling, femoral fracture, and narrowing of the introitus.

## *Chemotherapy*

Squamous cell carcinoma of the vulva is not particularly chemosensitive. Most agents that are active against squamous cell carcinomas from other sites like the lung and anal canal have limited activity in vulvar carcinoma. Several phase 2 studies have looked at single agents and have shown minimal responses to bleomycin[34] and doxorubicin.[35]

Chemoradiation has been explored in vulvar carcinoma after the positive results seen for carcinoma of the cervix. In cervical cancer the relative risk of death was reduced by 30–50% in multiple phase III trials when cisplatin was added to radiation therapy.[36,37] Patients who have inoperable vulvar tumor may benefit from neoadjuvant chemoradiation. The best evidence available comes from several prospective GOG phase II trials. In GOG 101, patients with unresectable advanced disease (T3 or T4 tumors) underwent preoperative chemoradiation consisting of two cycles of 5-fluorouracil, cisplatin, and radiation. Radiation was delivered to a dose of 47.6 Gy, using a planned split-course regimen. The patients then underwent either resection of the residual vulvar tumor, or in patients who responded completely, an incisional biopsy of the primary tumor site. Of 71 evaluable patients, 34 (48%) experienced a complete clinical tumor response. Of these patients, 31 underwent surgical assessment and 22 (70%) were confirmed to have no residual tumor in the pathologic specimens. Only two patients (3%) continued to have unresectable disease after neoadjuvant treatment. At median follow-up of 50 months, 11 patients (16%) developed locally recurrent disease involving the vulva.

A second group of patients were also evaluated in GOG 101, including patients with unresectable N2/N3 groin lymph nodes. Of the evaluable patients, 38 of 40 (95%) who completed neoadjuvant chemoradiation were considered surgical candidates after treatment. Of 37 patients who underwent radical vulvectomy with lymphadenectomy, 41% were histologically negative for disease in the lymph nodes.[38] The results of GOG 205 have not yet been reported, but this prospective trial will determine the efficacy of radiation and weekly cisplatin for the treatment of unresectable locally advanced squamous cell carcinoma of the vulva followed by excision of remaining tumor versus incisional biopsy.

### Recurrent Disease

Disease can recur regionally, in the groin, or at distant sites. Factors that are associated with an increased risk of local recurrence include tumor grade, lymphovascular space invasion, depth of stromal invasion (greater than 2.5 mm), stage of the tumor, and status of resection margin. When recurrence occurs locally, re-excision can result in disease-free survival for the majority of patients; patients with recurrent nodal disease and distant metastases have a much poorer prognosis and therapy generally consists of palliative chemotherapy and radiation.

### Outcome

Prognosis is primarily dependent on the stage at presentation and lymph node status. Fortunately, most patients present with early-stage disease. Five-year survival ranges from 78.5% for those with stage I disease, compared to only 13% for those with stage IV disease (see Table 2). However, if lymph nodes are negative, the survival rate is 96% regardless of stage. If inguinal nodes are involved, the five-year survival rate decreases dramatically to 50%. Survival for patients with pelvic lymph node involvement is as low as 10% at five-years.

## NON-SQUAMOUS VULVAR CANCERS

### Verrucous Carcinoma

Verrucous carcinoma is a variant of squamous cell carcinoma characterized as a fungating exophytic lesion with a gross appearance similar to condyloma acuminatum. It consists of well-differentiated squamous cells which are characteristically diploid. Verrucous tumors may be associated with HPV 6 or its variants.[39] These lesions are slow growing, and though lymph node metastasis is rare, these lesions are locally aggressive with bone involvement being reported.[40] These lesions require surgical resection with negative margins. Radiation therapy is not indicated, as the use of radiation has also been associated with worse outcome;[41] anaplastic transformation has also been reported.[42] Japaze *et al.* reported a five-year survival rate of only 42% for patients treated with surgery and radiation in comparison to 94% for those treated with surgery alone.[41] Recurrences should undergo repeat excision, with exenteration being necessary in some instances.

## Basal Cell Carcinoma

Basal cell carcinoma of the skin is the most common type of skin cancer; however, its counterpart in the vulva is rare, comprising only 2% of vulvar cancer cases.[43] Its gross appearance is described as having a pearly, raised edge with or without central ulceration. The only risk factor identified is increasing age. Mortality risk for basal cell carcinoma of the vulva is extremely low and metastases to the lymphatics are rarely seen. These lesions are locally invasive and may be adequately treated with local excision alone. Upon pathologic analysis, those containing a malignant squamous component, known as basosquamous carcinoma, display a more aggressive course, and should be treated in a similar fashion as squamous carcinomas.

## Vulvar Melanoma

Vulvar melanoma is a rare form of both skin melanoma and vulvar cancer, carrying a poorer prognosis compared to squamous cell carcinoma. Vulvar melanoma is the second most common histological type of vulvar cancer,[44] but comprises only 8–10% of vulvar cancers.[45] The incidence increases with age and reaches peak incidence in those over age 75.[46] Risk factors for developing vulvar melanoma are similar to those for skin melanoma: a family history of melanoma, poor tanning ability, and a history of sunburn in adolescence. The tumor is more prevalent in individuals with light versus dark skin, and presents as pigmented lesions in the vulvar area.[45,47] The most common presenting complaint is bleeding, but patients may also experience itching, a lump, or pain. On physical examination, suspicious findings include a raised, asymmetrical, pigmented lesion increasing in size with irregular borders and heterogeneous color.[48,49]

Similar to malignant melanoma of the skin, three histologic categories exist, including superficial spreading, nodular, and mucosal lentiginous melanoma. In most cases, vulvar melanoma consists of a mixed histological pattern which includes all three subtypes of tumor. They are most often pigmented but can be amelanotic in 25% of cases. Much like skin melanoma, vulvar melanoma is an aggressive disease and spreads to superficial inguinal lymph nodes much more readily when compared to squamous cell carcinoma. Prognosis for vulvar melanoma is determined by the size of the lesion and level of invasion.

FIGO staging is not relevant for vulvar melanoma. Various classification schemes exist, of which the Breslow technique[50] is the simplest, measuring the thickness of the invasive component. The Clark classification[47] utilizes histologic levels. Chung[51] described a third system measuring depth of invasion from the granular layer of the surface epithelium (see Table 7). As the level of invasion increases, so does the risk for metastasis and death (see Table 8).

Radical vulvectomy was originally recommended for management for malignant melanoma of the vulva; however, Trimble *et al.*[51] evaluated 80 patients and noted no difference in survival for radical surgery versus local excision. Resection goals for gross margins are 1–2 cm for thin

Table 7. Melanoma microstaging systems.

| Level | Breslow[1] | Clark[2] | Chung[3] |
|---|---|---|---|
| I | ≤0.75 mm | Epidermis | Intraepithelial |
| II | 0.76 to 1.50 mm | Into papillary dermis | Into dermis or lamina propria to depth of 1 mm or less |
| III | 1.51 to 2.25 mm | Filling papillary dermis | >1–2 mm invasion |
| IV | 2.26 to 3.0 mm | Into reticular dermis | >2 mm invasion |
| V | >3.0 mm | Into subcutaneous fat | Into subcutaneous fat |

[1]*Source*: Breslow A. Thickness, cross-sectional areas and depth of invasion in the prognosis of cutaneous melanoma. *Ann Surg* 1970;172:902–908.

[2]*Source*: Clark WH, *et al.* The histogenesis and biologic behavior of primary human malignant melanomas of the skin. *Cancer Res* 1969;29:705–727.

[3]*Source*: Chung AF, Woodruff JM, Lewis JL. Malignant melanoma of the vulva: a report of 44 cases. *Obstet Gynecol* 1975;45:638–646.

Table 8. Melanoma levels and prognosis in vulvar melanoma.

| Level | Clark 10 year survival (%)[1] | Chung 10 year survival (%)[2] |
|---|---|---|
| I | | 100 |
| II | 100 | 81 |
| III | 83 | 87 |
| IV | 65 | 11 |
| V | 23 | 23 |

[1]*Source*: Podratz KC, Gaffey TA, Symmonds RE, Johansen KL, O'Brien PC. Melanoma of the vulva: an update. *Gynecol Oncol* 1983;16(2):153–168.
[2]*Source*: Trimble EL, Lewis JL, Williams LL, Curtin JP, Chapman D, Woodruff JM, *et al*. Management of vulvar melanoma. *Gynecol Oncol* 1992;45(3):254–258.

lesions (less than 0.75 mm), 2 cm for lesions less than 2 mm, and 2–3 cm for thicker lesions. Obtaining margins greater than 3 cm affords no survival advantage. There does not appear to be therapeutic benefit associated with inguinal femoral lymphadenectomy, and pelvic lymphadenectomy is not justified.

## Bartholin's Gland Carcinoma and Adenocarcinoma

Most vulvar adenocarcinomas originate from, Bartholin's gland; however, vulvar sweat glands, other skin appendages, Skene's glands, endometriosis, and vulvar Paget's disease may also give rise to adenocarcinoma. Bartholin's glands are composed of vestibular glands with a main duct lined by transitional cell epithelium which switches to stratified squamous epithelium approaching the skin surface. These different cells give rise to a variety of histologies (see Table 1). Primary adenocarcinoma and squamous cell carcinoma each comprise about 40% of Bartholin's gland carcinoma, with adenoid cystic tumors contributing 15%, and adenosquamous carcinomas and transitional cell cancers occurring only in 5% of the cases.[52]

Delay in diagnosis is common. In some patients, diagnosis of malignancy is preceded by symptomatic inflammation of the gland, leading to the false diagnosis of abscess or cyst. Dyspareunia, mass, or ulceration are among the more common presenting complaints. Given that these tumors generally occur in older women, any enlargement in the posterior lateral vulva in a woman over the age of 50 should be aggressively investigated through biopsy. Biopsy or excision should be strongly considered for any solid mass that persists after drainage of a cyst. Because of their location deep in the vulva, these tumors may become quite large before being detected, often with local invasion into the ischiorectal fossa. Unfortunately, 20% have already metastasized to regional nodes at the time of diagnosis. Despite their tendency for a more advanced stage at presentation, outcomes are similar compared to primary vulvar squamous cell carcinomas when considered stage for stage.

The surgical management of Bartholin's gland adenocarcinoma is similar to that for squamous cell carcinoma of the vulva, consisting of radical vulvectomy and bilateral inguinal lymph node dissection. Posterior exenteration may be required in rare cases. Patients who have positive/close resection margins and positive nodal disease require radiotherapy; radiosensitizing chemotherapy may have a role in treatment. Interstitial implants may be used in selected cases. Five-year survival ranges from 52–89% for those with negative inguinal nodes to 18–20% for those with node-positive disease.

Adenoid cystic carcinomas tend to recur locally, and though they have a more favorable prognosis, distant metastases, particularly to the lungs, may still occur. Adenosquamous lesions are considered more aggressive, with a tendency towards not only local recurrence, but lymph node metastasis and perineural spread as well. Underwood *et al.* reported a five-year survival of 5.5% for patients with adenosquamous carcinomas compared to 62.3% for those with squamous cell carcinoma.[53]

## Sarcoma

Leiomyosarcoma of the vulva is an extremely rare form of vulvar cancer. It presents with pain and a mass generally greater than 5 cm. Histologically, it displays an infiltrating edge and consists of interlaced spindle cells with a high mitotic count greater than 10 mitoses per 10 high power fields. The tumor is treated with wide local excision or modified radical vulvectomy. Recurrence with distant metastases involving the lung and liver leads to death in 50–60% of cases.

Malignant fibrous histiocytoma presents with a growing painful nodule. Histologically, it has a "cartwheel" arrangement of malignant spindle cells with areas of marked pleomorphism and infiltrative margins. Resection and groin node dissection is recommended. Metastatic disease has been reported in the pleura, peritoneum and ventricles of the heart. Radiotherapy is indicated for nodal involvement.

## Vulvar Paget's Disease

Paget's disease of the vulva is a rare finding seen predominantly in postmenopausal women, accounting for less than 2% of vulvar tumors. It is often present in Caucasian women with longstanding symptoms of itching and pain. The affected skin is erythematous, excoriated, and inflamed with a sharply demarcated border. The area may be thick and smooth. A superficial white layer overlying the reddened tissue, the so-called "cake-icing effect", is pathognomonic for Paget's disease. Due to severe excoriation and inflammation, misdiagnosis as eczema or allergic dermatitis is common. The lesions may be localized to the labia, perineal body, or clitoral area, or may involve the entire vulva with extension to the perianal areas, groins, or mons. In contrast to perianal and breast Paget's disease which is continuous with an underlying primary or metastatic malignancy, vulvar Paget's occurs in isolation in small nests within the epithelium and can sometimes be associated with an underlying adenocarcinoma. Many patients with Paget's disease are diagnosed with associated adenocarcinomas of the breast, stomach, bladder, and other sites. Vigilance must be exercised to exclude underlying and distant malignancies.

Biopsy should be performed to establish the diagnosis. In particular, careful palpation is necessary in order to detect any thickening of the area, which may signal underlying adenocarcinoma. Fine-needle aspiration of suspicious nodules may be performed. Treatment comprises of wide local excision with clear margins. The margins of the specimen are frequently positive for disease even though clinically normal-appearing skin is present around the lesion. Surrounding normal-appearing skin may be infiltrated with neoplastic cells microscopically. Regardless of margin status, recurrences are common. If an underlying adenocarcinoma is diagnosed, then recommendations for therapy are similar to that for squamous cell

26. Oonk MHM, van Os MA, de Bock GH, de Hullu JA, Ansink AC, van der Zee AGJ. A comparison of quality of life between vulvar cancer patients after sentinel lymph node procedure only and inguinofemoral lymphadenectomy. *Gynecol Oncol* 2009;113(3):301–305.
27. Levenback CF. How safe is sentinel lymph node biopsy in patients with vulvar cancer? *J Clin Oncol* 2008;26(6):828–829.
28. Faul CM, Mirmow D, Huang Q, Gerszten K, Day R, Jones MW. Adjuvant radiation for vulvar carcinoma: improved local control. *Int J Radiat Oncol Biol Phys* 1997;38(2):381–389.
29. Stehman FB, Bundy BN, Thomas G, *et al.* Groin dissection versus groin radiation in carcinoma of the vulva: a Gynecologic Oncology Group study. *Int J Radiat Oncol Biol Phys* 1992;24(2):389–396.
30. Petereit DG, Mehta MP, Buchler DA, Kinsella TJ. A retrospective review of nodal treatment for vulvar cancer. *Am J Clin Oncol* 1993;16(1): 38–42.
31. Katz A, Eifel PJ, Jhingran A, Levenback CF. The role of radiation therapy in preventing regional recurrences of invasive squamous cell carcinoma of the vulva. *Int J Radiat Oncol Biol Phys* 2003;57(2):409–418.
32. Homesley HD, Bundy BN, Sedlis A, Adcock L. Radiation therapy versus pelvic node resection for carcinoma of the vulva with positive groin nodes. *Obstet Gynecol* 1986;68(6):733–740.
33. Kunos C, Simpkins F, Gibbons H, Tian C, Homesley H. Radiation therapy compared with pelvic node resection for node-positive vulvar cancer: a randomized controlled trial. *Obstet Gynecol* 2009;114(3):537–546.
34. Deppe G, Bruckner HW, Cohen CJ. Adriamycin treatment of advanced vulvar carcinoma. *Obstet Gynecol* 1977;50(1 Suppl):13s–14s.
35. Tropé C, Johnsson JE, Larsson G, Simonsen E. Bleomycin alone or combined with mitomycin C in treatment of advanced or recurrent squamous cell carcinoma of the vulva. *Cancer Treat Rep* 1980;64(4–5):639–642.
36. Rose PG, Bundy BN, Watkins EB, *et al.* Concurrent cisplatin-based radiotherapy and chemotherapy for locally advanced cervical cancer. *N Engl J Med* 1999;340(15):1144–1153.
37. Keys HM, Bundy BN, Stehman FB, *et al.* Cisplatin, radiation, and adjuvant hysterectomy compared with radiation and adjuvant hysterectomy for bulky stage IB cervical carcinoma. *N Engl J Med* 1999;340(15): 1154–1161.

38. Montana GS, Thomas GM, Moore DH, *et al.* Preoperative chemo-radiation for carcinoma of the vulva with N2/N3 nodes: a gynecologic oncology group study. *Int J Radiat Oncol Biol Phys* 2000;48(4):1007–1013.
39. Rando RF, Sedlacek TV, Hunt J, Jenson AB, Kurman RJ, Lancaster WD. Verrucous carcinoma of the vulva associated with an unusual type 6 human papillomavirus. *Obstet Gynecol* 1986;67(3 Suppl):70S–75S.
40. Gallousis S. Verrucous carcinoma. Report of three vulvar cases and review of the literature. *Obstet Gynecol* 1972;40(4):502–507.
41. Japaze H, van Dinh T, Woodruff JD. Verrucous carcinoma of the vulva: study of 24 cases. *Obstet Gynecol* 1982;60(4):462–466.
42. Demian SD, Bushkin FL, Echevarria RA. Perineural invasion and anaplastic transformation of verrucous carcinoma. *Cancer* 1973;32(2):395–401.
43. de Giorgi V, Salvini C, Massi D, Raspollini MR, Carli P. Vulvar basal cell carcinoma: retrospective study and review of literature. *Gynecol Oncol* 2005;97(1):192–194.
44. Ghurani GB, Penalver MA. An update on vulvar cancer. *Am J Obstet Gynecol* 2001;185(2):294–299.
45. Ronan SG, Eng AM, Briele HA, Walker MJ, Das Gupta TK. Malignant melanoma of the female genitalia. *J Am Acad Dermatol* 1990;22(3): 428–435.
46. Ragnarsson-Olding BK, Nilsson BR, Kanter-Lewensohn LR, Lagerlöf B, Ringborg UK. Malignant melanoma of the vulva in a nationwide, 25-year study of 219 Swedish females: predictors of survival. *Cancer* 1999;86(7): 1285–1293.
47. Podratz KC, Gaffey TA, Symmonds RE, Johansen KL, O'Brien PC. Melanoma of the vulva: an update. *Gynecol Oncol* 1983;16(2):153–168.
48. Ariel IM. Malignant melanoma of the female genital system: a report of 48 patients and review of the literature. *J Surg Oncol* 1981;16(4):371–383.
49. Phillips GL. Current management of vulvar melanoma. *Oncology (Williston Park)* 1990;4(9):61–64; discussion 66, 68.
50. Jaramillo BA, Ganjei P, Averette HE, Sevin BU, Lovecchio JL. Malignant melanoma of the vulva. *Obstet Gynecol* 1985;66(3):398–401.
51. Trimble EL, Lewis JL, Williams LL, *et al.* Management of vulvar melanoma. *Gynecol Oncol* 1992;45(3):254–258.
52. Woolcott RJ, Henry RJ, Houghton CR. Malignant melanoma of the vulva. Australian experience. *J Reprod Med* 1988;33(8):699–702.

53. Underwood JW, Adcock LL, Okagaki T. Adenosquamous carcinoma of skin appendages (adenoid squamous cell carcinoma, pseudoglandular squamous cell carcinoma, adenocanthoma of sweat gland of Lever) of the vulva: a clinical and ultrastructural study. *Cancer* 1978;42(4):1851–1858.

# 5

# VAGINAL CANCER

*Rajul Kothari and Peter A. Argenta*

## INTRODUCTION

Primary vaginal cancer is a relatively rare gynecologic malignancy, accounting for less than 2% of all gynecologic cancers or about 2,200 cases annually in the United States.[1] The incidence of primary vaginal cancer appears to be stable over the past decade. The vast majority of vaginal cancers are squamous carcinomas or adenocarcinomas, with sarcoma and melanoma comprising less than 10% of all cases.[2] Approximately 80% of cancers affecting the vagina simultaneously involve the cervix, vulva, bladder, or rectum; by convention these are categorized as non-vaginal primaries.

## ANATOMIC CONSIDERATIONS

The vagina is flanked anteriorly by the bladder, posteriorly by the rectum, proximally by the cervix, and distally by the vulva. The vagina is derived largely from the paramesonephric (müllerian) ducts which form the uterine body, cervix, and upper four fifths of the vagina. The lower one fifth is derived from endodermal sinovaginal bulbs which arise from the urogenital sinus. The vaginal tube starts as a solid organ and canalizes via central apoptosis, leaving a peripheral epithelium composed of modified, non-keratinized squamous epithelium. The surrounding muscle and stroma are of mesodermal origin. Glandular elements, including Bartholin's gland (located posteriorly and laterally) and Skene's glands (located periurethrally) are interspersed along the vaginal tube and with cervical secretions provide lubrication. Gartner's duct cysts, which are Wolffian duct remnants, can be present along the lateral aspects of the vagina.

The blood supply to the vagina is provided regionally by branches of the uterine, inferior vesical, and middle rectal arteries which anastomose to form an enveloping arcade around the vaginal tube. The venous and lymphatic drainage mimics the arterial flow with drainage from the proximal vagina flowing first to the parametria and then to the obturator and internal iliac nodes. Distally a "vulvar" drainage pattern predominates, placing the superficial and deep inguinal nodes at a relatively higher risk.

## EPIDEMIOLOGY

The etiologic agent of most squamous vaginal carcinomas is likely infection with the human papillomavirus (HPV). Not surprisingly, therefore, the risk factor profile for vaginal carcinoma largely reflects factors associated with acquisition of the virus (Table 1). As with other HPV-related

Table 1. Epidemiologic risk factors for *in situ* or invasive vaginal cancer.

| **Risk factor (Referent)** | **OR (95% CI)** |
|---|---|
| Prior HPV infection | |
| HPV 16 L1 antibody-positive (-negative) | 4.3 (2.1–8.7) |
| Genital warts ever (never) | 4.7 (3.1–7.3) |
| Prior HSV infection | 2.1 (1.4–3.2) |
| Previous anogenital cancer | 19.7 (12.2–32.0) |
| ≥5 sexual partners (=1) | 3.1 (1.9–4.9) |
| Sexual debut <17 years old (>21 years old) | 2.0 (1.2–3.5) |
| Smoking (never) | |
| Ever | 1.4 (1.0–2.0) |
| Current | 2.1 (1.4–3.1) |
| Low socio-economic status | |
| Immunosuppression | |
| Pelvic irradiation | |
| *In utero* exposure to diethylstilbestrol | |

*Source*: Adapted from Daling *et al.*[58] and Brinton *et al.*[59]

diseases, the incidence of both *in situ* and invasive cancer increases with age, with the peak of invasive carcinoma coming 1–2 decades later. In the United States the peak incidence of *in situ* and invasive vaginal carcinoma occurs in the sixth and eigth decades of life, respectively. Conversely, less than 1% of cancers occur before the age of 20, and these are almost exclusively adenocarcinomas (see below). Previous treatment for cervical carcinoma with radiation or surgery is a clear and significant risk factor for the development of vaginal carcinoma, likely due to the shared risk factor, acquisition of a high-risk HPV.

*In utero* exposure to synthetic nonsteroidal estrogens such as diethylstilbestrol (DES) prior to the 17th week of gestation has been linked to an increased risk of clear cell carcinoma, especially in young women.[3] The median age at presentation for DES-exposed patients is 19, with cases reported as young as 7; among non-exposed women vaginal clear cell carcinoma occurs almost exclusively among the elderly. Though the exact mechanism of carcinogenesis is unknown, DES is thought to induce the development of abnormal müllerian rests which in turn respond atypically to endogenous estrogens at puberty. Alternatively, some authors have suggested that the larger than normal transformation zones observed in DES-exposed women increases their receptiveness to HPV infection and that subsequent cancer risk can be attributed to these infections. Irrespective of the cause, the incidence of clear cell carcinoma in DES-exposed women is 0.1–1.4 per 1,000 by the age of 34, representing a 40-fold increase over the baseline population risk.[4] The US Food and Drug Administration issued an FDA Drug Bulletin advising against the use of DES in pregnant women; and in 1975 the common dosages (25 mg and 100 mg) were ordered to be withdrawn from the market.

Both melanomas and sarcomas of the vagina are sufficiently rare that the described epidemiologic risk factors are tenuous at best.

## PRESENTATION/NATURAL HISTORY

Most cases of vaginal intraepithelial neoplasia (VAIN) are asymptomatic at presentation and diagnosed cytologically as a result of routine cervical cancer screening or at follow-up after hysterectomy for cervical dysplasia or cancer.[5] As such, evaluation of the vagina should be a

Table 2. Presenting concern preceding diagnosis.

| | |
|---|---|
| Vaginal discharge | 62% |
| Palpable mass | 13% |
| Pain | 4% |
| Dysuria | 2% |
| Other | 3% |
| Asymptomatic/ Incidental cytology | 16% |

routine component of diagnostic colposcopy following abnormal screening. The threshold for biopsy of any visible vaginal lesion in this setting should be low. Conversely, identification of VAIN should prompt evaluation of the cervix and vulva, as additional lesions may be present in up to 50% of cases.

Symptoms are more common among patients with invasive cancer, but many are non-specific, and up to 20% of patients may remain asymptomatic (Table 2).[6] Bleeding is the most common symptom of clear cell carcinoma but, in the case of DES-exposed women, is frequently preceded by a vaginal discharge resulting from associated vaginal adenosis. Embryonal rhabdomyosarcoma (sarcoma botryoides) presents typically in infants (median age 2 years) as a protuberant, edematous mass with or without bleeding.

Most lesions involve the upper third of the vagina and many are multifocal. In addition to colposcopy, thorough palpation of the vaginal, paravaginal, and inguinal tissues should be performed prior to consideration of therapy. Approximately two thirds of patients will have disease overtly confined to the vagina or subvaginal tissues (stage I or II) at presentation; however, the incidence of nodal metastases even in low-stage disease is 6–32%.[7,8] Clinically palpable lymph nodes are present in 5–20% of patients at presentation.

The extent of invasion is the single most important predictor of outcome, and figures prominently in staging (Table 3). Creasman and colleagues identified a relatively even distribution of stage I, II, and III/IV disease at presentation; and though the overall incidence increases with age, the stage distribution remains similar across almost all ages.[2]

Table 3. Staging of vaginal cancer.

**FIGO Clinical Staging**

**Stage I**: Tumor confined to the vagina
**Stage II**: Tumor extends to the paravaginal tissues, but does not extend to the side wall
**Stage III**: Tumor extends to pelvic side wall or involved bladder without mucosal involvement (bullous edema only)
**Stage IV**: Tumor invades local organs or displays distant metastases
- **IVA**: Tumor invades the mucosa of bladder or rectum and/or extends directly beyond the true pelvis
- **IVB**: Distant metastases

**American Joint Committee on Cancer (AJCC) TNM System**

**Tumor extent (T)**
- **Tis**: Cancer cells are only in the most superficial layer of cells of the vagina without growth into the underlying tissues. This stage is also called *carcinoma in situ* (CIS) or *vaginal intraepithelial neoplasia 3* (VAIN 3)
- **T1**: The cancer is only in the vagina
- **T2**: The cancer extends to subvaginal tissues but not to the pelvic wall
- **T3**: The cancer is growing into the pelvic wall
- **T4**: The cancer is growing into the bladder or rectum or is out of the pelvis

**Lymph node spread of cancer (N)**
- **N0**: The cancer has not spread to lymph nodes
- **N1**: The cancer has spread to lymph nodes in the pelvis or groin (inguinal region)

**Distant spread of cancer (M)**
- **M0**: The cancer has not spread to distant sites
- **M1**: The cancer has spread to distant sites

**Staging**
- **Stage 0**: (Tis, N0, M0)
- **Stage I**: (T1, N0, M0)
- **Stage II**: (T2, N0, M0)
- **Stage III**: Either of the following:
  (T3, any N, M0) or
  (T1 or T2, N1, M0)
- **Stage IVA**: (T4, any N, M0)
- **Stage IVB**: (Any T, any N, M1)

# PATHOLOGY

## Childhood

### *Embryonal rhabdomyosarcoma*

Embryonal rhabdomyosarcoma (RMS) is the most common malignant neoplasm of the vagina in infants and children. Patients are less than five years at diagnosis in 90% of cases.[2] These tumors generally arise in the anterior wall of the vagina and appear as papillae, small nodules, or pedunculated or sessile soft, polypoid "grape-like" masses that may protrude from the vagina. Staging is per the Intergroup Rhabdomyosarcoma Study Group (IRSG) classification which is based on the extent of disease, resectability, and microscopic evaluation of margins of excision. Distinction microscopically is made by the presence of a cambium tumor cell layer underlying an intact epithelium.[9] The cambium layer is defined as the condensed subepithelial layer of rhabdomyoblasts that are scattered in a loose myxoid or dense collagenous stroma. Immunohistochemical staining for actin, desmin, MyoD1, or myogenin can help to distinguish RMS from other pathologies. Misdiagnosis of melanoma should be avoided as 20% of RMS cases have immunoreactivity for the S100 protein.[9]

Treatment options for RMS have traditionally been limited to exenterative procedures with modest survival expectations (20–30% at five years). Recent reports from the IRSG however suggest that RMS is sensitive to both chemotherapy and radiation, leading to multiple reports of multimodal therapy featuring induction chemotherapy (usually based on vincristine, actinomycin, and cyclophosphamide (VAC) with or without other agents) followed by tailored surgical resection with or without adjuvant radiation as indicated by the pathologic findings. Small series reporting the use of multimodal strategies have demonstrated overall survival rates of 85–100% with improved overall morbidity.

### *Endodermal sinus tumor*

Endodermal sinus tumor, also called yolk sac tumor, is another rare vaginal cancer with a propensity for development in infants and young children.[10,11] Though experience with this cancer is extremely limited, reported outcomes for patients receiving adjuvant chemotherapy (VAC, or bleomycin, etoposide, cisplatin (BEP), following tailored excision, appear greatly superior to patients receiving surgery alone. Adjuvant treatment with BEP has been favored by some authors owing to more favorable ovarian toxicity and significantly shorter treatment duration. While endodermal sinus tumors appear to be radiosensitive, potential ovarian toxicity limits its utility.

## Adolescence/Young Adult

### *Clear cell adenocarcinoma*

Vaginal cancers occurring in women less than 20 years of age are generally adenocarcinomas.[2] Historically, clear cell adenocarcinoma of the vagina is the most known because it occurs in young women with DES exposure *in utero* though cases in older women unrelated to DES exposure have been described.[12] Adenocarcinomas unrelated to DES exposure tend to have a poorer outcome.[12] Most clear cell tumors arise on the anterior wall, usually in the upper third, corresponding to the most frequent site of adenosis. Tumors have also been found on the wall opposite the main tumor, presumably as a result of implantation or "kissing lesion". The characteristic microscopic pattern for which the tumor is named consists of solid sheets of clear cells. The more frequent pattern (tubulocystic) is characterized by tubules and cysts lined by hobnail cells[11] and has a better prognosis.

## Adult

### *Squamous cell carcinoma*

Squamous cell carcinoma accounts for 80–90% of primary vaginal cancers. To be considered a primary tumor of the vagina, the neoplasm must be located in the vagina, without clinical or histologic evidence of involvement of the cervix or vulva. Squamous cell carcinoma occurring in the vagina within five years of therapy for cervical carcinoma is considered to be recurrent cervical carcinoma rather than a new primary carcinoma of the vagina.[13] Grossly these lesions may appear polypoid, fungating, indurated, or ulcerated and generally occur in the upper posterior wall of the vagina. Microscopically, vaginal cancer resembles squamous cell carcinoma of the cervix. Variants such as verrucous, warty, basaloid, keratinizing, and nonkeratinizing have been described, the nonkeratinizing type being the most common.[11]

## *Melanoma*

Malignant melanoma of the vagina is the second most common vaginal malignancy but represents less than 5% of vaginal neoplasms and less than 1% of all melanomas.[2] They appear as nodular, polypoid, or fungating gray or black soft masses that vary from 0.5 cm to 8 cm in diameter with frequent overlying ulceration. The lower third and anterior vaginal wall are the most common locations. Microscopically it is common to see junctional activity and atypical melanocytes either singly or in clusters extending through the squamous epithelium. Immunohistochemistry is generally positive for the S100 protein. Should S100 be negative, MART-1/Melan-A, HMB-45, and tyrosinase can help to distinguish melanoma from other histologies. Because of the mucosal location, Chung's classification, which is based on tumor thickness, is used to determine prognosis.[14] Five-year survival rates between 14% and 19% have been reported.[2,15]

## *Leiomyosarcoma*

The most common vaginal sarcoma in adults is leiomyosarcoma.[2] These tumors tend to arise from a submucosal location and are characterized by ≥5 mitoses per 10 high-power fields, moderate or marked cytologic atypia, and/or infiltrating margins. Gross appearance varies greatly. Radical resection of vaginal leiomyosarcoma, when possible, appears to offer the best chance for long-term survival. Like other sarcomas, these tumors are largely chemotherapy-refractory, though reports of gemcitabine-based treatments are lacking. The beneficial impact of adjuvant radiation on long-term survival is doubtful given the absence of benefit observed in uterine leiomyosarcomas.

## *Aggressive angiomyxoma*

Aggressive angiomyxioma is a rare mesenchymal neoplasm which occurs most commonly in the pelvis or perineum of reproductive-age women (peak incidence in the third/fourth decades of life). It is typically described as a slow-growing, gelatinous mass and can be mistaken for Gartner's duct or Bartholin's gland cysts. Histologically these tumors are typically highly vascular and demonstrate an infiltrative growth pattern. Though wide excision is typically recommended, the local recurrence rate after surgical extirpation has been reported as high as 72% and recurrences may occur years after primary excision, highlighting a need for prolonged surveillance. Recurrences have been treated alternately with surgery, radiation, and hormonal therapy without clear superiority of any particular strategy.

### *Secondary neoplasms*

Secondary spread of malignant neoplasms to the vagina is more common than primary neoplasms. The most common areas from which metastases occur are the cervix (32%), endometrium (18%), colon and rectum (9%), ovary (6%), vulva (6%), and urinary tract (4%).[16]

### *Other*

Other rarely reported pathologies include primary vaginal adenocarcinoma *in situ*, intestinal-type adenocarcinoma, adenosquamous carcinoma, adenocarcinoma arising in mesonephric duct remnants, adenoid basal cell carcinoma, adenoid cystic carcinoma, carcinoid tumor, neuroendocrine small cell carcinoma, and lymphomas. Endometrioid adenocarcinomas and malignant mixed müllerian tumors may arise in a background of endometriosis. Other reported sarcomas include stromal sarcoma, malignant schwannoma, fibrosarcoma, malignant fibrous histiocytoma, angiosarcoma, and alveolar soft part sarcoma.[11] Stromal sarcomas may also arise in a background of endometriosis.

## TREATMENT

## Surgery

### *Early stage (I and II)*

Treatment strategies in vaginal cancer rely mostly on retrospective data owing to the rarity of the disease. Although radiation is the mainstay of

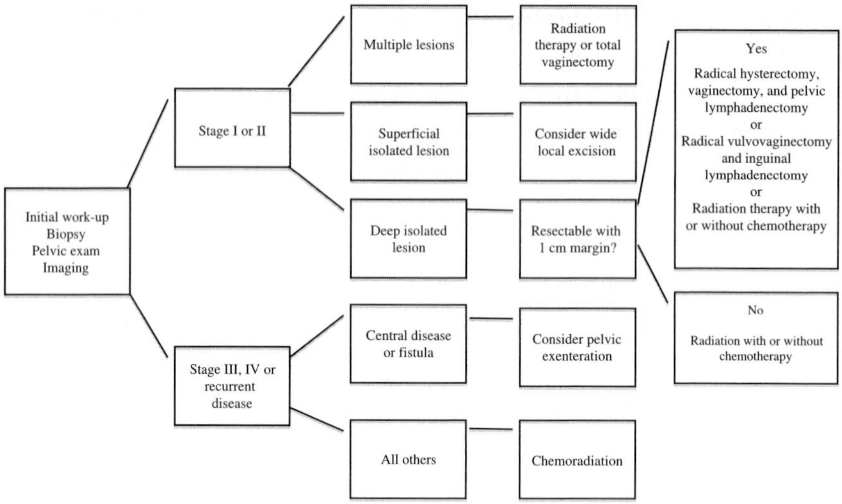


Figure 1. Management of vulvar cancer.

treatment, surgery can be performed for early-stage patients when adequate margins are obtainable (see Fig. 1). This would encompass superficial stage I lesions which can be removed by wide local excision as well as deeper lesions involving the upper third of the posterolateral vagina and the lower third of the vagina. The former can be adequately resected with radical hysterectomy, upper vaginectomy, and pelvic lymphadenectomy.[8] Lesions involving the lower third of the vagina may require vulvovaginectomy and inguinofemoral lymphadenectomy. Surgery can also be considered for verrucous carcinoma or when there is a desire to preserve ovarian function. Retrospective series reveal a survival rate of 56–91% in stage I lesions and 33–70% in stage II lesions with surgical treatment; however, a selection bias based on age and general health may have influenced results.[2,6,17]

Radiotherapy is generally preferred for all other lesions, or if surgical margins are positive. In the setting of positive margins, radiation can improve local control.[2,6,8,17–19] In patients who fail radiation with isolated central lesions, pelvic exenteration can be performed in appropriately selected patients.[17–21]

Neoadjuvant chemotherapy with cisplatin and paclitaxel followed by radical hysterectomy and upper vaginectomy has been studied in a series of 11 stage II patients. At 75 months of follow-up, two (18%) had disease that recurred.[22] Sentinel node techniques are feasible,[23] but should be considered investigational at this time.

### *Advanced stage (III and IV)*

Most advanced-stage patients are treated with chemoradiation, with pelvic exenteration reserved for those failing treatment. Exenteration is performed with curative intent and disease must be completely resectable with adequate margins and distant metastases ruled out. Berek *et al.* described a mixed series of persistent/recurrent cervical, vaginal, and uterine cancers treated with pelvic exenteration. Five-year survival for cervical and vaginal patients combined was 54% (all stages).[21] Primary pelvic exenteration in selected patients has been reported.[17–20] Neoadjuvant chemotherapy with cisplatin, vinblastine, and bleomycin followed by radical hysterectomy and lymphadenectomy has been successfully used to treat a stage III lesion in a case report.[24]

## Radiation

In patients with superficial stage I lesions, low-dose-rate (LDR) intracavitary brachytherapy (ICB) treating the entire vagina to 60 Gy with an additional mucosal dose of 20–30 Gy to the area of tumor involvement is adequate.[25] With thicker stage I lesions and selected cases of stage II lesions, a combination of ICB and interstitial brachytherapy (ITB) is utilized. ICB is used to treat the entire length of the vagina to 60–65 Gy with ITB used to give an additional 15–20 Gy to the site of tumor involvement.[26] Local control rates range from 95% to 100%.[17,27–29] External beam radiation therapy (EBRT) is appropriate for larger, more infiltrating, or poorly differentiated tumors.[26] The whole pelvis is treated with 10–20 Gy with an additional parametrial dose to give a total of 45–50 Gy to the parametrial and pelvic side walls.

For all other patients with stage II to IV disease, EBRT to approximately 50 Gy is used to shrink the primary tumor and treat the pelvic nodes, followed by intracavitary radiation with either ICB and/or ITB for a total dose of 75–80 Gy. Intrauterine tandem and vaginal ovoids or cylinders can be used to treat lesions in the upper third of the vagina. Multiple studies have shown that the combination of EBRT and brachytherapy is superior to either modality alone[17,30–31] at the expense of increased vaginal morbidity.[32] The groins should be irradiated bilaterally to 45–50 Gy for lesions involving the mid to lower vagina and when clinically involved for lesions involving the upper vagina.[31]

While most studies have shown no difference in outcome between LDR and high-dose-rate (HDR) brachytherapy,[33–35] one study showed an increased rate of late complications associated with HDR.[36] The advent of intensity-modulated radiation therapy (IMRT) may reduce radiation-associated complications affecting the bladder, rectum, and small bowel.[37–39] Some authors have suggested treating advanced stages with RT followed by vulvectomy and bilateral inguinofemoral lymphadenectomy.[39]

Borders of the radiation field for EBRT are as follows: true pelvis with 1.5–2.0 cm beyond the pelvic rim, superiorly L4–5 or L5–S1, inferiorly to the introitus, lateral fields if used should extend anteriorly to cover the external iliac nodes, anterior to the pubic symphysis and at least to the junction of S2–3 posteriorly.[26]

## Chemotherapy

Extrapolating from cervical cancer trials, chemopotentiation has improved local control in stage II–IV vaginal cancer with acceptable toxicity.[40] The most common agents used alone or in combination are cisplatin, 5-FU, and mitomycin C.[40–42] Mitoxantrone,[43] cisplatin,[44] and etoposide[45] have been used as single agents in advanced or recurrent disease with minimal activity. The combination of methotrexate, vinblastine, doxorubicin, and cisplatin (MVAC) achieved a complete response in three patients with advanced disease.[46] Some authors have suggested that multimodality therapy reduces the radiation dose required, thus improving complication rates.[41] Neoadjuvant therapy has been used prior to radical hysterectomy in a small Italian series. Combination regimens of irinotecan/cisplatin and cisplatin/vinblastine/bleomycin have been used successfully prior to radical surgery in case reports.[24,47]

## Recurrent Disease

The rate of locoregional recurrence is 10–20% in stage I, 30–40% in stage II, and 50–70% in advanced-stage patients. Most recurrences occur in the pelvis or vagina and prognosis with recurrence is generally poor.[48] The rate of distant metastasis is approximately 13% in stage I, 30% in stage IIA, 52% in stage IIB, 50% in stage III, and 47% in stage IV.[31] Nodal recurrence in the absence of local recurrence is uncommon. Appropriately selected patients with central recurrences in whom distant disease has been ruled out can be salvaged with pelvic exenteration.[21] Treatment of distant metastases is palliative with chemotherapy and/or radiation based on prior therapy.

## Complications

The immediate response to radiation is loss of most or all of the vaginal epithelium, particularly in areas that are in close proximity to brachytherapy sources, resulting in erythema, moist desquamation, and mucositis. These symptoms persist for three to six months followed by reepithelialization consisting of a thin layer of basal cells with progressive maturation after approximately two years. A fully developed stratified squamous epithelium, however, does not regenerate and thus there is absence of the small glands important for vaginal lubrication, narrowing or obliteration of the lumina of small blood vessels, and hyalinization and replacement of muscle fibers by fibrosis[49,50] with subsequent sexual dysfunction. Other chronic changes include thinning and atrophy of the vaginal epithelium and the development of telangiectasias. Some patients may also experience vascular damage and ischemia leading to epithelial sloughing, ulcer formation, and necrosis. Recurrent tumor should be ruled out in these patients. Severe radiation sequelae may result in fistula (rectovaginal, urethrovaginal, or vesicovaginal), small bowel obstruction, and fracture. Complication rate is correlated with radiation dose, FIGO stage, and history of smoking.[49]

Acute radiation vaginitis is managed with douching two to three times daily with a 1:10 mixture of hydrogen peroxide and water and is continued for two to three months or until the mucositis has resolved, after which douching can be continued on a weekly basis. Ulceration and necrosis are managed with debridement. Diligent use of vaginal dilators and intravaginal estrogen cream after the acute inflammatory phase post-radiation can ameliorate some of the symptoms of stenosis and allow for sexual function. Dilation during radiation is not supported by the literature. If healing response does not occur, it is not unreasonable to allow agglutination of the vagina in selected patients. Patients with late bowel or urinary complications may benefit from diversion or fistula repair.[49]

Direct effects of radiation are difficult to distinguish from secondary effects of chemotherapy on ovarian function. Chemotherapy appears to intensify the acute mucosal and late responses to radiotherapy.[49]

## OUTCOME/PROGNOSIS

Five-year overall survival rate is 78% for patients with stage I disease, 52% for stage II disease, 43% for stage III, and 13–21% for stage IV.[51] Prognosis is highly determined by stage of disease.[30–32,52] Stratifying stage II lesions into those without paravaginal infiltration (IIA) and those with paravaginal infiltration (IIB) appears to add prognostic value as patients with IIB lesions have a higher rate of local and distant recurrences.[31]

The prognostic significance of lesion size,[30,32,53] location, treatment time, and patient age remain controversial. Although some authors advocate that upper vaginal lesions tend to recur locally whereas lower lesions recur distally,[32,52] other studies have failed to show a difference in recurrences based on these factors.[54] Larger lesions in the posterior wall appear to have a poorer prognosis.[30,52] One study showed treatment time greater than nine weeks affected survival[55] while others have failed to confirm this.[30] Lymph node status[56] has also been shown to correlate with survival.

Histology has also been shown to affect prognosis. Clear cell adenocarcinomas have an increased tendency for distant metastases. Survival is superior in those with lower stage, tubulocystic pattern, size less than 3 cm, and depth of invasion less than 3 mm.[57] Nonclear cell adenocarcinomas have an extremely poor prognosis.[30] Melanoma is associated with a 1.5-fold increase in mortality[52] and has a propensity for distant metastases.

## REFERENCES


1. Jemal A, Siegel R, Ward E, Hao Y, Xu J, Thun MJ. Cancer statistics, 2009. *CA Cancer J Clin* 2009;59(4):225–249.
2. Creasman WT, Phillips JL, Menck HR. The National Cancer Database report on cancer of the vagina. *Cancer* 1998;83:1033–1040.
3. Herbst AL, Ulfelder H, Poskanzer DC. Adenocarcinomas of the vagina: association of maternal stilbestrol therapy with tumor appearance in young women. *N Engl J Med* 1971;284:878–881.
4. Melnick S, Cole P, Anderson D, Herbst A. Rates and risks of diethylstilbestrol-related clear cell adenocarcinomas of the vagina and cervix. *N Engl J Med* 1987;316:514–516.
5. Lenehan PM, Meffe F, Likrish GM. Vaginal intraepithelial neoplasia: biologic aspects and management. *Obstet Gynecol* 1986;68:333–337.
6. Tjalma WA, Monaghan JM, de Barros Lopes A, Naik R, Nordin AJ, Weyler JJ. The role of surgery in invasive squamous carcinoma of the vagina. *Gynecol Oncol* 2001;81(3):360–367.
7. Al-Kurdi M, Monaghan JM. Thirty-two years experience in the management of primary tumors of the vagina. *Br J Obstet Gynaecol* 1981;88: 115–150.
8. Davis KP, Stanhope CR, Garton GR, Atkinson EJ, O'Brien PC. Invasive vaginal carcinoma: analysis of early-stage disease. *Gynecol Oncol* 1991;42: 131–136.
9. Qualman SJ, Coffin CM, Newton WA, *et al*. Intergroup Rhabdomyosarcoma Study: update for pathologists. *Pediatr Dev Pathol* 1998;1(6):550–561.
10. Young RH, Scully RE. Endodermal sinus tumor of the vagina: a report of nine cases and review of the literature. *Gynecol Oncol* 1984;18:380–392.
11. Kurman R. *Blaustein's Pathology of the Female Genital Tract* 5th ed., New York: Springer.
12. Frank SJ, Deavers MT, Jhingran A, Bodurka DC, Eifel PJ. Primary adenocarcinoma of the vagina not associated with diethylstilbestrol (DES) exposure. *Gynecol Oncol* 2007;105(2):470–474.

13. Peters WA 3rd, Kumar NB, Morley GW. Carcinoma of the vagina. Factors influencing treatment outcome. *Cancer* 1985;55(4):892–897.
14. Chung AF, Casey MJ, Flannery JT, Woodruff JM, Lewis JL Jr. Malignant melanoma of the vagina — report of 19 cases. *Obstet Gynecol* 1980; 55(6):720–727.
15. Weinstock MA. Malignant melanoma of the vulva and vagina in the United States: patterns of incidence and population-based estimates of survival. *Am J Obstet Gynecol* 1994;171(5):1225–1230.
16. Fu Yao RJ. *Pathology of the Uterine Cervix, Vagina, and Vulva*. Philadelphia: Saunders, 1989.
17. Stock RG, Chen AS, Seski J. A 30-year experience in the management of primary carcinoma of the vagina: analysis of prognostic factors and treatment modalities. *Gynecol Oncol* 1995;56(1):45–52.
18. Ball HG, Berman ML. Management of primary vaginal carcinoma. *Gynecol Oncol* 1982;14(2):154–163.
19. Rubin SC, Young J, Mikuta JJ. Squamous carcinoma of the vagina: treatment, complications, and long-term follow-up. *Gynecol Oncol* 1985;20(3): 346–353.
20. Gallup DG, Talledo OE, Shah KJ, Hayes C. Invasive squamous cell carcinoma of the vagina: a 14-year study. *Obstet Gynecol* 1987;69(5):782–785.
21. Berek JS, Howe C, Lagasse LD, Hacker NF. Pelvic exenteration for recurrent gynecologic malignancy: survival and morbidity analysis of the 45-year experience at UCLA. *Gynecol Oncol* 2005;99(1):153–159.
22. Benedetti Panici P, Bellati F, Plotti F, *et al.* Neoadjuvant chemotherapy followed by radical surgery in patients affected by vaginal carcinoma. *Gynecol Oncol* 2008;111(2):307–311.
23. van Dam P, Sonnemans H, van Dam PJ, Verkinderen L, Dirix LY. Sentinel node detection in patients with vaginal carcinoma. *Gynecol Oncol* 2004;92(1):89–92.
24. Kim DS, Moon H, Hwang YY, Park MI. Histologic disappearance of locally advanced vaginal cancer after combination chemotherapy. *Gynecol Oncol* 1990;38(1):144–145.
25. Perez CA, Korba A, Sharma S. Dosimetric considerations in irradiation of carcinoma of the vagina. *Int J Radiat Oncol Biol Phys* 1977;2(7–8): 639–649.

26. Halperin EC, Perez CA, Brady LW. *Perez and Brady's Principles and Practice of Radiation Oncology*, 5th ed. Philadelphia: Lippincott Williams & Wilkins, 2008.
27. Kucera H, Vavra N. Radiation management of primary carcinoma of the vagina: clinical and histopathological variables associated with survival. *Gynecol Oncol* 1991;40(1):12–16.
28. Perez CA, Camel HM, Galakatos AE, *et al.* Definitive irradiation in carcinoma of the vagina: long-term evaluation of results. *Int J Radiat Oncol Biol Phys* 1988;15(6):1283–1290.
29. Urbanski K, Kojs Z, Reinfuss M, Fabisiak W. Primary invasive vaginal carcinoma treated with radiotherapy: analysis of prognostic factors. *Gynecol Oncol* 1996;60(1):16–21.
30. Chyle V, Zagars GK, Wheeler JA, Wharton JT, Delclos L. Definitive radiotherapy for carcinoma of the vagina: outcome and prognostic factors. *Int J Radiat Oncol Biol Phys* 1996;35(5):891–905.
31. Perez CA, Grigsby PW, Garipagaoglu M, Mutch DG, Lockett MA. Factors affecting long-term outcome of irradiation in carcinoma of the vagina. *Int J Radiat Oncol Biol Phys* 1999;44(1):37–45.
32. Lian J, Dundas G, Carlone M, Ghosh S, Pearcey R. Twenty-year review of radiotherapy for vaginal cancer: an institutional experience. *Gynecol Oncol* 2008;111(2):298–306.
33. Kucera H, Mock U, Knocke TH, Kucera E, Potter R. Radiotherapy alone for invasive vaginal cancer: outcome with intracavitary high dose rate brachytherapy versus conventional low dose rate brachytherapy. *Acta Obstet Gynecol Scand* 2001;80(4):355–360.
34. Nanavati PJ, Fanning J, Hilgers RD, Hallstrom J, Crawford D. High-dose-rate brachytherapy in primary stage I and II vaginal cancer. *Gynecol Oncol* 1993;51(1):67–71.
35. Mock U, Kucera H, Fellner C, Knocke TH, Potter R. High-dose-rate (HDR) brachytherapy with or without external beam radiotherapy in the treatment of primary vaginal carcinoma: long-term results and side effects. *Int J Radiat Oncol Biol Phys* 2003;56(4):950–957.
36. Tyree WC, Cardenes H, Randall M, Papiez L. High-dose-rate brachytherapy for vaginal cancer: learning from treatment complications. *Int J Gynecol Cancer* 2002;12(1):27–31.

37. Mundt AJ, Lujan AE, Rotmensch J, *et al.* Intensity-modulated whole pelvic radiotherapy in women with gynecologic malignancies. *Int J Radiat Oncol Biol Phys* 2002;52(5):1330–1337.
38. Mundt AJ, Mell LK, Roeske JC. Preliminary analysis of chronic gastrointestinal toxicity in gynecology patients treated with intensity-modulated whole pelvic radiation therapy. *Int J Radiat Oncol Biol Phys* 2003;56(5):1354–1360.
39. Boronow RC, Hickman BT, Reagan MT, Smith RA, Steadham RE. Combined therapy as an alternative to exenteration for locally advanced vulvovaginal cancer. II. Results, complications, and dosimetric and surgical considerations. *Am J Clin Oncol* 1987;10(2):171–181.
40. Samant R, Lau B, Choan E, Le T, Tam T. Primary vaginal cancer treated with concurrent chemoradiation using Cis-platinum. *Int J Radiat Oncol Biol Phys* 2007;69(3):746–750.
41. Dalrymple JL, Russell AH, Lee SW, *et al.* Chemoradiation for primary invasive squamous carcinoma of the vagina. *Int J Gynecol Cancer* 2004;14(1):110–117.
42. Roberts WS, Hoffman MS, Kavanagh JJ, *et al.* Further experience with radiation therapy and concomitant intravenous chemotherapy in advanced carcinoma of the lower female genital tract. *Gynecol Oncol* 1991;43(3):233–236.
43. Muss HB, Bundy BN, Christopherson WA. Mitoxantrone in the treatment of advanced vulvar and vaginal carcinoma. A gynecologic oncology group study. *Am J Clin Oncol* 1989;12(2):142–144.
44. Thigpen JT, Blessing JA, Homesley HD, Berek JS, Creasman WT. Phase II trial of cisplatin in advanced or recurrent cancer of the vagina: a Gynecologic Oncology Group Study. *Gynecol Oncol* 1986;23(1):101–104.
45. Slayton RE, Blessing JA, Beecham J, DiSaia PJ. Phase II trial of etoposide in the management of advanced or recurrent squamous cell carcinoma of the vulva and carcinoma of the vagina: a Gynecologic Oncology Group Study. *Cancer Treat Rep* 1987;71(9):869–870.
46. Long HJ 3rd, Monk BJ, Huang HQ, *et al.* Clinical results and quality of life analysis for the MVAC combination (methotrexate, vinblastine, doxorubicin, and cisplatin) in carcinoma of the uterine cervix: a Gynecologic Oncology Group study. *Gynecol Oncol* 2006;100(3):537–543.
47. Umesaki N, Kawamura N, Tsujimura A, Ichimura T, Tanaka T, Ogita S. Stage II vaginal cancer responding to chemotherapy with irinotecan and cisplatin: a case report. *Oncol Rep* 1999;6(1):123–125.

48. Tabata T, Takeshima N, Nishida H, Hirai Y, Hasumi K. Treatment failure in vaginal cancer. *Gynecol Oncol* 2002;84(2):309–314.
49. Grigsby PW, Russell A, Bruner D, *et al.* Late injury of cancer therapy on the female reproductive tract. *Int J Radiat Oncol Biol Phys* 1995;31(5): 1281–1299.
50. Pitkin RM, Bradbury JT. The effect of topical estrogen on irradiated vaginal epithelium. *Am J Obstet Gynecol* 1965;92:175–182.
51. Beller U, Benedet JL, Creasman WT, *et al.* Carcinoma of the vagina. FIGO 6th Annual Report on the Results of Treatment in Gynecological Cancer. *Int J Gynaecol Obstet* 2006;(95 Suppl) 1:S29–S42.
52. Shah CA, Goff BA, Lowe K, Peters WA 3rd, Li CI. Factors affecting risk of mortality in women with vaginal cancer. *Obstet Gynecol* 2009;113(5): 1038–1045.
53. Tewari KS, Cappuccini F, Puthawala AA, *et al.* Primary invasive carcinoma of the vagina: treatment with interstitial brachytherapy. *Cancer* 2001; 91(4):758–770.
54. Otton GR, Nicklin JL, Dickie GJ, *et al.* Early-stage vaginal carcinoma — an analysis of 70 patients. *Int J Gynecol Cancer* 2004;14(2):304–310.
55. Lee WR, Marcus RB Jr, Sombeck MD, *et al.* Radiotherapy alone for carcinoma of the vagina: the importance of overall treatment time. *Int J Radiat Oncol Biol Phys* 1994;29(5):983–988.
56. Pingley S, Shrivastava SK, Sarin R, *et al.* Primary carcinoma of the vagina: Tata Memorial Hospital experience. *Int J Radiat Oncol Biol Phys* 2000;46(1):101–108.
57. Herbst AL, Robboy SJ, Scully RE, Poskanzer DC. Clear-cell adenocarcinoma of the vagina and cervix in girls: analysis of 170 registry cases. *Am J Obstet Gynecol* 1974;119(5):713–724.
58. Daling JR, Madeleine MM, Schwartz SM, *et al.* A population-based study of squamous cell vaginal cancer: HPV and cofactors. *Gynecol Oncol* 2002;84:263–270.
59. Brinton LA, Nasca PC, Mallin K, *et al.* Case-control study of *in situ* and invasive carcinoma of the vagina. *Gynecol Oncol* 1990;38(1):49–54.

# 6

# CERVICAL CANCER

*Heidi J. Gray*

## INTRODUCTION

In 1951, a woman who was five months postpartum presented to the Johns Hopkins Hospital with severe vaginal bleeding and a cervical mass. A biopsy was performed confirming a locally advanced cervical cancer. As she began treatment with radium implants, this biopsy was given without her consent to the laboratory of Dr. Gordon Gey, as was common practice at that time. Unfortunately, the woman died from her disease several months after diagnosis. Ironically, her cancerous cells were discovered to be immortal and developed into the cell line known as HeLa, after her name Henrietta Lacks. HeLa cells have subsequently been used around the world in most major laboratories and have played an important role in developing many medical breakthroughs, such as the polio vaccine.[1]

Although her true story has many ethical lessons, it also highlights how often cervical cancer in the United States was commonly diagnosed at an advanced stage before the implementation of widespread cervical cytology screening. In the first of half of the 1900s, cervical cancer was the leading cause of cancer-related death for women in the United States. The development and subsequent use of cervical cytology screening, the Pap smear, has dramatically reduced the incidence of invasive cervical cancer in US women. Globally, however, cervical cancer remains a leading cause of death for women from cancer in developing countries. The discovery of HPV as the causative agent of cervical cancer has led to the development of HPV vaccines and their global implementation will with vaginal bleeding or discharge. Other common symptoms are back pain, bleeding after sexual intercourse, abnormal discharge, weight loss, leg pain, or swelling. The length of time from the last Pap test correlates with the stage of diagnosis: patients with no prior Pap test or more than 10 years since their last Pap test are at risk of having a higher stage at diagnosis.[9] Vaginal bleeding in a postmenopausal woman should be evaluated with a pelvic exam, cervical cytology screening, and/or cervical biopsy if a lesion is visible, and endometrial biopsy, if the cervix appears normal. If a symptomatic patient has never had a Pap test or a long interval has elapsed since the last test, a strong suspicion of cervical cancer should lead to performance of the Pap test or colposcopy.

### Cervical Biopsy Technique

If a visible lesion is present on the cervix, biopsy should be performed with Tischler or Kevorkian biopsy forceps. When obtaining a cervical biopsy in a lesion suspicious for cancer, Monsel's solution and vaginal packing material should be close at hand, as well as an assistant, to facilitate prompt control of potential heavy bleeding after biopsy. If the patient is too uncomfortable with an office biopsy or if excessive bleeding precludes visualization, examination under anesthesia in the operating room may provide a more controlled setting. In patients who have no visible lesion but a Pap test showing invasive cancer, cervical conization is recommended for evaluation of microinvasive disease.

## STAGING

Cervical cancer is staged clinically according to the International Federation of Gynecology and Obstetrics (FIGO) and TNM staging classification (Table 2). According to FIGO rules, cervical cancer is staged clinically using pelvic exam, colposcopy, cervical conization, cystoscopy, proctosigmoidoscopy intravenous pyelogram (IVP), and/or chest radiograph. Advanced imaging techniques such as computed axial tomography (CT), positron emission tomography (PET), and/or magnetic resonance imaging (MRI) are commonly utilized in developed countries to determine metastasis and aid in treatment planning, but are not allowed to alter FIGO staging.

Table 2. Staging of cervical carcinoma (FIGO 2009).[88]

| FIGO stages | | TNM categories |
|---|---|---|
| I | Cervical carcinoma confined to uterus | T1 |
| IA | Invasive carcinoma diagnosed only by microscopy | T1a |
| IA1 | Stromal invasion no greater than 3.0 mm in depth and 7.0 mm or less in horizontal spread | T1a1 |
| IA2 | Stromal invasion more than 3.0 mm in depth and not more than 5.0 mm with a horizontal spread of 7.0 mm or less | T1a2 |
| IB | Clinically visible lesion confined to cervix or microscopic lesion greater than IA2/T1a2 | T1b |
| IB1 | Clinically visible lesion 4 cm or less in greatest dimension | T1b1 |
| IB2 | Clinically visible lesion more than 4 cm in greatest dimension | T1b2 |
| II | Tumor invades beyond the uterus but not to pelvic wall or lower third of vagina | T2 |
| IIA | Without parametrial invasion | T2a |
| IIA1 | Clinically visible lesion ≤4 cm in greatest dimension | T2a1 |
| IIA2 | Clinically visible lesion >4 cm in greatest dimension | T2a2 |
| IIB | With parametrial invasion | T2b |
| III | Tumor extends to pelvic wall and/or involves lower third of vagina and/or causes hydronephrosis or nonfunctioning kidney | T3 |
| IIIA | Tumor involves lower third of vagina | T3a |
| IIIB | Tumor extends to pelvic wall and/or causes hydronephrosis or nonfunctioning kidney | T3b |
| IVA | Tumor invades mucosa of bladder or rectum and/or extends beyond true pelvis | T4 |
| IVB | Distant metastasis | M1 |

A subset of women presenting with cervical cancer will have disease with no visible lesion, which is only detected by Pap test or cervical biopsy. The term "microinvasive disease" or "stage IA" refers to early cervical cancer diagnosed microscopically on cervical conization — any gross lesion is automatically at least stage IB. There are two divisions of stage IA: IA1 lesions are ≤3 mm in depth and ≤7mm in width, and stage IA2 lesions have a depth of invasion between 3 mm and 5 mm and are <7 mm in width. The term "microinvasive disease" is traditionally applied to squamous lesions, and adoption of this nomenclature for adenocarcinoma is controversial. There is debate as to the accuracy and be a role for surgical nodal staging to assess the extent of disease, outline treatment portals, and improve response to treatment for debulking of positive lymph nodes found in imaging studies.

## TREATMENT

The main modalities of treatment for early cervical cancer are surgery or radiation with concurrent chemotherapy. Loco-regionally advanced cervical cancer is treated with primary radiation and chemotherapy. Patients presenting with distant metastatic cervical cancer are treated with systemic chemotherapy first, followed by local radiation therapy for select patients. An overview of treatment options by stage is presented in Table 3.

### Surgical Approaches

#### *Microinvasive disease (stage IA1 and IA2)*

Women presenting with microinvasive disease have options for conservative surgical management due to their low risk of recurrence and lymph node involvement.[31] Recommended treatment for stage IA1 (no greater than 3 mm in depth of invasion and no greater than 7 mm in horizontal spread) with negative cone biopsy margins is simple hysterectomy, with laparoscopic, abdominal, or vaginal approaches all being feasible. Since the risk of pelvic lymph node spread is minimal in stage IA1 (0.1–0.8%),[32,33] lymph node removal is usually not indicated. In cases with lymphovascular space invasion (LVSI), some recommend modified radical hysterectomy with lymph node dissection. Due to the low risk of ovarian involvement, ovarian preservation is recommended for premenopausal women. Emerging options for compliant women interested in fertility-sparing or medically compromised patients include large conization with negative margins and close observation[34] (see below: *Fertility-sparing surgical approaches*).

For stage IA2, the risk of pelvic lymph node spread is 2–7%, with low rates of para-aortic involvement.[35] Recommended treatment is radical or modified radical hysterectomy with pelvic lymph node dissection or radiation with concurrent cisplatin-based chemotherapy. Outcomes are

Table 3. Summary of primary treatment options by stage.

| FIGO Stage | Treatment |
|---|---|
| IA1 | Extrafascial simple hysterectomy +/– BSO<br>OR<br>Modified radical hysterectomy (+ pelvic LND if LVSI)<br>OR<br>Cone biopsy with negative margins (patient desires fertility or medically inoperable) |
| IA2 | Radical or modified radical hysterectomy, pelvic LND, +/– BSO<br>OR<br>WPXRT with concurrent cisplatin chemotherapy + brachytherapy<br>OR<br>Radical trachelectomy + laparoscopic pelvic LND +/– para-aortic LNS |
| IB1 and stage IIA (≤4 cm) | Radical hysterectomy, pelvic LND, +/– para-aortic LNS, +/– BSO<br>OR<br>WPXRT with concurrent cisplatin chemotherapy + brachytherapy<br>OR<br>Radical trachelectomy + laparoscopic pelvic LND, +/– para-aortic LNS (fertility desired, ≤ 2 cm) |
| IB2 and stage IIA (>4 cm) | Radical hysterectomy, pelvic and para-aortic LNS, +/– BSO<br>OR<br>WPXRT with concurrent cisplatin chemotherapy + brachytherapy, +/– adjuvant hysterectomy |
| Stage IIB, IIIA, IIIB, IVA | WPXRT + concurrent cisplatin chemotherapy + brachytherapy |
| Stage IVB | Systemic chemotherapy (paclitaxel + cisplatin), +/– WPXRT |

Abbreviations: LND, lymph node dissection; LNS, lymph node sampling; BSO, bilateral salpingo-oophorectomy; WPXRT, whole pelvic external radiotherapy. Based on the National Comprehensive Cancer Network (NCCN) Clinical Practice Guidelines in Oncology (available at www.nccn.org/professionals/physician_gls/default.asp).

excellent with a low risk of parametrial spread and a risk of recurrence around 3.6% in the absence of positive lymph nodes.[36,37] For select patients in whom fertility is desired, another option is radical vaginal trachelectomy with laparoscopic pelvic lymph node dissection (see *Fertility-sparing surgical approaches*).

## *Radical hysterectomy*

Stage IB patients can be offered treatment with radical hysterectomy with lymph node dissection or primary radiation with concurrent chemotherapy, with a similar overall survival of 87–92% for both treatment modalities.[38] Preference for surgical treatment is common for premenopausal women in whom ovarian preservation is important, given that pelvic radiation will cause ovarian failure. There is also data that radiation therapy causes more vaginal symptoms such as shortening, reduction in caliber and lubrication, as well as worse sexual functioning compared to surgery.[39] Other benefits of surgery are immediate treatment and surgical evaluation of lymph nodes.

Stage IB is divided into two subgroups based on tumor size; IB1 tumors are 4 cm or less and IB2 are greater than 4 cm in size. As the risk of nodal metastasis, recurrence risk, and need for post-surgical adjuvant therapy are all significantly higher for stage IB2, these patients tend to be grouped into the locally advanced disease for clinical trials and general treatment strategies.

In the early 1900s, Dr. Wertheim published a descriptive account of a surgical therapeutic approach to treatment of cervical cancer by removing the lateral tissues to the cervix (parametria), uterosacral ligaments, upper half of the vagina in addition to the pelvic lymph nodes. This revolutionized the surgical management of cervical cancer with improvement in local pelvic control for early-stage tumors. In addition to decreasing pelvic recurrence, the lymph node status was defined and identified a subset of women who were at higher risk of relapse as well. In 1974, Piver *et al.*, published a descriptive account of five classes of hysterectomy based on the degree of radicality of the procedure (Table 4).[40] Radical hysterectomy can be performed through a Pfannenstiel or low vertical incision as an open hysterectomy; or the minimally invasive laparoscopic or robotic-assisted radical hysterectomy which is being utilized increasingly.

Traditional class III or Wertheim radical hysterectomy was associated with high rates of bladder dysfunction, atony (15%), and urogenital fistula (2.5%).[41] The contemporary radical hysterectomy, which some term nerve-sparing, removes less uterosacral ligament and vagina (2–3 cm versus 4 cm) in order to reduce neurologic side effects. Bladder dysfunction still

Table 4. Classes of hysterectomy.[40]

| Type | Hysterectomy | Description | Lymph nodes |
|---|---|---|---|
| I | Extrafascial | Simple hysterectomy | No |
| II | Modified radical | Ligation of uterine artery medial to ureter, resection of medial half of cardinal ligaments and proximal uterosacral ligaments, upper one third of vagina removed | Pelvic |
| III | Radical | Ligation of uterine artery at origin from hypogastric artery, resection of cardinal and uterosacral ligaments at attachments to sacrum and sidewall, resection of upper one half of vagina | Pelvic and para-aortic |
| IV | Extended radical | Same as type III, but superior vesicle artery ligated, resection of three quarters of the vagina | Pelvic and para-aortic |
| V | Partial exenteration | Resection of portion of bladder and distal ureter with reimplantation | Pelvic and para-aortic |

remains one of the most common complications with long-term moderate to severe incontinence symptoms reported in 30–35% of women.[42]

Rates of ovarian metastasis in squamous lesions are low (<0.5%), therefore removal of the ovaries and fallopian tubes are generally performed in only post- or perimenopausal women (>45 years), with ovarian preservation for younger women. However, adenocarcinomas have higher rates of ovarian metastasis and therefore patients are usually counseled to undergo salpingo-oophorectomy.

### *Fertility-sparing surgical approaches: Radical trachelectomy and cervical conization*

Up to 15% of all cervical cancers and 45% of all surgically treated early stage cancers occur in women under 40 years of age.[43] This constitutes a large group of women who potentially desire fertility-sparing options. Radical vaginal trachelectomy with pelvic lymph node dissection was first described by Dr. Daniel Dargent in 1994 as a method of treating small invasive tumors (stage IA2 to IB1) while preserving the body of the uterus for future childbearing.[44] The procedure removes the entire cervix, up to the internal os, lateral parametria, and vaginal margins, with placement of a cervical cerclage. It can be performed vaginally or abdominally, with laparoscopic-assisted removal of pelvic and para-aortic lymph nodes.[45]

In a recent review of the published data on radical trachelectomy for early cervical cancer, recurrence rates appear to be low (5%). The highest rates of recurrence have been observed in patients whose tumor size is greater than 2 cm (17%) and have evidence of LVSI (12%).[46] Rates of surgical complications such as ureteral injury were similar compared to open radical hysterectomy. Pregnancy rates following radical trachelectomy are reported to be 40–52% at five years, but patients had higher miscarriage rates than expected.[47] For women with early-stage (IA2–IB1) small (<2 cm) tumors, who desire fertility, radical trachelectomy may be a reasonable option without compromise of outcome, although the presence of LVSI may be a relative contraindication.

For women with stage IA1 desiring fertility without LVSI, consideration may be given for treatment with large conization with negative margins.[34]

### *Minimally invasive surgery (laparoscopic- or robotic-assisted)*

With the increasing use of minimally invasive surgery, there is a growing body of literature describing the feasibility of laparoscopic-assisted radical hysterectomy as an alternative surgical approach in early-stage patients. There have been several large observational series published which have shown decreased surgical morbidity (less blood loss, decreased hospitalization, faster return to work) with laparoscopic-assisted radical hysterectomy.[48–50] A recent prospective study in 295 patients of attempted laparoscopic radical hysterectomy and pelvic/para-aortic lymph node dissection showed a mean operating time of 162 minutes with median blood loss of 230 mL. Conversion to laparotomy occurred 2% of the time, intraoperative injuries were 4%, and postoperative complications occurred in 11% of women. At three years' follow-up, disease-free survival was 95–96% for stage IA–IB patients.[49]

Many gynecologic oncologists are moving towards robotic-assisted technology for minimally invasive surgery. The robotic-assisted radical hysterectomy with pelvic lymph node dissection appears to have similar peri- and postoperative results with published laparoscopic-assisted data, with the potential advantage of decreased operative morbidity over open radical hysterectomy.[51] However, data on outcomes are still immature. Unfortunately, a prospective randomized trial comparing minimally invasive radical hysterectomy versus open abdominal radical hysterectomy is unlikely in the United States. Therefore, based on retrospective data, centers with expertise in this technique may consider offering laparoscopic- or robotic-assisted radical hysterectomy to early-stage cervical cancer patients.

## Radiation and Chemotherapy

Cervical cancer is highly radiosensitive. Radiation with concurrent cisplatin-based chemotherapy is the treatment of choice for locally advanced disease (stages IB2–IVA). There is also a role for adjuvant radiotherapy following radical hysterectomy for patients with tumors with high-risk or intermediate-risk features. Chemotherapy is used both as a sensitizing agent along with radiation (chemoradiation) and as treatment for metastatic or recurrent disease.

## Primary Radiation with Concurrent Chemotherapy

Primary treatment for locally advanced disease (stages IB2–IVA) is whole pelvic radiation with concurrent cisplatin-based chemotherapy. In the late 1990s, five randomized trials showed a significant improvement in progression-free and overall survival (30–50% reduction in risk of death) with the addition of cisplatin-based chemotherapy to radiation therapy in advanced cervical cancer.[52–56] The National Cancer Institute (NCI) issued a clinical alert recommending the use of cisplatin with or without 5-fluorouracil (5-FU) concurrently with radiation in locally advanced cervical cancer. Toxicities are greater with combination chemotherapy, leading many oncologists to treat with weekly single-agent cisplatin 40 mg/m$^2$.[57] There are data suggesting a threshold total dose of cisplatin of at least 200 mg/m$^2$ for tumoricidal effect.[58]

neoadjuvant chemotherapy followed by surgery, an improvement in progression-free survival was observed, though this did not translate into overall survival benefit.[65] Currently open and enrolling, EORTC protocol 55994 is a randomized phase III study of neoadjuvant chemotherapy with cisplatin followed by surgery (+/– radiation) versus chemoradiation for stages IB2–IIB cervical cancer (http://www.cancer.gov/clinicaltrials/EORTC-55994).

## OUTCOME

The two most important factors determining prognosis of cervical cancer are stage and lymph node status. Other important factors are depth of stromal invasion, tumor size, LVSI, histologic type, and grade of tumor. Table 5 shows the distribution of overall survival in cervical cancer by stage.

Within each stage, lymph node status is an important determination of the risk of recurrence. For instance, the rate of recurrence following radical hysterectomy for all stage IB patients is 20%, and overall survival is 87%.[66] However, when patients are classified by negative or positive pelvic lymph nodes, overall survival is 90–95% versus 65–74%. The data are more divergent for patients with positive para-aortic lymph nodes. Patients with positive para-aortic lymph

Table 5. Overall survival by stage.[89]

| FIGO stage | 5-Year survival (%) |
|---|---|
| IA1 | 98% |
| IA2 | 95% |
| IB1 | 89% |
| IB2 | 76% |
| IIA | 73% |
| IIB | 66% |
| IIIA | 40% |
| IIIB | 42% |
| IVA | 22% |
| IVB | 9% |

nodes have the highest recurrence risk and lowest overall survival rates within each stage.

## TREATMENT OF RECURRENT DISEASE

The risk of recurrent cervical cancer increases with stage. Determining whether the tumor is local or disseminated will guide treatment options and prognosis, with recurrent metastatic disease generally being considered incurable.

### Local or Isolated Recurrence

When patients present with recurrent pelvic disease, assessment of distant spread is important, as approximately half will also have metastatic disease. Imaging studies such as CT, PET/CT, or MRI can assess for the most common sites of metastasis: lung, liver, and lymph nodes. If the recurrence is isolated centrally in the pelvis without sidewall involvement, pelvic exenteration may be offered (see *Pelvic exenteration*). However, if the patient did not receive radiation therapy with primary treatment, she may also be a candidate for pelvic radiation therapy with concurrent cisplatin-based chemotherapy. There are some reported cases of long-term survivors of isolated liver or lung metastasis treated by surgical resection alone.

### Distant Recurrence

Patients who present with recurrent disease outside the pelvis are not generally considered curable in the long term. However, treatment options to prolong progression-free survival or palliation of symptoms include chemotherapy, biologic therapy, and radiation therapy. In rare cases, surgery is indicated.

#### *Single-agent chemotherapy*

There are a number of chemotherapy agents that have clinical activity in the recurrent or advanced-stage setting. As a single agent, cisplatin has the most activity, with response rates of around 25% at doses of 50–100 mg/m$^2$

Table 6. Single-agent chemotherapy for metastatic or recurrent cervical cancer.

| Study | Agent | N | RR (CR+PR) | Progression-free interval (median) |
|---|---|---|---|---|
| Bonomi *et al.* (1985)[67] | Cisplatin 50–100 mg/m$^2$ every 3 weeks | 497 | 21–31.5% | 3.7–4.6 months |
| Sutton *et al.* (1993)[71,72] | Ifosfamide 1.5 g/m$^2$ × 5d (1.2 g/m$^2$ if prior XRT) with mesna rescue | 92 | 15–16% | 4.2 months |
| McGuire *et al.* (1996)[69] Curtin *et al.* (2001)[70] | Paclitaxel 170 mg/m$^2$ (135 mg/m$^2$ prior XRT) every 3 weeks | 72 | 17–31% | 3.4–4.8 months |
| Muderspach *et al.* (2001)[73] | Topotecan 1.5 mg/m$^2$ × 5d every 4 weeks | 49 | 19% | 2.8 months |
| Arseneau *et al.* (1986)[90] | Carboplatin 400 mg/m$^2$ every 4 weeks | 39 | 28% | Not reported |
| Look *et al.* (1998)[74] | Irinotecan 125 mg/m$^2$ weekly | 45 | 13% | 4.8 months |
| Morris *et al.* (1998)[75] | Vinorelbine 30 mg/m$^2$ weekly | 33 | 18% | 5.2 months |

every three weeks in phase II trials.[67,68] A number of other single agents have been studied, including ifosfamide, paclitaxel, topotecan, carboplatin, irinotecan, and vinorelbine, with response rates of 13–28% and median progression-free survival of 3.5–4.5 months (see Table 6).[69–75] However, many of these trials were done in the era before cisplatin was given concurrently with radiation therapy in a primary setting. It is probable that women with recurrent disease following cisplatin-based chemoradiation will have lower response rates to retreatment with cisplatin. In addition, the site of the recurrent disease will predict the response, with lower rates of response if disease recurs in the prior radiated field.

### *Combination chemotherapy*

Multi-agent therapy for advanced or recurrent metastatic cervical cancer has been evaluated in several large randomized trials comparing against single-agent cisplatin (see Table 7). GOG 110 was a three-arm trial that

Table 7. Randomized trials of multi-agent chemotherapy for advanced or recurrent cervical cancer.

| Study | Agent | N | RR | Progression-free interval (median) |
|---|---|---|---|---|
| Omura *et al.* (1997)[76] GOG 110 | Cisplatin 50 mg/m$^2$ + ifosfamide 5 g/m$^2$ over 24 h v. cisplatin 50 mg/m$^2$ every 3 weeks | | 31% v. 18% | 4.6 v. 3.2 months |
| Moore *et al.* (2004)[77] GOG 169 | Cisplatin 50 mg/m$^2$ + paclitaxel 135 mg/m$^2$ over 24 h v. cisplatin 50 mg/m$^2$ every 3 weeks | 280 | 36% v. 19% | 4.6 v. 2.8 months |
| Long *et al.* (2005)[78] GOG 179 | Cisplatin 50 mg/m$^2$ + topotecan 0.75 mg/m$^2$ on days 1–3 v. cisplatin 50 mg/m$^2$ every 3 weeks | 293 | 27% v. 13% | 4.6 v. 2.9 months |
| Monk *et al.* (2009)[79] GOG 204 | Cisplatin 50 mg/m$^2$ + paclitaxel 135 mg/m$^2$ over 24 h | 513 | 29% | 5.8 months |
| | + vinorelbine 30 mg/m$^2$ on days 1 & 8 | | 26% | 4 months |
| | + gemcitabine 1000 mg/m$^2$ on days 1 & 8 | | 22% | 4.7 months |
| | + topotecan 0.75 mg/m$^2$ on days 1–3 | | 23.4% | 4.6 months |

randomized patients to receive single-agent cisplatin 50 mg/m$^2$ every three weeks versus cisplatin 50 mg/m$^2$ plus either dibromodulcitol 180 mg/m$^2$ on days 2–6 or ifosfamide 5 g/m$^2$ over 24 hours on day 1 with mesna every three weeks. The combination of cisplatin and ifosfamide had higher response rates than cisplatin alone (31% versus 18%) with median progession-free survival of 4.6 months; however, the hematologic, neurologic, and renal toxicities were significantly greater in the combination group.[76] Given its activity as a single agent, paclitaxel 135 mg/m$^2$ over 24 hours plus cisplatin 50 mg/m$^2$ every three weeks was evaluated against single-agent cisplatin 50 mg/m$^2$ in a phase III randomized trial (GOG 169). The multi-agent therapy had a higher response rate (36% versus 19%); median progression-free survival was higher (4.8 versus 2.8 months), but no survival benefit was seen.[77] Similar response rates were seen with the combination of cisplatin 50 mg/m$^2$ with topotecan 0.75 mg/m$^2$ days 1–3 every three weeks compared to cisplatin 50 mg/m$^2$ alone (27% versus 13%). Progression-free survival was 4.6 versus 2.9 months, but a survival benefit of 9.4 versus 6.5 months was also observed.[78]

GOG 204 was a large randomized phase III four-arm trial of doublet chemotherapy comparing cisplatin plus paclitaxel as the standard arm versus cisplatin plus vinorelbine, gemcitabine, or topotecan in the recurrent or stage IVB population. The paclitaxel and cisplatin combination was found to be favored, with the highest response rate of 29% and median PFS of 5.8 months, although it was not statistically different when compared to the other three arms.[79] Accordingly, the standard treatment for recurrent or advanced-stage IVB cervical cancer continues to be paclitaxel and cisplatin. There is some interest and rationale in substituting carboplatin for cisplatin, especially in patients with renal dysfunction, but there are no results from randomized trials comparing the two drugs. Improvement in long-term survival rates have not been noted in any drug combination trials (overall survival around 10 months).

### *Biologic therapy*

In order to improve the response rate and overall survival, there has been increasing interest in adding biologic agents alone or in combination with chemotherapy to the treatment of advanced or recurrent cervical cancer.

Several drugs have emerged with activity targeting the vascular endothelial growth factor (VEGF) and epidermal growth factor receptor (EGFR) pathways. In a phase II trial, 46 patients with recurrent cervical cancer were treated with bevacizumab, a humanized monoclonal antibody to the VEGF receptor, at 15 mg/kg every three weeks. Twenty-three percent of patients survived at least six months and median progression-free survival was 3.4 months.[80] Considering that three quarters of the patients had received one prior chemotherapy regimen and one quarter had received two, these data have led the GOG to add bevacizumab to advanced cervical cancer trials. The currently active GOG 240 is a randomized 2×2 study enrolling recurrent or stage IVB women with cervical cancer to paclitaxel/cisplatin +/– bevacizumab versus topotecan/paclitaxel +/– bevacizumab. Other drugs targeting VEGF in development for use in cervical cancer include pazopanib and sorafenib.

Cetuximab is a monoclonal antibody to the extracellular portion of the EGFR that has been shown to be active and approved for use in head and neck and colorectal cancer in conjunction with chemoradiation. Currently, there are several GOG clinical trials looking at cetuximab as monotherapy and in combination with chemotherapy in advanced cervical cancer. Other promising agents targeting EGFR include erlotinib, gefitinib, and lapatinib.[81]

## PELVIC EXENTERATION

In cases of central recurrence of cervical cancer, some women may be candidates for surgical removal of the pelvic organs as a potential treatment option, termed pelvic exenteration. This radical surgery may be offered to a select group of patients who have disease confined to the central pelvic when all other treatment options, such as radiation, have failed. Five-year survival rates are quoted at 50% for appropriately selected patients;[82] however, in women with a disease-free interval of less than one year or adenocarcinoma cell type, survival may be worse.[83]

The history of pelvic exenteration dates back to the 1940s when it was described by Brunschwig.[84] Morbidity and mortality rates were high from the procedure itself as modern resuscitation methods were not yet developed. A total pelvic exenteration generally refers to removal of the bladder, urethra, vagina, rectum, uterus/cervix (if still present), and portions of the levator ani en bloc with construction of urinary and bowel diversions. Anterior exenteration usually spares the rectum and posterior exenteration spares the bladder. There are variations in surgical techniques especially as to the urinary diversion with continent and incontinent urinary reservoirs possible.[85] Most commonly, a colostomy is created if resection of the anus and perineum is indicated; however, some cases have potential for low rectal reanastamosis. Myocutaneous flaps from the rectus or gracilis muscles are used to reconstruct the pelvis and some patients may be candidates for creation of a neovagina.[86]

Counseling the patient as to the risks of the surgery is critical. The surgery itself lasts 6–12 hours and hospital stay with ICU care can be upwards of three weeks. Over 50% will suffer major morbidities such as infectious complications, intestinal fistula, bowel obstruction, thromboembolic events, or hemorrhage.[87] Most patients will have one or two ostomy bags to learn to care for. Although reconstruction of a neovagina may be offered in some cases, many women will have little or no sexual function. Additionally, patients must be counseled about the 50% possibility of abandoning the procedure at the time of surgery due to unresectability of the tumor.

## REFERENCES

1. Skloot R. *The Immortal Life of Henrietta Lacks*. New York: Random House, 2010.
2. Jemal A, Siegel R, Xu J, Ward E. Cancer statistics, 2010. *CA Cancer J Clin* 2010;60:277–300.
3. Parkin DM, Bray F, Ferlay J, Pisani P. Global cancer statistics, 2002. *CA Cancer J Clin* 2005;55(2):74–108.
4. Berrington de González A. Comparison of risk factors for invasive squamous cell carcinoma and adenocarcinoma of the cervix: collaborative reanalysis of individual data on 8,097 women with squamous cell carcinoma and 1,374 women with adenocarcinoma from 12 epidemiological studies. *Int J Cancer* 2007;120(4):885–891.
5. Munoz N, Franceschi S, Bosetti C, *et al.* Role of parity and human papillomavirus in cervical cancer: the IARC multicentric case-control study. *Lancet* 2002;359(9312):1093–1101.

6. Appleby P, Beral V, Berrington de Gonzalez A, *et al.* Cervical cancer and hormonal contraceptives: collaborative reanalysis of individual data for 16,573 women with cervical cancer and 35,509 women without cervical cancer from 24 epidemiological studies. *Lancet* 2007;370(9599): 1609–1621.
7. Saraiya M, Ahmed F, Krishnan S, Richards TB, Unger ER, Lawson HW. Cervical cancer incidence in a prevaccine era in the United States, 1998–2002. *Obstet Gynecol* 2007;109(2 Pt 1):360–370.
8. Franco EL, Schlecht NF, Saslow D. The epidemiology of cervical cancer. *Cancer J* 2003;9(5):348–359.
9. Fox KV, Shah CA, Swisher EM, *et al.* An evaluation of cervical cancer in women age sixty and over. *Gynecol Oncol* 2008;109(1):53–58.
10. Ostor AG. Early invasive adenocarcinoma of the uterine cervix. *Int J Gynecol Pathol* 2000;19(1):29–38.
11. Bader AA, Winter R, Haas J, Tamussino KF. Where to look for the sentinel lymph node in cervical cancer. *Am J Obstet Gynecol* 2007;197(6):678 e1–7.
12. Lagasse LD, Creasman WT, Shingleton HM, Ford JH, Blessing JA. Results and complications of operative staging in cervical cancer: experience of the Gynecologic Oncology Group. *Gynecol Oncol* 1980;9(1):90–98.
13. Cosin JA, Fowler JM, Chen MD, Paley PJ, Carson LF, Twiggs LB. Pretreatment surgical staging of patients with cervical carcinoma: the case for lymph node debulking. *Cancer* 1998;82(11):2241–2248.
14. Goff BA, Muntz HG, Paley PJ, Tamimi HK, Koh WJ, Greer BE. Impact of surgical staging in women with locally advanced cervical cancer. *Gynecol Oncol* 1999;74(3):436–442.
15. Moore KN, Gold MA, McMeekin DS, Walker JL, Rutledge T, Zorn KK. Extraperitoneal para-aortic lymph node evaluation for cervical cancer via pfannenstiel incision: technique and peri-operative outcomes. *Gynecol Oncol* 2008;108(3):466–471.
16. Sonoda Y, Leblanc E, Querleu D, *et al.* Prospective evaluation of surgical staging of advanced cervical cancer via a laparoscopic extraperitoneal approach. *Gynecol Oncol* 2003;91(2):326–331.
17. Abu-Rustum NR, Chi DS, Sonoda Y, *et al.* Transperitoneal laparoscopic pelvic and para-aortic lymph node dissection using the argon-beam coagulator and monopolar instruments: an 8-year study and description of technique. *Gynecol Oncol* 2003;89(3):504–513.

18. Bipat S, Glas AS, van der Velden J, Zwinderman AH, Bossuyt PM, Stoker J. Computed tomography and magnetic resonance imaging in staging of uterine cervical carcinoma: a systematic review. *Gynecol Oncol* 2003;91(1):59–66.
19. Grigsby PW, Siegel BA, Dehdashti F. Lymph node staging by positron emission tomography in patients with carcinoma of the cervix. *J Clin Oncol* 2001;19(17):3745–3749.
20. Rose PG, Adler LP, Rodriguez M, Faulhaber PF, Abdul-Karim FW, Miraldi F. Positron emission tomography for evaluating para-aortic nodal metastasis in locally advanced cervical cancer before surgical staging: a surgicopathologic study. *J Clin Oncol* 1999;17(1):41–45.
21. Belhocine T, Thille A, Fridman V, *et al.* Contribution of whole-body 18FDG PET imaging in the management of cervical cancer. *Gynecol Oncol* 2002;87(1):90–97.
22. Lin WC, Hung YC, Yeh LS, Kao CH, Yen RF, Shen YY. Usefulness of (18)F-fluorodeoxyglucose positron emission tomography to detect para-aortic lymph nodal metastasis in advanced cervical cancer with negative computed tomography findings. *Gynecol Oncol* 2003;89(1):73–76.
23. Yen TC, Ng KK, Ma SY, *et al.* Value of dual-phase 2-fluoro-2-deoxy-d-glucose positron emission tomography in cervical cancer. *J Clin Oncol* 2003;21(19):3651–3658.
24. Reinhardt MJ, Ehritt-Braun C, Vogelgesang D, *et al.* Metastatic lymph nodes in patients with cervical cancer: detection with MR imaging and FDG PET. *Radiology* 2001;218(3):776–782.
25. Narayan K, Hicks RJ, Jobling T, Bernshaw D, McKenzie AF. A comparison of MRI and PET scanning in surgically staged loco-regionally advanced cervical cancer: potential impact on treatment. *Int J Gynecol Cancer* 2001;11(4):263–271.
26. Chou HH, Chang TC, Yen TC, *et al.* Low value of [18F]-fluoro-2-deoxy-D-glucose positron emission tomography in primary staging of early-stage cervical cancer before radical hysterectomy. *J Clin Oncol* 2006; 24(1):123–128.
27. Wright JD, Dehdashti F, Herzog TJ, *et al.* Preoperative lymph node staging of early-stage cervical carcinoma by [18F]-fluoro-2-deoxy-D-glucose-positron emission tomography. *Cancer* 2005;104(11):2484–2491.
28. Havrilesky LJ, Kulasingam SL, Matchar DB, Myers ER. FDG-PET for management of cervical and ovarian cancer. *Gynecol Oncol* 2005;97(1):183–191.

29. Loft A, Berthelsen AK, Roed H, *et al.* The diagnostic value of PET/CT scanning in patients with cervical cancer: a prospective study. *Gynecol Oncol* 2007;106(1):29–34.
30. Gold MA, Tian C, Whitney CW, Rose PG, Lanciano R. Surgical versus radiographic determination of para-aortic lymph node metastases before chemoradiation for locally advanced cervical carcinoma: a Gynecologic Oncology Group Study. *Cancer* 2008;112(9):1954–1963.
31. Creasman WT, Fetter BF, Clarke-Pearson DL, Kaufmann L, Parker RT. Management of stage IA carcinoma of the cervix. *Am J Obstet Gynecol* 1985;153(2):164–172.
32. Ostor AG. Pandora's box or Ariadne's thread? Definition and prognostic significance of microinvasion in the uterine cervix. Squamous lesions. *Pathol Annu* 1995;30 Pt 2:103–136.
33. Elliott P, Coppleson M, Russell P, *et al.* Early invasive (FIGO stage IA) carcinoma of the cervix: a clinico-pathologic study of 476 cases. *Int J Gynecol Cancer* 2000;10(1):42–52.
34. Koliopoulos G, Sotiriadis A, Kyrgiou M, Martin-Hirsch P, Makrydimas G, Paraskevaidis E. Conservative surgical methods for FIGO stage IA2 squamous cervical carcinoma and their role in preserving women's fertility. *Gynecol Oncol* 2004;93(2):469–473.
35. Sevin BU, Nadji M, Averette HE, Hilsenbeck S, Smith D, Lampe B. Microinvasive carcinoma of the cervix. *Cancer* 1992;70(8):2121–2128.
36. van Nagell JR Jr, Greenwell N, Powell DF, Donaldson ES, Hanson MB, Gay EC. Microinvasive carcinoma of the cervix. *Am J Obstet Gynecol* 1983;145(8):981–991.
37. Creasman WT, Zaino RJ, Major FJ, DiSaia PJ, Hatch KD, Homesley HD. Early invasive carcinoma of the cervix (3 to 5 mm invasion): risk factors and prognosis. A Gynecologic Oncology Group study. *Am J Obstet Gynecol* 1998;178(1 Pt 1):62–65.
38. Landoni F, Maneo A, Colombo A, *et al.* Randomised study of radical surgery versus radiotherapy for stage Ib–IIa cervical cancer. *Lancet* 1997;350(9077): 535–540.
39. Frumovitz M, Sun CC, Schover LR, *et al.* Quality of life and sexual functioning in cervical cancer survivors. *J Clin Oncol* 2005;23(30):7428–7436.
40. Piver MS, Rutledge F, Smith JP. Five classes of extended hysterectomy for women with cervical cancer. *Obstet Gynecol* 1974;44(2):265–272.

41. Lee YN, Wang KL, Lin MH, *et al.* Radical hysterectomy with pelvic lymph node dissection for treatment of cervical cancer: a clinical review of 954 cases. *Gynecol Oncol* 1989;32(2):135–142.
42. Brooks RA, Wright JD, Powell MA, *et al.* Long-term assessment of bladder and bowel dysfunction after radical hysterectomy. *Gynecol Oncol* 2009;114(1):75–79.
43. Covens A, Rosen B, Murphy J, *et al.* Changes in the demographics and perioperative care of stage IA(2)/IB(1) cervical cancer over the past 16 years. *Gynecol Oncol* 2001;81(2):133–137.
44. Dargent D, Martin X, Sacchetoni A, Mathevet P. Laparoscopic vaginal radical trachelectomy: a treatment to preserve the fertility of cervical carcinoma patients. *Cancer* 2000;88(8):1877–1882.
45. Abu-Rustum NR, Sonoda Y, Black D, Levine DA, Chi DS, Barakat RR. Fertility-sparing radical abdominal trachelectomy for cervical carcinoma: technique and review of the literature. *Gynecol Oncol* 2006;103(3):807–813.
46. Beiner ME, Covens A. Surgery insight: radical vaginal trachelectomy as a method of fertility preservation for cervical cancer. *Nat Clin Pract Oncol* 2007;4(6):353–361.
47. Shepherd JH, Spencer C, Herod J, Ind TE. Radical vaginal trachelectomy as a fertility-sparing procedure in women with early-stage cervical cancer-cumulative pregnancy rate in a series of 123 women. *BJOG* 2006;113(6):719–724.
48. Hertel H, Kohler C, Michels W, Possover M, Tozzi R, Schneider A. Laparoscopic-assisted radical vaginal hysterectomy (LARVH): prospective evaluation of 200 patients with cervical cancer. *Gynecol Oncol* 2003;90(3):505–511.
49. Chen Y, Xu H, Li Y, *et al.* The outcome of laparoscopic radical hysterectomy and lymphadenectomy for cervical cancer: a prospective analysis of 295 patients. *Ann Surg Oncol* 2008;15(10):2847–2855.
50. Pellegrino A, Vizza E, Fruscio R, *et al.* Total laparoscopic radical hysterectomy and pelvic lymphadenectomy in patients with Ib1 stage cervical cancer: analysis of surgical and oncological outcome. *Eur J Surg Oncol* 2009;35(1):98–103.
51. Boggess JF, Gehrig PA, Cantrell L, *et al.* A case-control study of robot-assisted type III radical hysterectomy with pelvic lymph node dissection compared with open radical hysterectomy. *Am J Obstet Gynecol* 2008;199(4):357 e1–e7.

52. Keys HM, Bundy BN, Stehman FB, *et al.* Cisplatin, radiation, and adjuvant hysterectomy compared with radiation and adjuvant hysterectomy for bulky stage IB cervical carcinoma. *N Engl J Med* 1999;340(15):1154–1161.
53. Whitney CW, Sause W, Bundy BN, *et al.* Randomized comparison of fluorouracil plus cisplatin versus hydroxyurea as an adjunct to radiation therapy in stage IIB–IVA carcinoma of the cervix with negative para-aortic lymph nodes: a Gynecologic Oncology Group and Southwest Oncology Group study. *J Clin Oncol* 1999;17(5):1339–1348.
54. Peters WA 3rd, Liu PY, Barrett RJ 2nd, *et al.* Concurrent chemotherapy and pelvic radiation therapy compared with pelvic radiation therapy alone as adjuvant therapy after radical surgery in high-risk early-stage cancer of the cervix. *J Clin Oncol* 2000;18(8):1606–1613.
55. Morris M, Eifel PJ, Lu J, *et al.* Pelvic radiation with concurrent chemotherapy compared with pelvic and para-aortic radiation for high-risk cervical cancer. *N Engl J Med* 1999;340(15):1137–1143.
56. Rose PG, Bundy BN, Watkins EB, *et al.* Concurrent cisplatin-based radiotherapy and chemotherapy for locally advanced cervical cancer. *N Engl J Med* 1999;340(15):1144–1153.
57. Monk BJ, Tewari KS, Koh WJ. Multimodality therapy for locally advanced cervical carcinoma: state of the art and future directions. *J Clin Oncol* 2007;25(20):2952–2965.
58. Ang KK. Concurrent radiation chemotherapy for locally advanced head and neck carcinoma: are we addressing burning subjects? *J Clin Oncol* 2004;22(23):4657–4659.
59. Petereit DG, Sarkaria JN, Chappell R, *et al.* The adverse effect of treatment prolongation in cervical carcinoma. *Int J Radiat Oncol Biol Phys* 1995;32(5):1301–1307.
60. Hareyama M, Sakata K, Oouchi A, *et al.* High-dose-rate versus low-dose-rate intracavitary therapy for carcinoma of the uterine cervix: a randomized trial. *Cancer* 2002;94(1):117–124.
61. Gothard L, Cornes P, Brooker S, *et al.* Phase II study of vitamin E and pentoxifylline in patients with late side effects of pelvic radiotherapy. *Radiother Oncol* 2005;75(3):334–341.
62. Green J, Kirwan J, Tierney J, *et al.* Concomitant chemotherapy and radiation therapy for cancer of the uterine cervix. *Cochrane Database Syst Rev* 2001;(4):CD002225.

63. Sedlis A, Bundy BN, Rotman MZ, Lentz SS, Muderspach LI, Zaino RJ. A randomized trial of pelvic radiation therapy versus no further therapy in selected patients with stage IB carcinoma of the cervix after radical hysterectomy and pelvic lymphadenectomy: a Gynecologic Oncology Group study. *Gynecol Oncol* 1999;73(2):177–183.
64. Rotman M, Sedlis A, Piedmonte MR, *et al.* A phase III randomized trial of postoperative pelvic irradiation in Stage IB cervical carcinoma with poor prognostic features: follow-up of a Gynecologic Oncology Group study. *Int J Radiat Oncol Biol Phys* 2006;65(1):169–176.
65. Rydzewska L, Tierney J, Vale CL, Symonds PR. Neoadjuvant chemotherapy plus surgery versus surgery for cervical cancer. *Cochrane Database Syst Rev* 2010;(1):CD007406.
66. Benedet JL, Odicino F, Maisonneuve P, *et al.* Carcinoma of the cervix uteri. *Int J Gynaecol Obstet* 2003;83 Suppl 1:41–78.
67. Bonomi P, Blessing JA, Stehman FB, DiSaia PJ, Walton L, Major FJ. Randomized trial of three cisplatin dose schedules in squamous-cell carcinoma of the cervix: a Gynecologic Oncology Group study. *J Clin Oncol* 1985;3(8):1079–1085.
68. Thigpen T. The role of chemotherapy in the management of carcinoma of the cervix. *Cancer J* 2003;9(5):425–432.
69. McGuire WP, Blessing JA, Moore D, Lentz SS, Photopulos G. Paclitaxel has moderate activity in squamous cervix cancer: a Gynecologic Oncology Group study. *J Clin Oncol* 1996;14(3):792–795.
70. Curtin JP, Blessing JA, Webster KD, *et al.* Paclitaxel, an active agent in nonsquamous carcinomas of the uterine cervix: a Gynecologic Oncology Group study. *J Clin Oncol* 2001;19(5):1275–1278.
71. Sutton GP, Blessing JA, DiSaia PJ, McGuire WP. Phase II study of ifosfamide and mesna in nonsquamous carcinoma of the cervix: a Gynecologic Oncology Group study. *Gynecol Oncol* 1993;49(1):48–50.
72. Sutton GP, Blessing JA, McGuire WP, Patton T, Look KY. Phase II trial of ifosfamide and mesna in patients with advanced or recurrent squamous carcinoma of the cervix who had never received chemotherapy: a Gynecologic Oncology Group study. *Am J Obstet Gynecol* 1993;168(3 Pt 1):805–807.
73. Muderspach LI, Blessing JA, Levenback C, Moore JL Jr. A Phase II study of topotecan in patients with squamous cell carcinoma of the cervix: a Gynecologic Oncology Group study. *Gynecol Oncol* 2001;81(2):213–215.

74. Look KY, Blessing JA, Levenback C, Kohler M, Chafe W, Roman LD. A phase II trial of CPT-11 in recurrent squamous carcinoma of the cervix:a Gynecologic Oncology Group study. *Gynecol Oncol* 1998; 70(3):334–338.
75. Morris M, Brader KR, Levenback C, *et al.* Phase II study of vinorelbine in advanced and recurrent squamous cell carcinoma of the cervix. *J Clin Oncol* 1998;16(3):1094–1098.
76. Omura GA, Blessing JA, Vaccarello L, *et al.* Randomized trial of cisplatin versus cisplatin plus mitolactol versus cisplatin plus ifosfamide in advanced squamous carcinoma of the cervix: a Gynecologic Oncology Group study. *J Clin Oncol* 1997;15(1):165–171.
77. Moore DH, Blessing JA, McQuellon RP, *et al.* Phase III study of cisplatin with or without paclitaxel in stage IVB, recurrent, or persistent squamous cell carcinoma of the cervix: a Gynecologic Oncology Group study. *J Clin Oncol* 2004;22(15):3113–3119.
78. Long HJ 3rd, Bundy BN, Grendys EC Jr, *et al.* Randomized phase III trial of cisplatin with or without topotecan in carcinoma of the uterine cervix: a Gynecologic Oncology Group study. *J Clin Oncol* 2005; 23(21): 4626–4633.
79. Monk BJ, Sill MW, McMeekin DS, *et al.* Phase III trial of four cisplatin-containing doublet combinations in stage IVB, recurrent, or persistent cervical carcinoma: a Gynecologic Oncology Group study. *J Clin Oncol* 2009;27(28):4649–4655.
80. Monk BJ, Sill MW, Burger RA, Gray HJ, Buekers TE, Roman LD. Phase II trial of bevacizumab in the treatment of persistent or recurrent squamous cell carcinoma of the cervix: a Gynecologic Oncology Group study. *J Clin Oncol* 2009;27(7):1069–1074.
81. del Campo JM, Prat A, Gil-Moreno A, Perez J, Parera M. Update on novel therapeutic agents for cervical cancer. *Gynecol Oncol* 2008;110(3 Suppl 2): S72–S76.
82. Berek JS, Howe C, Lagasse LD, Hacker NF. Pelvic exenteration for recurrent gynecologic malignancy: survival and morbidity analysis of the 45-year experience at UCLA. *Gynecol Oncol* 2005;99(1):153–159.
83. Morley GW, Hopkins MP, Lindenauer SM, Roberts JA. Pelvic exenteration, University of Michigan: 100 patients at 5 years. *Obstet Gynecol* 1989;74(6):934–943.

84. Brunschwig A. Complete excision of pelvic viscera for advanced carcinoma; a one-stage abdominoperineal operation with end colostomy and bilateral ureteral implantation into the colon above the colostomy. *Cancer* 1948;1(2):177–183.
85. Hancock KC, Copeland LJ, Gershenson DM, Saul PB, Wharton JT, Rutledge FN. Urinary conduits in gynecologic oncology. *Obstet Gynecol* 1986; 67(5):680–684.
86. Copeland LJ, Hancock KC, Gershenson DM, Stringer CA, Atkinson EN, Edwards CL. Gracilis myocutaneous vaginal reconstruction concurrent with total pelvic exenteration. *Am J Obstet Gynecol* 1989;160(5 Pt 1):1095–1101.
87. Salom EM, Penalver MA. Pelvic exenteration and reconstruction. *Cancer J* 2003;9(5):415–424.
88. Pecorelli S. Revised FIGO staging for carcinoma of the vulva, cervix, and endometrium. *Int J Gynaecol Obstet* 2009;105(2):103–104.
89. Quinn MA, Benedet JL, Odicino F, *et al.* Carcinoma of the cervix uteri. FIGO 6th Annual Report on the Results of Treatment in Gynecological Cancer. *Int J Gynaecol Obstet* 2006;95 Suppl 1:S43–S103.
90. Arseneau J, Blessing JA, Stehman FB, McGehee R. A phase II study of carboplatin in advanced squamous cell carcinoma of the cervix (a Gynecologic Oncology Group Study). *Invest New Drugs* 1986;4(2):187–191.

# 7

# ENDOMETRIAL CANCER

*Evelyn B. Marsh*

## INTRODUCTION

Endometrial cancer is the most common gynecologic malignancy diagnosed in the United States, and the fourth most common malignancy in women overall, behind breast, colorectal, and lung cancers. Worldwide, the only gynecologic malignancy more prevalent than endometrial cancer is cervical cancer. Endometrial cancer is most often diagnosed in the sixth and seventh decades of life, and is very rare in young women.

The majority of endometrial cancers are diagnosed at an early stage, while still confined to the uterus. A favorable prognosis is therefore associated with many endometrial cancers. However, patients who present with high-risk features, including specific histology, advanced stage, and higher-grade tumors, are faced with significantly worse outcomes.

Current management of early endometrial cancer generally consists of surgical therapy, including staging, followed by adjuvant therapy in some high-risk cases. Significant controversy exists over the role of nodal dissection in this disease, as well as over the appropriate chemotherapeutic and radiation treatments. Endocrine agents are also being explored as a possible treatment option.

## EPIDEMIOLOGY

It is estimated that there were 42,160 new cases of endometrial carcinoma in the United States in 2009, and 7,780 deaths due to the disease.[1] It is the most common gynecologic malignancy in the United States, and the fourth most common cancer overall following breast, lung, and colorectal cancers. Its incidence varies significantly by country, with rates four to five times lower in Japan, India, and South Asia than in the United States and other Western industrialized nations. For American women, the lifetime risk of developing endometrial cancer is 2.6%.

There are two distinct clinicopathologic categories of endometrial cancer[2] (Table 1).

Type I endometrial cancers are related to increased exposure to estrogen, whereas type II endometrial cancers are largely unrelated to hormone exposure. Approximately 80% of endometrial carcinomas diagnosed in the United States are type I, largely due to the high rate of obesity in that population.[3] In comparison to type II cancers, type I cancers are typically of endometrioid histology, are better differentiated, occur at a younger age, and are less aggressive. They carry a more favorable prognosis than type II cancers. The average age at diagnosis of patients with endometrioid cancers is 63 years, with approximately 70% being stage I or stage II. The Five-year survival rate for these cancers is 83%. By contrast, type II cancers are generally non-endometrioid (e.g., papillary serous, clear cell), tend to be poorly differentiated, and are more often diagnosed at a late stage. The average age at diagnosis is 67 years, and 50% are diagnosed at stage III or IV. The five-year survival rate for these cancers is between

Table 1. Type I and Type II endometrial cancer.

| | **Type I** | **Type II** |
|---|---|---|
| Prevalence | 80% | 20% |
| Risk Factor | Unopposed estrogen exposure (obesity, nulliparity) | Advancing age |
| Histology | Endometrioid | Non-endometrioid (clear cell, papillary serous) |
| Differentiation | Well-differentiated | Poorly differentiated |
| Stage at Diagnosis | Early | Late |
| Prognosis | More favorable | Not favorable |
| Genetic Alterations | PTEN, KRAS, PIK3CA microsatellite instability | p53, Her-2/neu and K-ras overexpression |

53% and 62%. There are distinct genetic alterations associated with each subtype. Type I cancers show microsatellite instability at PTEN, KRAS, and PIK3CA, whereas type II cancers have p53, Her-2/neu, and K-ras overexpression.[4,5]

Multiple factors have been identified that confer an increased risk of endometrial cancer (see Table 2). Most of these factors are related to increased lifetime exposure to estrogen, which leads to an excess of type I cancers. Obese nulliparous patients who reach menopause at age 52 or later appear to have a five times greater risk for endometrial cancer over those without these risk factors.[6] Hereditary non-polyposis colorectal cancer syndrome (HNPCC, or Lynch II) occurs in families with clusters of early-onset colon, ovarian, and endometrial cancers. Other associated tumors include kidney, bladder, liver, stomach, gall bladder, and small bowel. HNPCC has been linked to several mutations in the DNA mismatch repair (MMR) genes, which lead to the inability of cells to correct mismatched DNA nucleotides, resulting in microsatellite instability, accumulated mutations in oncogenes and tumor suppressor genes, and ultimately to the development of invasive cancers.[7,8] Though mutations in five genes have been documented, the two responsible for over 90% of cases are mutations in MLH1 on chromosome 3 and MSHS on chromosome 2.[9] Carriers of mutations in the MMR genes carry a 40–60% lifetime risk of endometrial cancer.[10]

## PRESENTATION

The most common presenting symptom of endometrial carcinoma is abnormal vaginal bleeding. Abnormal bleeding can be caused by a

Table 2. Risk factors for endometrial cancer.[6]

| |
|---|
| Obesity |
| Nulliparity |
| Late menopause |
| Unopposed exogenous estrogen |
| Tamoxifen use |
| Hereditary non-polyposis colon cancer syndrome (HNPCC or Lynch II) |

The cell types typically associated with endometrial adenocarcinoma are endometrioid, serous, clear cell, and mucinous. Mixed carcinomas, those that include two or more of the cell types, are defined as those in which the less prevalent component comprises at least 10% of the tumor.

### *Endometrioid*

The most common type of endometrial adenocarcinoma is the endometrioid type, which comprises 75–80% of cases. The glands of the carcinoma are characterized by tall, columnar cells that share a common apical border. This type of adenocarcinoma can range from well-differentiated to undifferentiated, with decreasing differentiation associated with increasing solid growth and less gland formation. Approximately 25% of endometrioid endometrial adenocarcinomas include foci of squamous differentiation. These tumors behave similarly to endometrioid carcinomas without such differentiation.

### *Serous*

Serous endometrial adenocarcinomas are the second most common cell type, representing approximately 10% of these tumors. This carcinoma is generally found in older women at an advanced stage, and is considered to be more aggressive than endometrioid endometrial adenocarcinoma. It commonly arises in a background of atrophy, rather than hyperplasia, and is not associated with unopposed estrogen exposure. Histologically, its papillary growth and cellular features resemble serous carcinoma of the ovary. This tumor has a high likelihood of spreading throughout the peritoneal cavity, and the risk of recurrence is high even with apparently minimally invasive disease.

### *Clear cell*

Clear cell adenocarcinoma comprises approximately 4% of endometrial adenocarcinoma. It is characterized by the distinctive clearing of the neoplastic cells. This is a particularly aggressive tumor type, associated with high recurrence rates and a five-year survival rate of 20–65%.

### *Other cell types*

Approximately 1% of endometrial adenocarcinomas are of a mucinous type. These tumors behave similarly to endometrioid endometrial adenocarcinomas.

The endometrium is a potential site of metastasis of malignancies from other organs. The most common pelvic source of metastasis is the ovary. However, malignancies of the breast, stomach, colon, pancreas, and kidney have also been reported to metastasize to the endometrium.

## DIAGNOSIS

The most common presenting symptom of endometrial cancer is abnormal vaginal bleeding, particularly in postmenopausal women. However, all women with symptoms which are concerning for endometrial adenocarcinoma should be evaluated with biopsy. The gold standard method for assessing these symptoms is a fractional dilation and curettage, where an endocervical curettage is performed, followed by cervical dilation and endometrial curettage. Less invasive biopsy methods, such as endometrial biopsy or aspiration curettage, may also be used. However, it should be noted that these methods are only considered definitive if positive for cancer. If the results of these tests are inconclusive or insufficient, a fractional dilation and curettage should be performed.

Following a histologic diagnosis of endometrial carcinoma, further evaluation is warranted. Extensive metastatic workup is not generally necessary for well-differentiated tumors. However, CA-125 levels and imaging studies should be checked for patients with higher-grade tumors.

For a select group of patients who are considered medically inoperable, or who wish to preserve future fertility, conservative management may be indicated. In these cases, decision making may be informed by both ultrasonography and MRI, which may be useful in determining lymph node involvement and depth of myometrial invasion.

# PROGNOSTIC FACTORS

## Stage

In 2009, FIGO revised the staging for endometrial carcinoma[13] (Table 4). Prior to this revision, two staging methods had been used. The FIGO staging system of 1971[14] was entirely clinical, whereas the subsequent staging system of 1988[15] included pathologic factors as well (Table 5). The 1988 staging system is included for reference, given that all studies reported hereafter were performed prior to the 2009 change in staging.

Comparisons of the two staging methods demonstrated the superiority of surgico-pathologic staging over clinical staging in prognostic significance. In multiple multivariate studies, FIGO stage is the strongest predictor of outcome for patients with endometrial adenocarcinoma.[16,17]

## Histology

The histologic cell type of endometrial adenocarcinoma is a well-recognized predictor of survival and tumor behavior. The endometrioid subtype of endometrial adenocarcinoma, which comprises the large

Table 4. Revised FIGO staging for endometrial adenocarcinoma (2009).

| | |
|---|---|
| **Stage I** | **Tumor confined to the corpus uteri** |
| IA | No myometrial invasion or invasion of less than half of the myometrial thickness |
| IB | Invasion equal to or more than half of the myometrial thickness |
| **Stage II** | **Tumor invades cervical stroma but does not extend beyond the uterus** |
| **Stage III** | **Local and/or regional spread of tumor** |
| IIIA | Tumor invades the serosa of the corpus uteri and/or the adnexae |
| IIIB | Vaginal and/or parametrial involvement |
| IIIC | Metastases to pelvic and/or para-aortic lymph nodes |
| IIIC1 | Positive pelvic nodes |
| IIIC2 | Positive para-aortic nodes |
| **Stage IV** | **Tumor invades bladder and/or bowel mucosa, and/or distant metastases** |
| IVA | Tumor invasion of bladder and/or bowel mucosa |
| IVB | Distant metastases, including intra-abdominal metastases and/or inguinal lymph nodes |

Table 5. FIGO surgical staging for endometrial cancer (1988).

| | |
|---|---|
| Stage 1A | Tumor limited to endometrium |
| Stage 1B | Tumor invades less than half of the myometrial thickness |
| Stage IC | Tumor invades more than half of the myometrial thickness |
| Stage IIA | Endocervical glandular involvement |
| Stage IIB | Cervical stromal invasion |
| Stage IIIA | Invasion of uterine serosa or adnexae, or positive peritoneal cytology |
| Stage IIIB | Vaginal involvement |
| Stage IIIC | Metastases to pelvic or para-aortic lymph nodes |
| Stage IVA | Invasion of bladder or bowel mucosa |
| Stage IVB | Distant metastases, including intra-abdominal or inguinal lymph nodes |

majority of cases, has a relatively good prognosis. Clear cell carcinoma is a very aggressive disease, with five-year survival rates of 30–75%. Serous carcinoma has similarly poor five-year survival rates, ranging from 40% to 60%. Adenocarcinoma with squamous differentiation behaves similarly to endometrioid adenocarcinoma in terms of epidemiologic distribution and distribution by stage, but with a slightly improved five-year survival rate.

Histologic grade has also been consistently related to survival rates. A GOG study of patients with stage I or occult stage II endometrioid adenocarcinoma revealed a five-year survival rate of 94% for grade 1, 84% for grade 2, and 72% for grade 3.[17] Additionally, histologic grade is a very good indicator of the risk of tumor spread. The incidence of deep myometrial invasion is significantly higher with less differentiated tumors. Therefore, there is a higher rate of pelvic and para-aortic lymph node metastasis with higher-grade tumors as well.

## Myometrial Invasion

Deep myometrial invasion is strongly correlated with an increased probability of extrauterine tumor spread, treatment failure, and recurrence. Therefore, it is strongly associated with a decreased probability of survival. A GOG study of patients with clinical stage I and occult stage II endometrioid adenocarcinoma revealed that the five-year survival rate was 94% when the tumor did not invade the myometrium, 91% when the tumor involved papillary serous adenocarcinoma, a complete omentectomy and peritoneal biopsies should be performed even in the absence of gross disease. Traditionally, this surgery has been performed abdominally, through a midline vertical incision. However, more recent advances have brought laparoscopic and now robotic surgical techniques into use. Based on the histologic and cytologic features determined by the surgical evaluation, risk of recurrence can be determined. Those cases with significant risk of recurrence are then offered adjuvant therapy.

## *Nodal dissection*

There is significant debate over the value and extent of nodal dissection as it relates to the surgical staging of endometrial adenocarcinoma. Those in favor of routine nodal dissection offer that knowledge of the presence of microscopic disease spread to the nodes is the most accurate way to determine the risk of recurrence, and affects the choice of adjuvant treatments. Specifically, the information gained may result in decreased use of radiation, and replacing whole pelvic radiation with more directed vaginal cuff brachytherapy. Those who opt out of routine surgical staging cite the risks associated with the procedure. These risks include increased blood loss, lymphedema, lymphocyst formation, vascular injury, genitofemoral nerve injury resulting in medial thigh neuropathy, and increased operative time. In general, these risks occur infrequently and are considered acceptable. Nonetheless, at this time each physician determines for his or herself whether surgical staging is valuable enough to perform routinely, or whether it is reserved for those patients with specific high-risk risk factors such as high tumor grade or outer half myometrial invasion as determined on intraoperative frozen section.

The questions that raise the most discussion regarding nodal dissection include which patients should be offered the procedure (none, only those with high-risk features, or all patients), the appropriate extent of the dissection (excision of enlarged nodes or complete lymphadenectomy), and whether or not para-aortic nodes should be sampled in addition to pelvic nodes.

### No nodal dissection

The strongest argument for not performing nodal dissection in patients with endometrial cancer may be that most patients with the disease do not present with high-risk features for nodal metastases.[19] The GOG study reporting the disease patterns of over 600 patients with clinical stage I and occult stage II disease showed that 59% had either absent or <1/3 myometrial invasion. Seventy-five percent had grade I or II tumors. Nine percent had positive lymph node metastases. In 2003, the Post Operative Radiation Therapy in Endometrial Cancer (PORTEC) trial compared postoperative observation to pelvic radiation in patients with stage IC, grade 1; stages IB and IC, grade 2; and stage IB, grade 3 disease. These patients' initial surgery consisted of hysterectomy without lymph node dissection. The results of the study revealed favorable outcomes in both groups: 85% five-year survival in the observation group and 81% five-year survival in the pelvic radiation group.[20]

A Study in the Treatment of Endometrial Cancer (ASTEC) was published in 2009, and is the only randomized control trial comparing lymphadenectomy to no lymphadenectomy to date.[21] In it, endometrial cancer patients were randomized to hysterectomy with or without pelvic lymphadenectomy. After surgical treatment, those patients with stage I and IIA disease with high-risk features (i.e., grade 3 tumors, serous or clear cell histology, endocervical glandular invasion, or greater than 50% myometrial invasion) were randomized to observation or pelvic radiation therapy. In the study, vaginal cuff brachytherapy was permitted in all groups. Follow-up showed no benefit of lymphadenectomy in terms of disease-free survival or overall survival in patients with stage I and IIA endometrial cancer.

### Selective nodal dissection

Pelvic and para-aortic lymph node status has been a part of endometrial cancer staging since the FIGO staging criteria of 1988. The latest revision of the staging criteria continues to involve the presence or absence of lymph node metastases. Multiple studies have shown that simple palpation of the pelvic lymph nodes is not sufficient to accurately predict the presence of lymph node disease.[22] Pathologic evaluation of the nodal tissue is required. In GOG 33, the rate of para-aortic nodal metastases was found to be approximately half of the rate of pelvic metastases, across various tumor grades and depths of invasion.[19] Only 2% of patients had isolated para-aortic nodal involvement in the absence of pelvic nodal involvement. The argument has been made, therefore, to perform para-aortic nodal dissection only on those patients in whom high-risk features are present. For example, inspection of the uterus at the time of surgery could be performed to roughly estimate the depth of myometrial invasion. Additionally, in patients with preoperative tissue sampling, presence of a high-grade tumor would prompt thorough nodal evaluation.

### Routine nodal dissection

Many arguments have been made for routinely performing a comprehensive nodal dissection as part of surgical staging of endometrial cancer. These include the relative infrequency of patients with no risk factors for lymph node metastases, the relative imprecision of preoperative techniques (i.e., endometrial sampling to evaluate tumor grade) and intraoperative techniques (i.e., gross evaluation of the uterus to evaluate depth of invasion), the significant difference in treatment modalities and outcomes in patients with presence or absence of nodal metastases, and the relatively low rate of risks of the procedure. Since nodal disease status appears to be a significant predictor of disease recurrence, and therefore a primary determinant of the need for adjuvant therapy, routine nodal dissection would seem to be indicated as a method of determining appropriate postoperative treatments. In fact, most gynecologic oncologists now perform some degree of nodal dissection for all of their patients with endometrial cancer.

## *Laparoscopic surgical management*

Historically, the primary management of endometrial cancer has been with an abdominal surgical approach. However, more recent advances have brought laparoscopic surgical management into use. As primary treatment, laparoscopic surgery may be used in the form of a laparoscopic-assisted vaginal hysterectomy or total laparoscopic hysterectomy. Pelvic and para-aortic lymph node dissections may be performed laparoscopically, either as part of the primary procedure or in patients with prior incomplete staging procedures.

The LAP 2 trial, a GOG study published in 2009, was a large, prospective, randomized trial designed to determine equivalency in outcomes of early-stage endometrial cancer treated with laparoscopic-assisted vaginal hysterectomy and lymph node dissection compared to that treated with laparotomy.[23] The outcomes that were measured were completion of the staging procedure, safety of the procedure, short-term outcomes, and long-term survival and recurrence rates. The data on the long-term outcomes is still maturing. There were 920 patients enrolled in the laparotomy arm, and 1,696 enrolled in the laparoscopy arm. Twenty-six percent of the laparoscopic procedures were converted into laparotomies, for indications such as poor visibility, extrauterine disease, and excessive bleeding. The laparoscopic success rate increased with decreasing BMI. Complication rates, including vascular, urinary, bowel, and nerve injury, were slightly higher in the laparoscopy arm (9.5%) than in the laparotomy arm (7.6%). The number of nodes removed and incidence of positive nodes was similar in both arms. In patients for whom the procedure was completed laparoscopically, surgical time was 70 minutes longer but hospital stay two days shorter than in patients in the laparotomy arm. The conclusion of the study was that laparoscopic surgical treatment for endometrial cancer is an equivalent, if not better, option than laparotomy. The findings underscored the importance of appropriate patient selection for laparoscopic surgical techniques, as the benefits were far superior in the group for whom laparoscopy could be successfully completed.

## Nonsurgical Management

Although the primary treatment for endometrial cancer is generally surgical, there are a select few groups of patients for whom nonsurgical management may be appropriate. These groups of patients include those no significant difference in overall survival between the two arms, for a subset of patients with deep myometrial invasion and grade 3 disease, an overall survival benefit was noted (18% versus 7%). A similar study compared pelvic radiation alone to pelvic radiation with the addition of vaginal brachytherapy.[28] In this study, 270 patients with stage I–II endometrial cancer were treated with pelvic radiation alone or pelvic radiation with vaginal brachytherapy, without evidence of benefit in terms of either recurrence rates or disease-free survival at five years. Finally, as surgical lymph node dissection has become more common, many have advocated the use of vaginal brachytherapy alone as adjuvant treatment. In this setting, the absence of lymph node metastases could obviate the need for whole pelvic radiation, while vaginal brachytherapy could be used to decrease vaginal cuff recurrence rates. Many studies have evaluated this approach, and found very low recurrence rates, both at the vaginal cuff or elsewhere in the pelvis.[29,30] All of this evidence suggests that there are numerous, diverse radiation options for patients with early-stage endometrial cancer. All factors, including stage and grade of disease, the risk of local or nodal recurrence, and whether lymph node staging was performed, need to be considered when planning adjuvant radiation therapy for these patients.

## *Radiation therapy for advanced-stage disease*

Pelvic radiation is often used in patients with advanced-stage endometrial cancer, with relatively good results. In patients with isolated adnexal involvement (stage IIIA), reported disease-free survival at five-years is 70.9%.[31] Patients with isolated serosal involvement have somewhat less favorable outcomes when treated with pelvic radiation, with a reported five-year overall survival of 41.5%.[32] In cases of stage IIIC1 disease (positive pelvic lymph nodes without positive para-aortic nodes) treated with pelvic radiation, overall survival rates of 60–72% have been reported.[33,34] There is also a role for extended field radiation in patients with positive para-aortic lymph node metastases. In these patients, treatment with a radiation field encompassing the pelvic and para-aortic regions has yielded a 30–40% overall survival rate.[35]

### *Chemotherapy for advanced-stage disease*

The GOG 122 trial randomized 396 patients with stage III and stage IV disease (optimally debulked) to either whole abdominal radiation ($n = 202$) or chemotherapy with doxorubicin and cisplatin ($n = 194$).[36] The results showed a significant improvement in progression-free and overall survival, in favor of the chemotherapy arm. With a median of 74 months of follow-up, the rate of progression-free survival was 50% in the chemotherapy arm versus 38% in the radiation arm ($p = 0.007$), and the rate of overall survival was 55% versus 42% ($p = 0.004$). The Japanese Gynecologic Oncology Group conducted a randomized trial comparing whole pelvic radiation to combination chemotherapy with cisplatin, doxorubicin, and paclitaxel (CAP).[37] This trial included patients with stage III disease as well as those with high-risk early-stage disease (stage IC and II). Overall, there was no difference between the two arms in terms of both progression-free survival (84% vs. 82%, $p = 0.73$) and overall survival (85% vs. 87%, $p = 0.46$). When analyzing patients with stage IC, II, or IIIA disease with >50% myometrial invasion, there was a significant advantage for chemotherapy, though this same advantage was not observed in patients with other stage III disease.

GOG 184 randomized patients with advanced disease who had undergone surgery and prior tumor volume-directed adjuvant radiation to either AP or CAP every three weeks.[38] Overall three-year PFS was statistically similar for the two groups (64% vs. 62%), though CAP was noted to be superior in women with gross residual disease at the time of study entry. CAP conferred a 50% reduction in the risk of relapse or death compared to AP in these women. Chemotherapy is at least equivalent to radiation in patients with some advanced-stage endometrial cancers, and may be used in combination with tumor-directed radiation in these cases.

## TREATMENT OF RECURRENT DISEASE

Close follow-up of patients with endometrial cancer is warranted after surgery and primary adjuvant therapy. Appropriate follow-up includes routine pelvic exams and Pap smears. In the setting of recurrent disease, treatment is warranted either for palliation or cure. Possible treatment modalities include surgery, radiation, chemotherapy, and endocrine therapy. These treatments may be used individually or in combination with one another.

## *Radiation therapy for recurrent disease*

In patients who have not previously been irradiated, radiation therapy may be used for treatment of local recurrence. Reported five-year recurrence-free survival rates after salvage radiation treatment range from 42% to 65%.[39,40] Reported overall survival rates in this group range from 31% to 53%.

## *Chemotherapy for recurrent disease*

While there is a role for chemotherapy in the treatment of recurrent endometrial cancer, it is primarily palliative. Responses have been reported to both single-agent and combination chemotherapy regimens in this setting. However, the overall survival of patients with recurrent endometrial cancer is less than one year, and the average progression-free survival of patients receiving chemotherapy for recurrent disease is less than six months. Therefore, when selecting a chemotherapy regimen for recurrent endometrial cancer, significant attention should be paid to minimizing side effects of the treatment.

### Single agent chemotherapy

Many studies have evaluated single chemotherapeutic agents as possible treatments for recurrent endometrial cancer.[41–43] The most commonly used agents include carboplatin, cisplatin, docetaxel, paclitaxel, doxorubicin, epirubicin, and ifosfamide. These agents have reported response rates of approximately 14–25% in this setting. Multiple reports have shown significant variation in response rates to a single agent, probably having to do with a number of patient-specific factors. Dosing and treatment schedules are often individually adjusted to minimize toxicity, given the lack of data supporting a specific regimen.

## Combination chemotherapy

A number of GOG trials have studied combination chemotherapy in recurrent endometrial cancer.[44–47] In 2004, Fleming *et al.* reported the results of GOG 177 which randomized patients with advanced and recurrent disease to treatment with AP versus CAP.[48] CAP was noted to confer improved progression-free (8.3 versus 5.3 months, $p < 0.01$) as well as overall survival (15.3 versus 12.3 months, $p = 0.037$) when compared to AP. However, patients receiving triple-agent therapy experienced significantly more peripheral neuropathy. The results of GOG 209, a phase III randomized study comparing CAP to the less toxic carboplatin/paclitaxel regimen, are eagerly awaited.

### *Endocrine therapy for recurrent disease*

Treatment with hormonal agents in patients with recurrent endometrial cancer has been modestly successful, and is the topic of much ongoing research. Potentially useful agents include progestins, antiestrogens, and aromatase inhibitors. In general, the response rate of recurrent endometrial cancer to progestin therapy is approximately 25%.[49] However, multiple studies have revealed that the response rate to progestins is not dose-dependent.[50] The response rate to tamoxifen, an antiestrogenic compound, is significantly lower — reportedly in the 10–15% range.[51] Studies are ongoing to evaluate other hormonal treatments, alone and in combination.

## REFERENCES

1. Jemal A, Siegel R, Ward E, *et al.* Cancer statistics, 2009. *CA Cancer J Clin* 2009;59(4):225–229.
2. Bokhman JV. Two pathologenic types of endometrial carcinoma. *Gynecol Oncol* 1983;10:237–246.
3. Schottenfeld D. Epidemiology of endometrial neoplasia. *J Cell Biochem Suppl* 1995;23:151–159.
4. Kovalev S, Marchenko ND, Gngliotta BG, Chalas E, Chumas J, Moll UM. Loss of p53 function in uterine papillary serous carcinoma. *Hum Pathol* 1998;23:613–619.

5. Cao QJ, Belbin T, Socci N, *et al.* Distinctive gene expression profiles by cDNA microarrays in endometrioid and serous carcinomas of the endometrium. *Int J Gynecol Pathol* 2004;23:321–329.
6. Creasman WT. Adenocarcinoma of the uterus. In: DiSaia JP, Creasman WT, eds. *Clinical Gynecologic Oncology*, 7th ed. Philadelphia: Mosby Elsevier, 2007, pp. 147–184.
7. Aaltonen LA, Peltomäki P, Leach FS, *et al.* Clues to the pathogenesis of familial colorectal cancer. *Science* 1993;260:812–816.
8. Leach FS, Nicolaides NC, Papadopoulas, *et al.* Mutations of a mutS homolog in hereditary nonpolyposis colorectal cancer. *Cell* 1993;75:1215–1225.
9. Bellacosa A, Genuardi M, Anti M, Viel A, Ponz de Leon M. Hereditary nonpolyposis colorectal cancer: review of clinical, molecular genetics, and counseling aspects. *Am J Med Genet* 1996;62:353–364.
10. Aarnio M, Mecklin JP, Aaltonen LA, *et al.* Life-time risk of different cancers in hereditary non-polyposis colorectal cancer (HNPCC) syndrome. *Int J Cancer* 1995;64:430–433.
11. Gredmark T, Kvint S, Havel G, Mattsson LA. Histopathologic findings in women with postmenopausal bleeding. *Br J Obstet Gynaecol* 1995;102: 133–136.
12. Kurman RJ, Kaminski PF, Norris HJ. The behavior of endometrial hyperplasia. A long-term study of "untreated" hyperplasia in 170 patients. *Cancer* 1985; 56(2):403–412.
13. Pecorelli S. Revised FIGO staging for carcinoma of the vulva, cervix, and endometrium. *Int J Gynaecol Obstet* 2009;105:103–104.
14. International Federation of Gynecology and Obstetrics: classification and staging of malignant tumors in the female pelvis. *Int J Gynaecol Obstet* 1971;9:172.
15. Mikuta JJ. FIGO staging of endometrial cancer — 1988. *Cancer* 1993; 71:1460–1463.
16. Abeler V, Kjorstad KE, Barle E. Carcinoma of the endometrium in Norway: a histopathological and prognostic survey of a total population. *Int J Gynecol Cancer* 1992;2:9–22.
17. Morrow CP, Bundy BN, Kurman RJ, *et al.* Relationship between surgical-pathological risk factors and outcome in clinical stages I and II carcinoma of the endometrium: a Gynecologic Oncology Group study. *Gynecol Oncol* 1991;40:55.

18. Barakat RR, Lev G, Hummer AJ, *et al.* Twelve-year experience in the management of endometrial cancer: a change in surgical and postoperative radiation approaches. *Gynecol Oncol* 2007;105:150–156.
19. Creasman WT, Morrow CP, Bundy BN, Homesley HD, Graham JE, Heller PB. Surgical pathologic spread patterns of endometrial cancer: a Gynecologic Oncology Group study. *Cancer* 1987;60:2035–2041.
20. Creutzbert CL van Putten WL, Koper PC, *et al.* Surgery and postoperative radiotherapy versus surgery alone for patients with stage-1 endometrial carcinoma: multicentre randomized trial. PORTEC Study Group. Post Operative Radiation Therapy in Endometrial Carcinoma. *Lancet* 2000;355: 1404–1411.
21. ASTEC study group, Kitchener H, Swart AM, Qian Q, Amos C, Parmar MR. Efficacy of systematic pelvic lymphadenectomy in endometrial cancer (MRC ASTEC trial): a randomised study. *Lancet* 2009;373(9658):125–136.
22. Franchi M, Ghezzi F, Melpignano M, *et al.* Clinical value of intraoperative gross examination in endometrial cancer. *Gynecol Oncol* 2000;76:357–361.
23. Walker JL, Piedmonke MR, Spirtos NM, *et al.* Laparoscopy compared with laparotomy for comprehensive surgical staging of uterine cancer: Gynecologic Oncology Group Study LAP2. *J Clin Oncol* 2009;27(32): 5331–5336.
24. Wright J, Powell MA, Herzog TJ, *et al.* Panniculectomy: improving lymph node yield in morbidly obese patients with endometrial neoplasms. *Gynecol Oncol* 2004;94:436–441.
25. Ramirez P, Frumovitz M, Bodurka DC, Sun CC, Levenback C. Hormonal therapy for the management of grade 1 endometrial adenocarcinoma: a literature review. *Gynecol Oncol* 2004;95:133–138.
26. Roberts JA, Brunetto VL, Keys HM, *et al.* A phase III randomized study of surgery vs. surgery plus adjunctive radiation therapy in intermediate risk endometrial adenocarcinoma (GOG#99) *Gynecol Oncol* 1998;68:135.
27. Aalders J, Abeler V, Kolstad P, Onsrud M. Postoperative external irradiation and prognostic parameters in stage I endometrial carcinoma: clinical and histopathologic study of 540 patients. *Obstet Gynecol* 1980;56:419–427.
28. Greven KM, D'Agostino RB Jr, Lanciano RM, Corn BW. Is there a role for a brachytherapy vaginal cuff boost in the adjuvant management of patients with uterine-confined endometrial cancer? *Int J Radiat Oncol Biol Phys* 1998;42:101–104.

29. Horowitz NS, Peters WA 3rd, Smith MR, Drescher CW, Atwood M, Mate TP. Adjuvant high dose rate vaginal brachytherapy as treatment of stage I and II endometrial carcinoma. *Obstet Gynecol* 2002;99:235–240.
30. Anderson JM, Stea B, Hallum AV, Rogoff E, Childers J. High-dose-rate postoperative vaginal cuff irradiation alone for stage IB and IC endometrial cancer. *Int J Radiat Oncol Biol Phys* 2000:46:417–425.
31. Connell PP, Rofmensch J, Waggoner S, Mundt AJ. The significance of adnexal involvement in endometrial carcinoma. *Gynecol Oncol* 1999;74:74–79.
32. Ashman JB, Connell PP, Yamada D, Rotmensch J, Waggoner SE, Mundt AJ. Outcome of endometrial carcinoma patients with involvement of the uterine serosa. *Gynecol Oncol* 2001;82:338–343.
33. Greven K, Lanciano RM, Corn B, Case D, Randall ME. Pathologic stage III endometrial carcinoma. *Cancer* 1993;71:3697–3702.
34. Mariana A, Webb MJ, Keeney GL, Haddock MG, Aletti G, Podratz KC. Stage IIIC endometrioid corpus cancer includes distinct subgroups. *Gynecol Oncol* 2002;87:12–17.
35. Corn BW, Lanciano RM, Greven KM, *et al.* Endometrial cancer with para-aortic adenopathy: patterns of failure and opportunities for cure. *Int J Radiat Oncol Biol Phys* 1992;24:223–227.
36. Randall, M, Filiaci VL, Muss H, *et al.* Randomized phase III trial of whole-abdominal radiation therapy versus doxorubicin and cisplatin chemotherapy in advanced endometrial carcinoma: a Gynecologic Oncology Group study. *J Clin Oncol* 1006:24:36–44.
37. Susumu H, Sagae S, Udagawa Y, *et al.* Randomized phase III trial of pelvic radiotherapy versus cisplatin-based combined chemotherapy in patients with intermediate- and high-risk endometrial cancer: a Japanese Gynecologic Oncology Group study. *Gynecol Oncol* 2008;108:226–233.
38. Homesley HD, Filiaci V, Gibbors SK, *et al.* A randomized phase III trial in advanced endometrial carcinoma of surgery and volume directed radiation followed by cisplatin and doxorubicin with or without paclitaxel: a Gynecologic Oncology Group study. *Gynecol Oncol* 2009;112:543–552.
39. Sears J, Greven KM, Hoen HM, Randall ME. Prognostic factors and treatment outcome for patients with locally recurrent endometrial cancer. *Cancer* 1994;74:1303–1308.
40. Wylie J, Irwin C, Pintilie M, *et al.* Results of radical radiotherapy for recurrent endometrial cancer. *Gynecol Oncol* 2000;77:66–72.

41. Ball H, Blessing JA, Lentz SS, Mutch DG. A phase II trial of Taxol in advanced and recurrent adenocarcinoma of the endometrium: a Gynecologic Oncology Group study. *Gynecol Oncol* 1996;62:278–281.
42. von Hoff DD, Kronmal R, O'Toole RV, Surwit EA, Hutton JJ, Alberts DS. Phase II study of fludarabine phosphate in patients with advanced endometrial cancer. A Southwest Oncology Group study. *Am J Clin Oncol* 1991;14:193–194.
43. Gunthert AR, Ackermann S, Beckmann MW, *et al.* Phase II study of weekly docetaxel in patients with recurrent or metastatic endometrial cancer: AGO Uterus-4. *Gynecol Oncol* 2007;104:86–90.
44. Thigpen JT, Brady MF, Homesley HD, *et al.* Phase III trial of doxorubicin with or without cisplatin in advanced endometrial carcinoma: a Gynecologic Oncology Group study. *J Clin Oncol* 2004;22:3902–3908.
45. Gallion HH, Brunetto VL, Cibull M, *et al.* Randomized phase III trial of standard timed doxorubicin plus cisplatin versus circadian timed doxorubicin plus cisplatin in stage III and IV or recurrent endometrial carcinoma: a Gynecologic Oncology Group study. *J Clin Oncol* 2008;21:3808–3813.
46. Fleming GF, Filiaci VL, Bentley RC, *et al.* Phase III randomized trial of doxorubicin + cisplatin versus doxorubicin + 24-h paclitaxel + filgrastim in endometrial carcinoma: a Gynecologic Oncology Group study. *Ann Oncol* 2004;15:1173–1178.
47. Fleming GF, Brunetto VL, Cella D, *et al.* Phase III trial of doxorubicin plus cisplatin with or without paclitaxel plus filgrastim in advanced endometrial carcinoma: a Gynecologic Oncology Group study. *J Clin Oncol* 2004;22:2159–2166.
48. Lentz SS, Brady MF, Major FJ, Reid GC, Soper JT. High-dose megestrol acetate in advanced or recurrent endometrial carcinoma: a Gynecologic Oncology Group study. *J Clin Oncol* 1996;14:357–361.
49. Thigpen JT, Brady MF, Alvarez RD, *et al.* Oral medroxyprogesterone acetate in the treatment of advanced or recurrent endometrial carcinoma: a dose-response study by the Gynecologic Oncology Group. *J Clin Oncol* 1999;17:1736–1744.
50. Thigpen JT, Brady MF, Homesley HD, Soper JT, Bell J. Tamoxifen in the treatment of advanced or recurrent endometrial carcinoma: a Gynecologic Oncology Group study. *J Clin Oncol* 2001;19:364–367.

# 8

# UTERINE SARCOMA

*Andrea R. Hagemann*

## INTRODUCTION

Uterine sarcomas comprise a varied group of rare smooth muscle and connective tissue tumors, accounting for only 1% of female genital tract malignancies and 3–7% of uterine cancers.[1] As a whole, these tumors behave more aggressively, have a greater tendency to develop distant recurrences, and carry a poorer prognosis compared to endometrial carcinoma.[2] Because of their rarity, uterine sarcomas have traditionally been grouped together in the literature, but differences in histopathology and tumor biology translate into important differences in clinical management, and our understanding of this group of tumors is still evolving. In this chapter, we will review the histopathologic classifications, clinical manifestations, diagnosis, and current staging and treatment options for each of these tumors.

## CLASSIFICATION AND TERMINOLOGY

Advances in our knowledge of the biology of these rare tumors have led to reclassification by the World Health Organization (WHO) in 2003 (Table 1) and new staging criteria by the International Federation of Gynecology and Obstetrics (FIGO) in 2009 (Table 2).[3]

The uterus is composed of myometrial smooth muscle, endometrial stroma and epithelium, and connective tissue and vascular elements. Together, the smooth muscle and stromal elements of the uterus are referred to as the mesenchyma. With this in mind, the WHO and

elevated in patients with uterine sarcoma, but this does not seem to correlate with histologic subtype.[6] Preoperative full-body imaging with ultrasonography, chest X-ray, computed tomography, or magnetic resonance imaging (MRI) should also be performed to exclude metastatic disease in the workup of a suspicious pelvic or uterine mass. Even when appropriate workup does not reveal a malignancy, the possibility should be discussed if conservative measures such as hormonal therapy, endometrial ablation, myomectomy, or morcellation are considered.

## SMOOTH MUSCLE TUMORS: STUMP AND LEIOMYOSARCOMA

### Smooth Muscle Tumor of Uncertain Malignant Potential

#### *Histopathology*

STUMPs are uterine smooth muscle tumors that are not unequivocally benign or malignant on microscopic examination. The borderline nature of these tumors does not allow for definite prediction of their clinical behavior. These tumors include the following microscopic features: (1) tumor cell necrosis as the only worrisome finding, (2) necrosis of uncertain type and either marked diffuse atypia or more than 10 mitotic figures per 10 high-power fields, or (3) greater than 15 mitotic figures per 10 high-power fields as the only worrisome finding.[7]

#### *Diagnosis and treatment*

STUMPs are often diagnosed after myomectomy or hysterectomy. Removal of the uterus after a diagnosis of STUMP in a myomectomy specimen should be considered, but is not required. Close follow-up with pelvic exams, a baseline chest radiograph, and abdominal imaging is suggested. Adjuvant chemotherapy is not recommended.

#### *Recurrence*

In a recent study of 41 patients with STUMP from a single institution, the overall recurrence rate was 3 out of 41 (7%), with a mean recurrence-free interval of 42 months. One quarter of patients were diagnosed following a myomectomy; none of these patients had a subsequent hysterectomy and none recurred.[8] One recurrence was consistent with LMS and two with STUMP, all occurring in patients who had undergone total abdominal hysterectomy whose recurrences were as retroperitoneal masses. Another case report has documented diffuse lung metastases with biopsy-proven STUMP recurrence nine years following initial diagnosis, with treatment for recurrence including both GnRH agonists and an aromatase inhibitor.[9]

### *Prognosis*

Although data are limited to small case series and case reports, patients with uterine STUMP generally have a favorable prognosis. In contrast to LMS, race and ethnicity do not seem to play a role in the recurrence or prognosis of STUMP.[8] Despite the overall favorable prognosis, it is still recommended that patients with STUMP undergo close surveillance and follow-up, especially since case reports have shown recurrence to occur, albeit rarely, as LMS.

## Leiomyosarcoma

### *Epidemiology*

With the exclusion of carcinosarcoma from the category of uterine sarcomas, LMS accounts for at least 80% of uterine sarcomas,[7] but only 1–2% of uterine malignancies. The mean age at diagnosis is 60, but ranges in age from the third to ninth decades; they are twice as common in African American women as compared to Caucasian women.[10] It is a common misconception that LMS originates from benign leiomyoma. Different karyotypic anomalies in leiomyoma and leiomyosarcoma do not suggest a common pathogenesis.[11,12] The incidence of sarcomas in patients operated on for presumed benign leiomyomas is low (0.23%), even for rapidly growing fibroids (0.27%).[13] However, most caution should be taken for postmenopausal patients with symptomatic fibroids or a pelvic mass, where the incidence of LMS is 1–2%.[14]

## *Histopathology*

Leiomyosarcomas are typically solitary, but can be associated with fibroids. The mean diameter of LMS is 10 cm, and less than 5% arise in the cervix. Microscopically, they are a smooth muscle neoplasm characterized by (1) hypercellularity, (2) diffuse moderate to marked nuclear atypia, (3) high mitotic rate, and (4) tumor cell necrosis[7] (see Fig. 1).

On a molecular level, LMS is known to be genetically unstable with multiple complex karyotypes, several of which have potential therapeutic implications. Mutations or overexpression of p53 have been described.[15] Most leiomyosarcomas express platelet-derived growth factor receptor

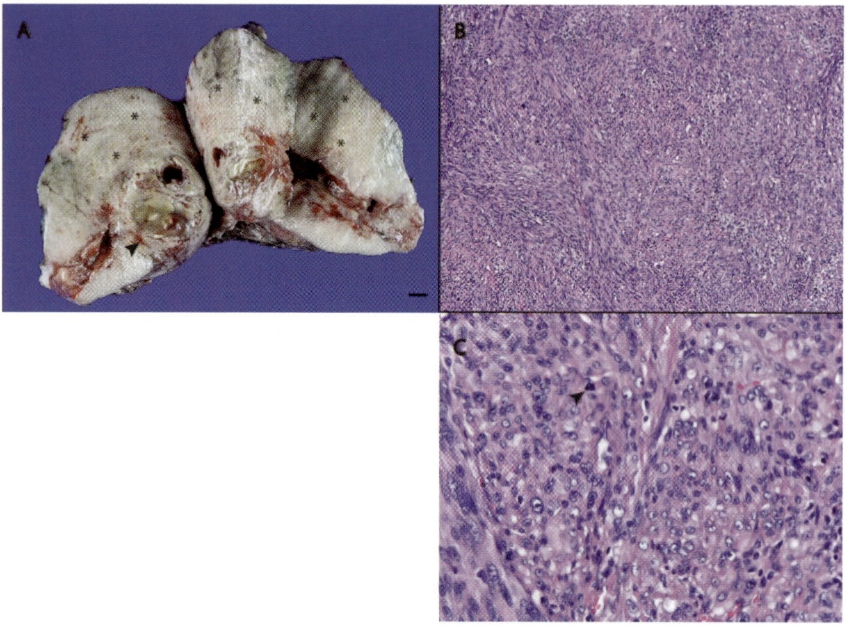


Figure 1. Leiomyosarcoma in a 62-year-old woman with postmenopausal bleeding and a biopsy diagnosis of high-grade spindle and epithelioid cell neoplasm. (A) Bivalved gross specimen demonstrating typical appearance for leiomyosarcoma: a dominant intramural lesion with frank hemorrhage and necrosis. Although the main mass was measured at 4.3 cm, microscopically the lesion permeated the rest of the myometrium (asterisks). Scale bar, 1 cm. (B) Microscopically, the tumor demonstrates fascicles of myoid cells intersecting at right angles. Even at low magnification, nuclear atypia and pleomorphism are apparent. (C) Mitoses (arrowhead) numbered at least 36 per 50 high-power fields. 400x.

alpha (PDGFR-$\alpha$), Wilms' tumor gene (*WT1*), aromatase, and gonadotropin-releasing hormone receptor.[16] Seventy-five percent will show immunoreactivity for c-KIT, but no mutations have been identified.[15,17] They are also characterized by a lack of expression of epidermal growth factor receptor (EGFR) and epidermal growth factor receptor 2 (ErbB2). The genetic instability of LMS is likely a result of an accumulation of multiple genetic defects, and leads to its aggressive clinical phenotype.

## *Diagnosis and treatment*

The standard treatment for LMS is hysterectomy with bilateral salpingo-oophorectomy. Lymphadenectomy is not part of the staging criteria for sarcomas and is only indicated for cytoreductive effect. In a large study of almost 1,400 patients with LMS, neither routine lymphadenectomy nor oophorectomy in premenopausal women were found to have a significant impact on overall survival.[18] However, oophorectomy is usually performed in postmenopausal patients given the small chance of ovarian metastases, or the potential for hormone sensitivity in a low-grade tumor.

Given the high rate of recurrence for LMS, systemic chemotherapy is recommended in most settings, especially for advanced-stage disease. Older studies for adult soft-tissue sarcoma, which have included uterine sarcomas in some but not all, have shown the combination of an anthracycline, such as doxorubicin, and ifosfamide to be an active systemic regimen for this group of tumors.[2] However, only two randomized trials of adjuvant treatment specific to uterine sarcomas have been performed, one using adjuvant doxorubicin, and the other examining postoperative pelvic radiation;[19–21] neither has shown a survival benefit.

Gemcitabine has now emerged as an active agent against LMS. A small prospective study of 25 patients has recently shown promise for adjuvant therapy with gemcitabine (900 mg/m$^2$ on days 1 and 8) and docetaxel (75 mg/m$^2$ on day 8) every three weeks for four cycles. Gemcitabine is given at a fixed-dose-rate infusion of 10 mg/m$^2$/min to optimize the concentration (20 $\mu$mol/l) for formation of the active gemcitabine metabolite.[22] After a median follow-up of 49 months, 10 (45%) of the 23 evaluable patients remained progression-free at two years, with a median progression-free survival of 13 months, and median overall survival not reached at the time of publication.[23]

There is growing support in the literature that for early-stage LMS, a tumor-free interval of six months after initial treatment predicts a less aggressive tumor biology, which may be responsive to hormonal treatment. To that end, close follow-up, followed by targeted therapy or resection of metastatic disease for patients with recurrence more than six months following hysterectomy, is a reasonable approach to management of early-stage LMS.[16,24] Targeted and other new therapies under recent or current investigation include medroxyprogesterone (targeting progesterone receptor),[25] sunitinib (targeting receptor tyrosine kinases including PDGFRs), letrozole (targeting aromatase),[26] deforolimus (targeting mammalian target of rapamycin [mTOR]),[16] and trabectedin (ecteinascidin 743).[27] A summary of treatment options can be found in Table 4.

## *Prognosis*

Uterine LMS has a worse prognosis stage for stage compared to other sarcomas, and certainly compared to endometrial cancer. However, a wide span of survival rates ranging anywhere from 4% to 76% can be found in the literature.[18,28] A recent analysis of 219 patients with LMS at a single institution using the previous FIGO staging system showed the five-year overall survival for stages I, II, III, and IV to be 57%, 29%, 35%, and 16%[29] (see Table 5). A larger SEER database analysis of 1,396 patients recently found that five-year overall disease-specific survival (DSS) was 76%, with DSS for stages I, II, III, and IV being 76%, 60%, 45%, and 29%, respectively.[18] As reflected in the 2009 FIGO staging system, tumor size and degree of spread outside the pelvis are the most important prognostic factors. Increasing age, African American race, higher grade, and lack of primary surgery have also been found to portend a worse prognosis. A GOG study noted mitotic rate to be a significant predictor of progression-free interval.[30] Because of the high risk of recurrence, the National Comprehensive Cancer Network (NCCN) recommends that surveillance for recurrent disease should include a physical exam every three months for two years following completion of initial treatment, with

Table 4. Summary of adjuvant treatment options for LMS, ESS, and carcinosarcoma.

| Uterine tumor | Treatment options |
|---|---|
| Endometrial stromal sarcoma | |
| Early stage (I–II) | Observation alone<br>Consider hormonal therapy |
| Advanced stage | Hormonal therapy<br>• Progestins<br>— Medroxyprogesterone acetate 250 mg q day<br>— Megestrol 160 mg q day<br>• Aromatase inhibitors<br>— Letrozole 2.5 mg q day<br>— Anastrozole<br>• Gonadotropin-releasing hormone agonists<br>±Radiation therapy |
| Leiomyosarcoma | |
| Early stage | Observation alone<br>Targeted therapy<br>• If ER+: Aromatase inhibitor[26]<br>• If PR+: Medroxyprogesterone[25]<br>Consider systemic chemotherapy<br>• Ifosfamide + doxorubicin |
| Advanced stage | Systemic chemotherapy<br>• Gemcitabine + docetaxel[59]<br>±Radiation therapy |
| Carcinosarcoma | |
| Stages I–II | Systemic chemotherapy<br>• Cisplatin + doxorubicin + etoposide<br>• Ifosfamide + cisplatin |
| Advanced stage | Systemic chemotherapy<br>• Ifosfamide + cisplatin<br>• Ifosfamide + paclitaxel<br>• Carboplatin + paclitaxel<br>Consider radiation therapy |

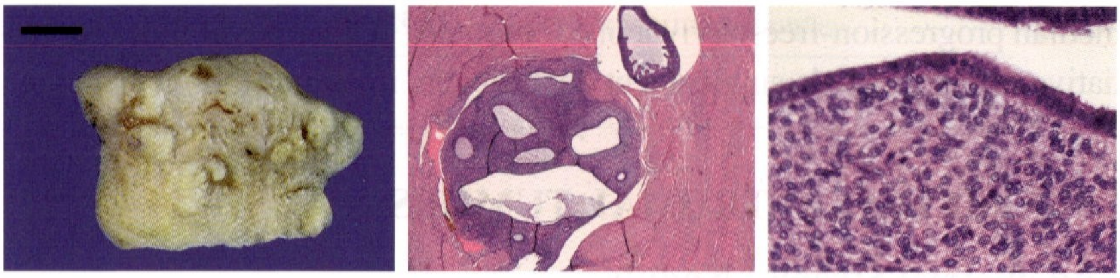

(A) (B) (C)

Figure 2. Endometrial Stromal Sarcoma in a 50-year-old woman. (A) Cross section of endomyometrium. Worm-like intravascular plugs are present; this is the presentation that was formerly referred to as "endolymphatic stromal myosis". The uterine serosa is at the bottom. Scale bar, 1 cm. (B) Lymphatic vessels of the myometrium contain macroscopic plugs of mildly atypical stroma with intermixed benign glands, most likely the result of divergent differentiation. There are subtle periglandular hypocellular cuffs, not to be confused with the hypercellular "cambium" layer of adenosarcoma. Additionally, the vascular invasion and failure to form a discrete mass argue against the diagnosis of adenosarcoma here. Identical lesions were found in the lungs. 40x. (C) At high power, occasional stromal mitoses are seen. The epithelium is benign. 200x.

myometrium, or both, with characteristic "worm-like" plugs of tumor that fill and distend the myometrial vessels.[7] Microscopically, they exhibit mild nuclear atypia and rarely necrosis (see Fig. 2).

## *Diagnosis*

ESS may be suspected on the basis of imaging obtained for the workup of hormonal irregularities or pelvic pain symptoms. Ultrasound may reveal a hypoechogenic mass with irregular margins, with irregular central or circular vascularization. Compared to endometrial cancer, MRI for ESS will more often show nodular lesions at the margin, intramyometrial nodular extension, and multiple nodular masses.[35] Preoperative full-body imaging is mandatory, as up to one third of cases will present with peritoneal or lung extension.

## *Treatment*

The preferred treatment for ESS is hysterectomy. The roles of oophorectomy and lymphadenectomy, however, have been debated. Oophorectomy has historically been recommended, as ESS is a hormone-sensitive treatment, but has not been shown to have a survival advantage or to improve recurrence rates.[33,36] Furthermore, smaller studies have correlated estrogen replacement with worsened outcome.[37] Therefore, ovarian preservation is reasonable especially in young, premenopausal women with small tumors. As reflected in the new staging system, lymphadenectomy is not mandated (Table 2). Several retrospective studies have failed to show a survival benefit for lymphadenectomy. If there is obvious transperitoneal spread at the time of surgery, cytoreductive surgery may help to improve treatment response.

Data on treatment outcomes for ESS are limited, but the mainstay of adjuvant treatment is hormonal therapy with either progestins or aromatase inhibitors. Adjuvant therapy with medroxyprogesterone (250 mg) or megestrol (160 mg) daily for two years following initial surgery has been shown to have some benefit.[37,38] Aromatase inhibitors such as letrozole, aminoglutethimide, or anastrozole can be used as well. Tamoxifen and estrogen replacement should be avoided, as their long-term use has been associated with recurrence of ESS.[39]

## *Prognosis*

Endometrial stromal sarcomas are notable for their indolent course and overall favorable prognosis. The five-year overall survival (OS) for all women with ESS is 80–100%; 100% OS for stage Ia and 93% for stage Ib.[36] Long-term follow-up is recommended, as late recurrences are common even in patients with early-stage disease. Approximately one third to half of patients will develop recurrence, most commonly in the pelvis and abdomen. Less frequent sites of recurrence include the lung and vagina.[34] In a recent multivariate analysis performed from SEER data, older patients, black race, advanced stage, higher grade, lack of primary surgery, and nodal metastasis were independent poor prognostic factors.[33]

## *Recurrence*

The median time to recurrence is 65 months for stage I disease and nine months for higher stages.[34] Because of its indolent nature, repeated surgical strongest prognostic factor.[42] Myometrial invasion and sarcomatous overgrowth also portend a worse prognosis. Recurrences occur most often in the vagina or pelvis, most often more than five years after hysterectomy. Five percent of patients will present with local or distant recurrence, and biopsies of these recurrences almost always show a transition to a pure sarcomatous element.[7,43]

# CARCINOSARCOMA

## Epidemiology

Uterine carcinosarcomas (CS) have historically been referred to as malignant mixed müllerian tumors, and have until recently been classified among uterine sarcomas. They are rare, accounting for 1.2% of uterine neoplasms and affecting 7 per 100,000 women over the age of 35 in the United States per year.[10] The median age at diagnosis is 62–67.

Carcinosarcomas are now categorized as carcinomas, because they appear to derive from a monoclonal cancer cell with sarcomatous metaplasia. These tumors behave more similarly to endometrial carcinoma than to sarcomas, and are staged according to the FIGO criteria for endometrial cancer. Like endometrial cancer, nulliparity, obesity, and use of exogenous estrogen and tamoxifen are known risk factors.[44] However, they are still felt to represent a distinct biologic entity. A recent SEER comparison of almost 5,000 women with grade 3 endometrial cancer and 4,000 women with CS showed that women with CS were more likely to be older, more often non-white, more likely to present with advanced-stage disease, and carried a worse survival.[45] A prior history of pelvic radiation may be a risk factor.

## Histopathology

Grossly, carcinosarcomas typically have a soft, polypoid tumor filling the endometrial cavity, often with evidence of myometrial invasion. Microscopically, the carcinomatous and sarcomatous elements are intimately mixed. The carcinomatous element is usually high-grade endometrioid or serous histology. Likewise, the sarcomatous component

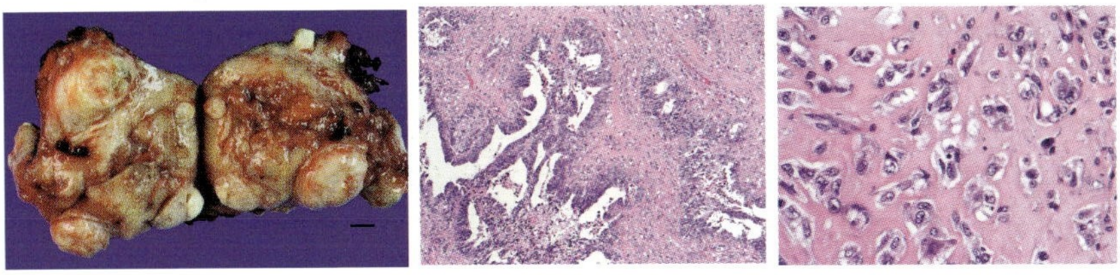

(A) (B) (C)

Figure 3. Carcinosarcoma, FIGO grade III, in a 72-year-old woman with a preoperative diagnosis of poorly differentiated uterine cancer. (A) Gross specimen bivalved in the coronal plane to demonstrate cavity filled with polypoid, necrotic material. Scale bar, 1 cm. (B) Mixed malignant epithelial and mesenchymal elements. Epithelial elements show endometrioid histology with cytologic atypia and architectural disturbances including cribriforming and nuclear stratification. In stromal elements, cytologic atypia is prominent. 100x original magnification. (C) High-power view of heterologous elements (nested cells growing in a chondroid matrix). 400x.

is also usually high-grade, with 50–75% presenting with heterologous elements such as rhabdomyosarcoma, chondrosarcoma, or osteosarcoma[7] (see Fig. 3).

## Diagnosis and Treatment

Diagnosis is made based on histology, often on biopsy, with confirmation following surgery with total abdominal hysterectomy, bilateral salpingo-oophorectomy, and staging lymphadenectomy. The incidence of regional lymph node metastasis is 20%, and lymphadenectomy is indicated, as its performance has been associated with significantly improved survival.[46] Optimal cytoreduction is recommended, as benefits are likely to be similar to those found with debulking of advanced high-grade endometrial cancer.

Regardless of stage, carcinosarcomas have a high risk of recurring (up to 60%), and although it has been difficult to identify a superior regimen for the treatment of both the epithelial and sarcomatous components of CS, adjuvant chemotherapy is recommended, and radiation may also be of some benefit. For all stages, ifosfamide, platinum, and doxorubicin have been the agents most examined in clinical trials. A phase II trial of ifosfamide and mesna in patients with CS previously untreated with chemotherapy showed a 32.3% response rate (compared to a 17.2% rate in LMS).[47] For early-stage CS (stages I and II), the combination of cisplatin, doxorubicin, and etoposide has been reported to have a two-year overall survival of 92%,[48] while ifosfamide and cisplatin together was reported by the GOG to have a 69% PFS and 82% OS[49] (see Table 7).

A randomized trial for postoperative radiation versus observation in early-stage (stages I and II) uterine sarcoma patients was recently published by the European Organisation for Research and Treatment of Cancer (EORTC) group and showed a trend towards improved local control but no improvement in survival, likely due to the development of extra-pelvic metastases.[20] It is still reasonable to consider a combination approach with chemotherapy followed by pelvic irradiation. In a retrospective review, ifosfamide and cisplatin followed by pelvic irradiation was associated with a decreased mortality compared to either chemotherapy or radiation therapy alone.[50]

For those diagnosed at an advanced stage, a combination of either platinum or ifosfamide with a taxane is recommended. GOG 108 included patients with measurable advanced or recurrent CS who were randomized to ifosfamide with or without cisplatin. The combination arm was highly toxic, and showed a higher response rate (54% versus 34%) and a longer progression-free survival (6 months versus 4 months), but no difference in overall survival (9 months versus 8 months).[51] GOG 161 compared ifosfamide and paclitaxel to ifosfamide alone, and found a superior overall survival benefit with the combination regimen (13.5 months vs. 8.4 months).[52] Toxicity was improved by reducing the ifosfamide to a three-day infusion time. These encouraging results with paclitaxel may make sense given the predominance of the epithelial component of CS, and the known activity of paclitaxel in endometrial adenocarcinoma. Retrospective reviews and a recent phase II GOG study have shown a reasonable antitumor effect of carboplatin and paclitaxel for advanced or recurrent disease.[53,54] While phase III data are not available, carboplatin and paclitaxel may be as effective and have fewer dose-limiting toxicities than ifosfamide and paclitaxel. This combination also offers the advantages of a more convenient dosing schedule, decreased cost, and ease of delivery.[54]

Table 7. Summary of important Gynecologic Oncology Group trials for uterine sarcomas.

| GOG protocol | Patient population | Agents tested | Result | Reference |
|---|---|---|---|---|
| 20 | Stages I and II uterine sarcoma | Adriamycin v. no adjuvant therapy | No significant difference | Omura *et al.* 1983, 1985[19,21] |
| | Advanced uterine sarcoma | Adriamycin ± dacarbazine | Combination 24% response rate (ns) | |
| 40 | Early-stage uterine sarcomas (LMS and CS) | — | Defining prognostic indicators (see text) | Silverberg *et al.* 1990[60] |
| 42 | Recurrent or advanced uterine sarcomas (LMS and CS) | Phase III: Doxorubicin ± cyclophosphamide | No significant difference | Muss *et al.* 1985[61] |
| 108 | Advanced, persistent, or recurrent carcinosarcoma | Phase III: Ifosfamide ± cisplatin | Slight prolongation of PFS with combination, no change in OS | Sutton *et al.* 2000[51] |
| 117 | Stages I and II carcinosarcoma | Ifosfamide and cisplatin | Tolerable toxicity profile; 2-yr PFS 69%; 2-yr OS 82%; 7-yr PFS 54%; 7-yr OS 52%; | Sutton *et al.* 2005[49] |
| 150 | Stages I–IV carcinosarcoma s/p complete resection | Phase III: Adjuvant whole abdominal irradiation (WAI) v. cisplatin, ifosfamide, mesna (CIM) | Recurrence 21% lower in CIM than WAI | Wolfson *et al.* 2007[62] |
| 161 | Advanced or recurrent carcinosarcoma | Ifosfamide ± paclitaxel | Improved OS with combination | Homesley *et al.* 2007[52] |

## Prognosis

Carcinosarcomas are highly aggressive and carry a poor prognosis. The overall five-year survival is approximately 30%, and only 50% for even those with stage I disease.[30,55] The presence of clear cell or serous features, or heterologous elements such as muscle, cartilage, or bone, are particularly poor prognostic factors for stage I tumors. The depth of myometrial invasion and lymphovascular space invasion are also important prognostic factors. Compared to ovarian carcinosarcomas, uterine CS typically present at an earlier stage, but have a more aggressive course and shorter progression-free interval.[56]

## Recurrence

Treatment for recurrent disease is mainly palliative, rarely curative, and as such, quality of life considerations should play a role in decision-making. Paclitaxel has been shown to have a response rate of 18.2% in patients with persistent or recurrent CS who have failed other treatments.[57] Weekly docetaxel and gemcitabine were recently studied as a potential combination for recurrent CS, but toxicities were great, and progressive disease was seen in 50% of patients.[58]

## REFERENCES

1. Jemal A, Siegel R, Ward E, Hao Y, Xu J, Thun MJ. Cancer statistics, 2009. *CA Cancer J Clin* 2009;59(4):225–249.
2. Gadducci A, Cosio S, Romanini A, Genazzani AR. The management of patients with uterine sarcoma: a debated clinical challenge. *Crit Rev Oncol Hematol* 2008;65(2):129–142.
3. Prat J. FIGO staging for uterine sarcomas. *Int J Gynaecol Obstet* 2009;104(3):177–178.
4. Bell SW, Kempson RL, Hendrickson MR. Problematic uterine smooth muscle neoplasms. A clinicopathologic study of 213 cases. *Am J Surg Pathol* 1994;18(6):535–558.
5. Bansal N, Herzog TJ, Burke W, Cohen CJ, Wright JD. The utility of preoperative endometrial sampling for the detection of uterine sarcomas. *Gynecol Oncol* 2008;110(1):43–48.

6. Duk JM, Bouma J, Burger GT, Nap M, De Bruijn HW. CA 125 in serum and tumor from patients with uterine sarcoma. *Int J Gynecol Cancer* 1994;4(3):156–160.
7. Clement PY, Young RH. Mesenchymal and mixed epithelial-mesenchymal tumors of the uterine corpus and cervix. In: *Atlas of Gynecologic Surgical Pathology*. Philadelphia: Elsevier, 2008, pp. 194–235.
8. Guntupalli SR, Ramirez PT, Anderson ML, Milam MR, Bodurka DC, Malpica A. Uterine smooth muscle tumor of uncertain malignant potential: a retrospective analysis. *Gynecol Oncol* 2009;113(3):324–326.
9. Berretta R, Rolla M, Merisio C, Giordano G, Nardelli GB. Uterine smooth muscle tumor of uncertain malignant potential: a three-case report. *Int J Gynecol Cancer* 2008;18(5):1121–1126.
10. Brooks SE, Zhan M, Cote T, Baquet CR. Surveillance, epidemiology, and end results analysis of 2677 cases of uterine sarcoma 1989–1999. *Gynecol Oncol* 2004;93(1):204–208.
11. Packenham JP, du Manoir S, Schrock E, *et al.* Analysis of genetic alterations in uterine leiomyomas and leiomyosarcomas by comparative genomic hybridization. *Mol Carcinog* 1997;19(4):273–279.
12. Quade BJ, Pinto AP, Howard DR, Peters WA 3rd, Crum CP. Frequent loss of heterozygosity for chromosome 10 in uterine leiomyosarcoma in contrast to leiomyoma. *Am J Pathol* 1999;154(3):945–950.
13. Parker WH, Fu YS, Berek JS. Uterine sarcoma in patients operated on for presumed leiomyoma and rapidly growing leiomyoma. *Obstet Gynecol* 1994;83(3):414–418.
14. Leibsohn S, d'Ablaing G, Mishell DR Jr, Schlaerth JB. Leiomyosarcoma in a series of hysterectomies performed for presumed uterine leiomyomas. *Am J Obstet Gynecol* 1990;162(4):968–974; discussion 74–76.
15. D'Angelo E, Prat J. Uterine sarcomas: a review. *Gynecol Oncol* 2010; 116(1):131–139.
16. Amant F, Coosemans A, Debiec-Rychter M, Timmerman D, Vergote I. Clinical management of uterine sarcomas. *Lancet Oncol* 2009;10(12): 1188–1198.
17. D'Angelo E, Spagnoli LG, Prat J. Comparative clinicopathologic and immunohistochemical analysis of uterine sarcomas diagnosed using the World Health Organization classification system. *Hum Pathol* 2009; 40(11):1571–1585.

18. Kapp DS, Shin JY, Chan JK. Prognostic factors and survival in 1396 patients with uterine leiomyosarcomas: emphasis on impact of lymphadenectomy and oophorectomy. *Cancer* 2008;112(4):820–830.
19. Omura GA, Blessing JA, Major F, *et al.* A randomized clinical trial of adjuvant adriamycin in uterine sarcomas: a Gynecologic Oncology Group study. *J Clin Oncol* 1985;3(9):1240–1245.
20. Reed NS, Mangioni C, Malmstrom H, *et al.* Phase III randomised study to evaluate the role of adjuvant pelvic radiotherapy in the treatment of uterine sarcomas stages I and II: an European Organisation for Research and Treatment of Cancer Gynaecological Cancer Group Study (protocol 55874). *Eur J Cancer* 2008;44(6):808–818.
21. Omura GA, Major FJ, Blessing JA, *et al.* A randomized study of adriamycin with and without dimethyl triazenoimidazole carboxamide in advanced uterine sarcomas. *Cancer* 1983;52(4):626–632.
22. Grunewald R, Kantarjian H, Keating MJ, Abbruzzese J, Tarassoff P, Plunkett W. Pharmacologically directed design of the dose rate and schedule of 2',2'-difluorodeoxycytidine (Gemcitabine) administration in leukemia. *Cancer Res* 1990;50(21):6823–6826.
23. Hensley ML, Ishill N, Soslow R, *et al.* Adjuvant gemcitabine plus docetaxel for completely resected stages I-IV high grade uterine leiomyosarcoma: results of a prospective study. *Gynecol Oncol* 2009;112(3): 563–567.
24. Giuntoli RL 2nd, Garrett-Mayer E, Bristow RE, Gostout BS. Secondary cytoreduction in the management of recurrent uterine leiomyosarcoma. *Gynecol Oncol* 2007;106(1):82–88.
25. Uchida T, Nakakawaji K, Sakamoto J, *et al.* The effectiveness of medroxyprogesterone in the treatment of multiple metastasizing leiomyosarcomas: report of a case. *Surg Today* 1996;26(2):138–141.
26. O'Cearbhaill R, Zhou Q, Iasonos A, *et al.* Treatment of advanced uterine leiomyosarcoma with aromatase inhibitors. *Gynecol Oncol* 2010;116(3): 424–429.
27. Le Cesne A, Blay JY, Judson I, *et al.* Phase II study of ET-743 in advanced soft tissue sarcomas: a European Organisation for the Research and Treatment of Cancer (EORTC) soft tissue and bone sarcoma group trial. *J Clin Oncol* 2005;23(3):576–584.

28. Livi L, Paiar F, Meldolesi E, *et al.* Treatment of uterine sarcoma at the University of Florence from 1980–2001. *Tumori* 2005;91(2):139–143.
29. Zivanovic O, Leitao MM, Iasonos A, *et al.* Stage-specific outcomes of patients with uterine leiomyosarcoma: a comparison of the International Federation of Gynecology and Obstetrics and American Joint Committee on Cancer staging systems. *J Clin Oncol* 2009;27(12):2066–2072.
30. Major FJ, Blessing JA, Silverberg SG, *et al.* Prognostic factors in early-stage uterine sarcoma. A Gynecologic Oncology Group study. *Cancer* 1993; 71(4 Suppl):1702–1709.
31. Hensley ML, Blessing JA, Degeest K, Abulafia O, Rose PG, Homesley HD. Fixed-dose rate gemcitabine plus docetaxel as second-line therapy for metastatic uterine leiomyosarcoma: a Gynecologic Oncology Group phase II study. *Gynecol Oncol* 2008;109(3):323–328.
32. Oliva E, Clement PB, Young RH. Endometrial stromal tumors: an update on a group of tumors with a protean phenotype. *Adv Anat Pathol* 2000; 7(5):257–281.
33. Chan JK, Kawar NM, Shin JY *et al.* Endometrial stromal sarcoma: a population-based analysis. *Br J Cancer* 2008;99(8):1210–1215.
34. Chang KL, Crabtree GS, Lim-Tan SK, Kempson RL, Hendrickson MR. Primary uterine endometrial stromal neoplasms. A clinicopathologic study of 117 cases. *Am J Surg Pathol* 1990;14(5):415–438.
35. Ueda M, Otsuka M, Hatakenaka M, *et al.* MR imaging findings of uterine endometrial stromal sarcoma: differentiation from endometrial carcinoma. *Eur Radiol* 2001;11(1):28–33.
36. Shah JP, Bryant CS, Kumar S, Ali-Fehmi R, Malone JM Jr, Morris RT. Lymphadenectomy and ovarian preservation in low-grade endometrial stromal sarcoma. *Obstet Gynecol* 2008;112(5):1102–1108.
37. Chu MC, Mor G, Lim C, Zheng W, Parkash V, Schwartz PE. Low-grade endometrial stromal sarcoma: hormonal aspects. *Gynecol Oncol* 2003; 90(1):170–176.
38. Amant F, de Knijf A, van Calster B, *et al.* Clinical study investigating the role of lymphadenectomy, surgical castration and adjuvant hormonal treatment in endometrial stromal sarcoma. *Br J Cancer* 2007;97(9):1194–1199.
39. Pink D, Lindner T, Mrozek A, *et al.* Harm or benefit of hormonal treatment in metastatic low-grade endometrial stromal sarcoma: single center

experience with 10 cases and review of the literature. *Gynecol Oncol* 2006;101(3):464–469.

40. Sutton G, Blessing J, Hanjani P, Kramer P. Phase II evaluation of liposomal doxorubicin (Doxil) in recurrent or advanced leiomyosarcoma of the uterus: a Gynecologic Oncology Group study. *Gynecol Oncol* 2005;96(3):749–752.
41. McCluggage WG, Haller HU, Kurman RJ, Kubick-Huch RA. Mixed epithelial and mesenchymal tumors. In: Tavassoli FA, Devilee P, eds., *Pathology and Genetics of Tumours of the Breast and Female Genital Organs*. Lyon: IARC Press, 2003, pp. 245–249.
42. Abeler VM, Royne O, Thoresen S, Danielsen HE, Nesland JM, Kristensen GB. Uterine sarcomas in Norway. A histopathological and prognostic survey of a total population from 1970 to 2000 including 419 patients. *Histopathology* 2009;54(3):355–364.
43. Clement PB, Scully RE. Mullerian adenosarcoma of the uterus: a clinicopathologic analysis of 100 cases with a review of the literature. *Hum Pathol* 1990;21(4):363–381.
44. Zelmanowicz A, Hildesheim A, Sherman ME, *et al*. Evidence for a common etiology for endometrial carcinomas and malignant mixed mullerian tumors. *Gynecol Oncol* 1998;69(3):253–257.
45. Bansal N, Herzog TJ, Seshan VE, *et al*. Uterine carcinosarcomas and grade 3 endometrioid cancers: evidence for distinct tumor behavior. *Obstet Gynecol* 2008;112(1):64–70.
46. Nemani D, Mitra N, Guo M, Lin L. Assessing the effects of lymphadenectomy and radiation therapy in patients with uterine carcinosarcoma: a SEER analysis. *Gynecol Oncol* 2008;111(1):82–88.
47. Sutton GP, Blessing JA, Rosenshein N, Photopulos G, DiSaia PJ. Phase II trial of ifosfamide and mesna in mixed mesodermal tumors of the uterus (a Gynecologic Oncology Group study). *Am J Obstet Gynecol* 1989;161(2):309–312.
48. Resnik E, Chambers SK, Carcangiu ML, Kohorn EI, Schwartz PE, Chambers JT. A phase II study of etoposide, cisplatin, and doxorubicin chemotherapy in mixed mullerian tumors (MMT) of the uterus. *Gynecol Oncol* 1995;56(3):370–375.
49. Sutton G, Kauderer J, Carson LF, Lentz SS, Whitney CW, Gallion H. Adjuvant ifosfamide and cisplatin in patients with completely resected stage I or II carcinosarcomas (mixed mesodermal tumors) of the uterus: a Gynecologic Oncology Group study. *Gynecol Oncol* 2005;96(3):630–634.

50. Menczer J, Levy T, Piura B, *et al.* A comparison between different postoperative treatment modalities of uterine carcinosarcoma. *Gynecol Oncol* 2005;97(1):166–170.
51. Sutton G, Brunetto VL, Kilgore L, *et al.* A phase III trial of ifosfamide with or without cisplatin in carcinosarcoma of the uterus: a Gynecologic Oncology Group study. *Gynecol Oncol* 2000;79(2):147–153.
52. Homesley HD, Filiaci V, Markman M, *et al.* Phase III trial of ifosfamide with or without paclitaxel in advanced uterine carcinosarcoma: a Gynecologic Oncology Group study. *J Clin Oncol* 2007;25(5):526–531.
53. Powell MA, Filiaci VL, Rose PG, *et al.* Phase II evaluation of paclitaxel and carboplatin in the treatment of carcinosarcoma of the uterus: a Gynecologic Oncology Group study. *J Clin Oncol* 2010;28(16):2727–2731.
54. Hoskins PJ, Le N, Ellard S, *et al.* Carboplatin plus paclitaxel for advanced or recurrent uterine malignant mixed mullerian tumors. The British Columbia Cancer Agency experience. *Gynecol Oncol* 2008;108(1):58–62.
55. Yamada SD, Burger RA, Brewster WR, Anton D, Kohler MF, Monk BJ. Pathologic variables and adjuvant therapy as predictors of recurrence and survival for patients with surgically evaluated carcinosarcoma of the uterus. *Cancer* 2000;88(12):2782–2786.
56. Garg G, Shah JP, Kumar S, Bryant CS, Munkarah A, Morris RT. Ovarian and uterine carcinosarcomas: a comparative analysis of prognostic variables and survival outcomes. *Int J Gynecol Cancer* 2010;20(5):888–894.
57. Curtin JP, Blessing JA, Soper JT, DeGeest K. Paclitaxel in the treatment of carcinosarcoma of the uterus: a gynecologic oncology group study. *Gynecol Oncol* 2001;83(2):268–270.
58. Miller BE, Blessing JA, Stehman FB, *et al.* A phase II evaluation of weekly gemcitabine and docetaxel for second-line treatment of recurrent carcinosarcoma of the uterus: a Gynecologic Oncology Group study. *Gynecol Oncol* 2010;118:139–144.
59. Hensley ML, Blessing JA, Mannel R, Rose PG. Fixed-dose rate gemcitabine plus docetaxel as first-line therapy for metastatic uterine leiomyosarcoma: a Gynecologic Oncology Group phase II trial. *Gynecol Oncol* 2008;109(3): 329–334.
60. Silverberg SG, Major FJ, Blessing JA, *et al.* Carcinosarcoma (malignant mixed mesodermal tumor) of the uterus. A Gynecologic Oncology Group pathologic study of 203 cases. *Int J Gynecol Pathol* 1990;9(1):1–19.

Table 1. FIGO Staging system for ovarian and fallopian tube carcinomas.

| | |
|---|---|
| **Stage I** | **Limited to the ovaries** |
| IA | Limited to one ovary, no capsular or surface involvement, negative ascites & peritoneal washings |
| IB | Limited to both ovaries, no capsular or surface involvement, negative ascites & peritoneal washings |
| IC | IA or IB with surface involvement, capsular rupture, malignant ascites or positive peritoneal washings |
| **Stage II** | **Pelvic extension** |
| IIA | Extension to the uterus &/or tubes |
| IIB | Extension to other pelvic organs |
| IIC | IIA or IIB with surface involvement, capsular rupture, malignant ascites or positive peritoneal washings |
| **Stage III** | **Tumor implants outside the pelvis, positive retroperitoneal or inguinal lymph nodes, or superficial liver metastases** |
| IIIA | Microscopic seeding of abdominal peritoneal surfaces, small bowel or mesentery or omentum |
| IIIB | Tumor implants outside the pelvis of <2 cm in diameter |
| IIIC | Tumor implants outside the pelvis of >2 cm in diameter, or positive retroperitoneal or inguinal lymph nodes |
| **Stage IV** | **Distant metastases, positive pleural effusion, parenchymal liver metastases** |

omentectomy, pelvic and para-aortic lymph node sampling, random peritoneal biopsies, and complete abdominal exploration should be performed. Stage IV disease may be confirmed with cytologically positive pleural fluid, histologically positive parenchymal liver lesions or supraclavicular lymph nodes. The FIGO staging system, revised in 1985, is presented in Table 1.

## TREATMENT

### Surgery

Surgery is not only the method by which patients with ovarian and fallopian tube carcinoma are staged, but is also the primary means of treatment.[1]

### *Early-stage disease*

Despite the lack of gross visual disease present in early-stage ovarian and fallopian tube cancer, complete surgical staging is still of utmost importance.[1] Young *et al.* found that in patients with presumed stage I and II disease who were surgically staged, 31% were upstaged, and of those, 77% were truly stage III.[9]

### *Advanced disease*

When advanced disease is present, the goal is not only appropriate staging but also surgical cytoreduction or debulking, as the volume of residual disease is directly associated with survival.[10] Optimally cytoreduced patients show a significant survival benefit over those patients who are suboptimally debulked, and there is a significant survival advantage in patients who are able to be debulked to less than 2 cm of residual disease.[11] Even patients with stage IV disease have shown an improvement in survival when optimal cytoreduction is performed.[12]

## Chemotherapy

### *Adjuvant chemotherapy*

For patients with stage IA or IB, grade 3 disease and greater, adjuvant chemotherapy is the standard of care. For early-stage disease (stages IA or IB, grade 3, or IC) a platinum/taxane doublet is given every 21 days for three to six cycles. GOG 157, a comparison of three versus six cycles of carboplatin (AUC 7.5) and paclitaxel (175 mg/m$^2$) in stage IA or IB, grade 3, and stage IC patients, demonstrated a lower but non-significant recurrence rate in the group receiving six cycles, as well as similar death rates, but an 11% versus 3% incidence of grade 3 or 4 neurotoxicity in the group receiving six versus three cycles.[13]

For patients with advanced disease (stage II and greater) the standard of care became six cycles of carboplatin (AUC 6) and paclitaxel (175 mg/m$^2$) every 21 days in 2003 when GOG 158, a non-inferiority study comparing cisplatin (75 mg/m$^2$) and paclitaxel (135 mg/m$^2$ over 24 hours) to carboplatin (AUC 7.5) and paclitaxel (175 mg/m$^2$ over 3 hours), showed that carboplatin and paclitaxel were not inferior to cisplatin and paclitaxel, and resulted in less toxicity.[14] A new era in chemotherapy began with intraperitoneal (IP) chemotherapy. GOG 172, a randomized phase III trial of patients with optimally debulked stage III ovarian carcinoma or primary peritoneal carcinoma comparing IP chemotherapy to intravenous (IV) chemotherapy, demonstrated progression-free and overall survival of 23.8 and 65.6 months, respectively, in patients receiving IP therapy while progression-free and overall survival were 18.3 and 49.7 months, respectively, in patients receiving IV therapy.[15] There is some controversy surrounding this trial given that the control arm used cisplatin (75 mg/m$^2$) instead of carboplatin, which is considered the platinum standard of care. There are also concerns regarding the toxicity of the IP regimen, as only 42% of patients completed all six cycles. The Japanese GOG has reported improved progression-free survival and overall survival using a dose-dense regimen consisting of paclitaxel (80 mg/m$^2$; 1 hour IV infusion) given on days 1, 8, and 15 plus carboplatin (AUC 6) given on day 1 of a 21-day cycle. The median progression-free survival was 28.0 months versus 17.2 months in patients receiving the dose-dense regimen in comparison to the conventional regimen, and the three-year overall survival was 72.1% versus 65.1% in the dose-dense regimen group compared with the conventional treatment group.[16] Higher rates of grade 3 or 4 neutropenia were reported in the dose-dense group, and less than half were able to complete the dose-dense regimen.

### *Neoadjuvant chemotherapy*

Neoadjuvant chemotherapy is usually given to patients with advanced disease at presentation who have surgically unresectable disease, or to those patients who may be too ill for aggressive primary cytoreduction.[1] In a retrospective study by Everett *et al.* patients with upfront debulking were compared to patients receiving neoadjuvant chemotherapy, and it was found that optimal cytoreduction, rather than type of treatment, was related to median survival.[17] However, patients who were initially cytoreduced had longer progression-free periods. The European Organisation for Research and Treatment of Cancer (EORTC) is currently conducting a randomized phase III study comparing upfront debulking surgery with neo-adjuvant chemotherapy in patients with stage IIIC or IV epithelial ovarian carcinoma (EORTC 55971), and these results are much anticipated.[1]

### *Targeted/novel therapies*

The GOG is currently examining the effects of bevacizumab, a VEGF inhibitor, in the treatment of advanced ovarian, fallopian tube, and primary peritoneal carcinomas.[18] Preliminary results of GOG 218 indicate improved progression-free survival in patients receiving carboplatin and paclitaxel plus bevacizumab followed by maintenance bevacizumab, compared with patients receiving only carboplatin and paclitaxel, or patients who received bevacizumab only during the treatment phase.

For patients with BRCA1/2 mutations, poly(adenosine diphosphate [ADP]-ribose) polymerase (PARP) inhibitors are being used for targeted therapy.[19] PARP has an important role in the repair of DNA single-strand breaks, and therefore PARP inhibitors cause accumulation of DNA single-strand breaks at replication forks. These single-strand breaks are usually repaired by a homologous-recombination double-stranded DNA repair pathway; BRCA1 and BRCA2 tumor suppression proteins are important components of this pathway. BRCA mutations result in defective DNA repair, which triggers carcinogenesis. Therefore the tumor cells have a DNA repair defect that is not found in normal cells, and inhibiting repair of DNA breaks in tumor cells results in preferential tumor cell toxicity, while sparing normal cells.

## FOLLOW-UP

### Surveillance

Patients in clinical remission are generally seen every three months for the first two years, then every six months for the following three years. Patients are followed by symptoms, pelvic exams, CT imaging, and CA-125 levels.[1] Rustin *et al.* stated that a doubling of CA-125 to twice the upper limit of normal was predictive of recurrence, and the median lead time to clinical progression was 63 days following an elevated CA-125.[20]

Preliminary data presented from a randomized trial of immediate treatment of patients with CA-125 levels twice the upper limit of normal versus treatment at the time of clinical or symptomatic recurrence demonstrated no increase in overall survival.[21]

## Consolidation Chemotherapy

It is controversial whether consolidation chemotherapy is effective for prolonging disease-free intervals and survival. In patients with advanced ovarian cancer who achieved a complete response to primary chemotherapy, GOG 178 demonstrated a 22-month versus a 14-month progression-free survival in patients receiving 3 versus 12 monthly cycles of paclitaxel (175 mg/$m^2$ over 3 hours).[22] However, the trial was stopped early by the Data and Safety Monitoring Committee when there was a clear benefit shown for 12 cycles, and at that time it was too early to assess overall survival. Follow-up data was recently published, which demonstrated no significant increased overall survival in the patients receiving 12 cycles.[23] This may be explained by the fact that the trial was stopped early which resulted in a smaller than planned sample size or possible crossover of patients from 3 to 12 cycles once progression-free survival was found to be superior. To answer this question, the GOG is currently conducting a trial (GOG 212) comparing polyglutamate paclitaxel versus paclitaxel as consolidation/maintenance therapy versus no further treatment until disease progression.[24]

## Role of Second-look Surgery

Second-look laparotomies were traditionally performed to assess response to chemotherapy.[1] However, second-look laparotomies are very invasive and expensive, and there has been no survival difference shown in patients receiving second-look laparotomies compared with those who do not.[25]

# TREATMENT OF RECURRENT DISEASE

## Secondary Cytoreduction

Several small studies have reported improved survival in patients who are optimally cytoreduced at secondary debulking.[26] Favorable prognostic indicators were found to be extended disease-free interval, single or very few sites of intra-abdominal recurrence, and good performance status. The GOG is conducting a trial examining the role of secondary cytoreduction in platinum-sensitive patients (GOG 213): appropriate candidates are randomized to secondary debulking or not, followed by a second randomization to carboplatin and paclitaxel alone or in combination with bevacizumab plus bevacizumab maintenance.[27]

## Second-Line Chemotherapy

### *Platinum sensitivity*

Response to chemotherapy can be divided into those with platinum-sensitive and platinum-refractory disease, which are defined as recurrences after more than six months and fewer than six months, respectively, from the completion of primary platinum-based chemotherapy.[1] Patients with platinum-refractory tumors generally have a worse prognosis and are less likely to respond to any subsequent chemotherapy.[28] Patients with platinum-sensitive tumors, however, will likely have a shorter disease-free interval following secondary chemotherapy than the first disease-free interval following initial platinum-based chemotherapy. ICON-4 showed that platinum plus paclitaxel had a superior two-year progression-free survival rate (57% versus 50%), and median survival (29 months versus 24 months) compared to a platinum agent alone.[29] However, 60% of the patients had not received prior paclitaxel as part of their first-line chemotherapy regimen, so there remains the question of whether the effect was due to the successful administration of paclitaxel as a second-line agent, or simply improved tumor response in taxane-naïve patients.

### *Other FDA-approved agents*

Weekly paclitaxel at a dose of 80 mg/m$^2$ has a 20–30% response rate in patients with platinum-refractory disease.[30] This regimen is much less myelosuppressive than other regimens.

Liposomal doxorubicin, which acts by binding to DNA as an anthracycline, is another chemotherapeutic agent that is given at 40 mg/m$^2$ every four weeks.[1] It has been shown to have a response rate of 8–9%.[31,32] Its

# 10

# SEX CORD-STROMAL AND GERM CELL TUMORS OF THE OVARY

*John B. Liao*

## INTRODUCTION

Germ cell and sex cord-stromal tumors of the ovary comprise a small minority of ovarian cancers, but encompass a diverse group of tumors with very distinct natural histories from the more common epithelial ovarian cancers. The surgical approach and chemotherapeutic agents used for these tumors will vary given the demographics of these patients and their unique tumor biology. An understanding of the clinical nuances of these groups of tumors is necessary to guide appropriate management.

## GERM CELL TUMORS

### Epidemiology

While ovarian germ cell tumors make up nearly a quarter of all ovarian neoplasms, *malignant* germ cell tumors comprise barely 5% of ovarian cancers. Ovarian germ cell tumors make up approximately 70% of all ovarian neoplasms in young women aged 10 to 30 and appear to be more common in Asian and Hispanic women than in Caucasians for reasons that are not yet clear.[1,2]

## Presentation

Malignant ovarian germ cell tumors, unlike epithelial ovarian cancers, typically present in girls and young women. The mean age at presentation ranges from 16 to 20 years of age.[1] The signs and symptoms seen in the majority of cases of these tumors are abdominal pain associated with a large, palpable abdominal mass. Indeed, 10% of these patients may present with an acute abdomen due to rupture of the mass or ovarian torsion with subsequent peritoneal signs.[2] Other presenting signs and symptoms include abdominal distension, fever, vaginal bleeding, precocious puberty, and signs of pregnancy.

Germ cell tumors produce characteristic serum tumor markers that may be used to provide assistance in the initial diagnosis. They also serve to monitor the progress of therapy, and provide a means of surveillance after treatment (Table 1). Choriocarcinomas characteristically produce elevated serum hCG, while yolk sac tumors feature elevated AFP. LDH may be elevated in dysgerminomas. CA-125 may also be elevated nonspecifically.[3]

The initial workup of a patient suspected to have a malignant germ cell tumor, after a history and physical exam, should then include routine blood studies along with the serum tumor markers described above. Imaging studies should include chest radiographs, pelvic ultrasonography, and CT scans of the abdomen and pelvis. Karyotyping is indicated if, based on these studies, there is a suspicion of dysgenetic gonads.

Table 1. Serum tumor marker elevations in malignant germ cell tumors.

| | **AFP** | **hCG** | **LDH** |
|---|---|---|---|
| Dysgerminoma | No | Possible | YES |
| Yolk sac tumor | YES | NO | YES |
| Embryonal carcinoma | Possible | YES | Possible |
| Polyembryoma | Possible | YES | NO |
| Immature teratoma | Possible | NO | Possible |
| Mixed germ cell tumor | Possible | Possible | Possible |
| Choriocarcinoma | NO | YES | Possible |

*Notes*: AFP: alpha-fetoprotein; hCG: human chorionic gonadotropin; LDH: lactate dehydrogenase.

## Histology

As a further consequence of being rare tumors, malignant germ cells tumors have historically suffered from shifting nomenclature in describing their many histologic patterns. In recent years, greater standardization has been achieved with the adoption of the WHO classification system (Table 2).[4] This system divides malignant germ cell tumors into three groups: primitive germ cell tumors, biphasic or triphasic teratomas, and monodermal teratoma and somatic-type tumors associated with biphasic or triphasic teratomas. However, when viewed clinically, it is more useful to consider them in terms of dysgerminomas and nondysgerminomas given their distinct clinical characteristics.

Table 2. WHO classification of malignant ovarian germ cell tumors.

I. Primitive germ cell tumors
   a. Dysgerminoma
   b. Yolk sac tumor
   c. Embryonal carcinoma
   d. Polyembryoma
   e. Nongestational choriocarcinoma
   f. Mixed germ cell tumor

II. Biphasic or triphasic teratoma
   a. Immature teratoma
   b. Mature teratoma

III. Monodermal teratoma and somatic-type tumors associated with biphasic or triphasic teratoma
   a. Thyroid tumor group
   b. Carcinoid group
   c. Neuroectodermal tumor group
   d. Carcinoma group
   e. Melanocytic group
   f. Sarcoma group
   g. Sebaceous tumor group
   h. Pituitary-type tumor group
   i. Retinal anlage tumor group
   j. Others

Dysgerminoma is the most common malignant ovarian germ cell tumor and is the most common tumor in women with dysgenetic gonads. Dysgerminomas are usually large, white, fleshy, lobulated masses. Twenty percent will have gross or microscopic involvement of the contralateral ovary. Tumors contain glycogen, which can be seen with periodic acid-Schiff (PAS) staining, and they also display diffuse staining for placenta-like alkaline phosphatase. Dysgerminomas are the only malignant germ cell tumor to stain positive for c-kit.

Yolk sac tumors or endodermal sinus tumors are the second most common malignant germ cell tumor and are notable for their rapid growth. They are usually unilateral with a smooth surface and have a tan and gray appearance on cut section, often featuring hemorrhage and necrosis. Microscopically these tumors display a number of histologic features, commonly flattened or cuboidal epithelial cells with atypia and the diagnostic Schiller-Duval bodies, papillary structures with a central blood vessel.

Embryonal carcinomas and polyembryomas are rarely found in the ovary. They are more commonly reported to be associated with yolk sac tumors in mixed germ cell tumors. Embryonal carcinomas feature crowded cells with pleomorphic nuclei and a high mitotic rate. Polyembryomas have characteristic "embryoid" bodies, embryonic discs separating yolk sacs and amniotic cavities.

Choriocarcinomas have abundant hemorrhage and necrosis that can often be appreciated grossly. Microscopically, these tumors display a mixture of syncytiotrophoblasts, which produce hCG, and cytotrophoblasts. It is important to distinguish gestational choriocarcinomas by identifying paternal DNA, because nongestational choriocarcinomas carry a worse prognosis and consequently demand more aggressive therapy.

Mixed germ cell tumors contain two or more types and are usually unilateral. A thorough pathologic sampling of these tumors is vital as the particular cellular components will dictate therapy and provide prognostic information. Teratomas are germ cell tumors that are derived from two or more embryonic layers. Most teratomas are mature cystic teratomas and are benign neoplasms unless a somatic malignancy arises from the differentiated elements. Immature teratomas are usually unilateral and have a soft, fleshy, and encephaloid appearance on cut surface.

Microscopically, mature and immature tissue components are present. The immature components feature blue cells organized in rosettes and tubules. These tumors are graded 1 to 3, with grade 3 representing high-grade tumor containing immature neural tissue occupying more than three low-power fields on a single slide. High-grade tumors are approached more aggressively with adjuvant therapy due to their poor prognosis.[5]

## Treatment

### *Surgery*

Primary surgery should be performed for both diagnosis and therapy. The extent of the surgery should take into consideration the patient's desire for future fertility given the expected age range of patients with these tumors. Surgical exploration should be performed with a laparotomy that would allow inspection of all peritoneal surfaces and adequate evaluation and exploration of the upper abdomen. A laparoscopic approach could theoretically be feasible, but is not universally accepted. Removal of any ascites or peritoneal washings and removal of the mass, cyst, or ovary and tube is performed to allow frozen section diagnosis. If a malignancy is confirmed, then salpingo-oophorectomy with staging would be the minimum recommended surgery. When patients have not had comprehensive surgical staging, the value of surgical restaging must be evaluated against data from the Pediatric Oncology Group and the Children's Cancer Study Group showing that deviations from standard surgical guidelines did not have an impact on overall survival.[6] For these clinical scenarios, MD Anderson Cancer Center advocates using postoperative CT imaging and tumor markers to guide further treatment.[2]

If childbearing is completed, then the uterus and both ovaries and tubes should be removed. Peritoneal biopsies and pelvic and para-aortic lymph node sampling should be performed as with surgical staging for epithelial ovarian cancer and then reported using the same FIGO system. For patients who wish to preserve fertility, a unilateral salpingo-oophorectomy with preservation of a normal-appearing uterus and contralateral tube and ovary is acceptable. When advanced disease is present, surgical debulking should be performed according to the principles used for epithelial ovarian cancer, although the benefits of this for germ cell tumors are not as well established. The surgeon should carefully weigh the known sensitivity of this group of tumors to chemotherapy when considering aggressive cytoreduction. Nevertheless, a number of studies have suggested that optimally debulked patients attain better outcomes.[7–9]

## *Chemotherapy*

Many of the advances in the chemotherapeutic treatment of malignant germ cell tumors of the ovary have emerged from the treatment of testicular germ cell tumors. Prior to the introduction of combination chemotherapy, the prognosis for patients with malignant germ cell tumors of the ovary, outside of patients with dysgerminomas, was bleak. Combination chemotherapy in the 1970s utilizing vincristine, dactinomycin, and cyclophosphamide began to yield some modest improvements for patients with early-stage disease, but the cure rates for patients with metastatic disease remained below 50%.[1,8] However, the breakthrough in the treatment of testicular cancer with the advent of platinum-based regimens led to a new chemotherapy standard for malignant germ cell tumors of the ovary: cisplatin, vinblastine, and bleomycin.[10,11] The regimen of choice then shifted again with the discovery of single-agent activity of etoposide in testicular cancer patients, leading to the adoption of the combination of bleomycin, etoposide, and cisplatin (BEP), which showed equal efficacy and less toxicity in testicular cancer patients.[12] Used in malignant germ cell tumors of the ovary, this regimen has brought cure rates of early-stage disease to nearly 100% and has approached 75% even in advanced-stage disease.[13,14] In the largest trial reported to date by the Gynecologic Oncology Group (GOG), 93 patients with completely resected ovarian germ cell tumors, stage I, II, and III disease, were treated with three courses of BEP chemotherapy. Of the 93 patients, 91 were completely disease-free after an average follow-up of more than two years. However, two patients developed secondary hematologic malignancies.[14] Secondary malignancies are among the late effects of BEP chemotherapy seen in men treated with testicular cancer, and they also include renal and gonadal dysfunction, cardiotoxicity, neurotoxicity, and bleomycin-induced pulmonary fibrosis.

Experience with completely resected nondysgerminomas has shown that even stage I endodermal sinus tumors, embryonal carcinoma, nongestational choriocarcinoma, high-grade immature teratoma, and mixed tumors containing these elements had a high rate of recurrence and mortality when treated with surgery alone.[5] Subsequent case series and prospective studies have demonstrated the effectiveness of platinum-based chemotherapy in preventing recurrence and improving progression-free survival. The GOG's prospective study reported no recurrences among its patients who received three cycles of BEP as adjuvant treatment after surgery.[14] The most commonly used regimen, and the one recommended by the National Comprehensive Cancer Network (NCCN) guidelines, is three cycles of bleomycin 30 units IV on days 1, 8, 15, etoposide 100 mg/m$^2$ IV days 1 through 5, and cisplatin 20 mg/m$^2$ IV days 1 through 5,[14] but the optimal number of cycles has not been rigorously established. While there have been reports suggesting that the substitution of carboplatin for cisplatin may have comparable therapeutic efficacy,[15–17] and could be considered in patients with pre-existing renal disease or neuropathy, current guidelines still recommend BEP.[2]

Treatment of dysgerminomas has historically included radiation therapy due to the exquisite sensitivity of this tumor to radiation. However, the introduction of effective platinum-based chemotherapy regimens and concomitant concerns regarding impact on future fertility has led to a shift away from the use of radiation. Stage IB or higher tumors are treated with three or four cycles of BEP, with four cycles used for patients with more advanced disease. Platinum-based chemotherapy regimens have successfully prevented recurrence even in series reporting incompletely resected disease.[13,18–20] More recently, data from the GOG has suggested that a regimen of carboplatin and etoposide may have equivalent activity in dysgerminomas. In 42 patients with completely resected stage IB to stage III dysgerminomas treated with carboplatin and etoposide, there were no recurrences in a median follow-up period of 7.8 years.[21]

Although the overall effectiveness of the BEP chemotherapy regimen has now been well established, the selection of patients for adjuvant chemotherapy versus surveillance alone remains an area of controversy. Only patients with stage IA dysgerminomas and stage IA, grade I immature teratomas have historically been treated with surgery alone.[22] Recent studies have proposed this approach with other substages of stage I disease and stage II disease, and even in selected patients with other stage IA nondysgerminomas; however; this is still not the standard approach. In a prospective trial, 22 patients with stage I or stage II, grade 1 or grade 2, immature teratomas of the ovary were treated with surgery alone. Patients were then followed with either ultrasonography or with at least one second-look surgery. Two patients subsequently recurred (stage IA, grade 2, and stage IC, grade 2) with bulky abdominal disease and were salvaged with a secondary cytoreductive surgery. All patients were alive and disease-free with a follow-up of nearly four years.[23] As more studies emerge regarding reliable prognostic factors, appropriate risk stratification may allow more judicious use of adjuvant chemotherapy.[5,24]

The movement toward more limited use of chemotherapy in malignant germ cell tumors would likely have an impact on the incidence of late effects of chemotherapy and on the effects of chemotherapy on reproductive function given the age of patients commonly afflicted with these tumors. While a proportion of women treated with fertility-sparing surgery and adjuvant platinum-based chemotherapy may experience premature menopause, up to 80% of women have been reported to resume normal menstrual function, with several documented normal pregnancies.[18,25–27] Secondary malignancies such as acute myelogenous leukemia are another late effect and are related to the cumulative dose of etoposide.[28]

## Outcome

The evolution of treatment for malignant germ cell tumors of the ovary has been one of the great success stories in the field of gynecologic oncology. The majority of patients with malignant germ cell tumors are cured. Cure rates approach 100% for early-stage disease and exceed 75% even for patients with advanced-stage disease. The approach to patients who recur, usually within the first two years, is individualized, due to limited experience gleaned from the rarity of these cases. A number of combination chemotherapy regimens have been employed as salvage therapy, primarily three-drug regimens employing cisplatin and ifosfamide.[29,30] For male germ cell tumor patients with persistent, refractory, or platinum-resistant disease, high-dose chemotherapy with stem cell rescue has been attempted, but an advantage over conventional chemotherapy has not yet been established.[31]

## SEX CORD-STROMAL TUMORS

### Epidemiology

Sex cord-stromal tumors originate from cells of the ovarian sex cords and stroma or mesenchyme surrounding oocytes. These tumors are rare and account for about 7% of all cancers arising from the ovary.[32] Sex cord-stromal tumors generally have a very favorable long-term prognosis and an indolent course. Unlike epithelial ovarian cancers, malignant sex cord-stromal tumors are usually diagnosed at an early stage. They have no known association with BRCA mutations or any other genetic associations with breast and ovarian cancer.[33]

Sex cord-stromal tumors can be thought of in a classification scheme that groups them according to their cell type of origin and their functional status (Table 3).[34] Granulosa-stromal cell tumors represent 70% of ovarian sex cord-stromal tumors. Within this group, fibromas are the most common tumor and can occur in both pre- and postmenopausal women. They are most often benign and do not produce hormones. Granulosa cell tumors are the most common sex cord-stromal tumor with malignant potential. Average age at diagnosis is 52 years.[35] Adult granulosa cell tumors are commonly isolated to the ovary, with 90% found in stage I at the time of diagnosis.[36] These tumors are also noted for their extremely indolent growth rate. Sertoli-Leydig tumors are extremely rare and are more often found in younger women, with a mean age of 25–30 years at the time of presentation.

### Presentation

Sex cord-stromal tumors of the ovary may present with nonspecific symptoms, abdominal pain, distension, or bloating. Because many sex cord-stromal tumors produce steroid hormones, their presentation is often further characterized by either estrogen or androgen excess associated with an adnexal mass. Estrogen excess may present as precocious puberty,

Table 3. Classification of sex cord-stromal tumors of the ovary.

I. Granulosa-stromal cell tumors
   a. Granulosa cell tumor
      i. Adult type
      ii. Juvenile type
   b. Thecoma-fibroma group
      i. Thecoma
      ii. Fibroma-fibrosarcoma
      iii. Sclerosing stromal tumor

II. Sertoli-stromal cell tumors
   a. Sertoli cell tumor
   b. Leydig cell tumor
   c. Sertoli-Leydig cell tumor
      i. Well differentiated
      ii. Intermediate differentiation
      iii. Poorly differentiated
      iv. Heterologous elements
      v. Retiform
      vi. Mixed

III. Gynandroblastoma
IV. Sex cord tumor with annular tubules
V. Unclassified

abnormal uterine bleeding, and endometrial hyperplasia or carcinoma, while androgen excess may cause virilization. Due to the functional status of these tumors, serum tumor markers, such as inhibin,[37,38] may be used to help establish diagnosis, track therapeutic responses, and as a component of subsequent surveillance (Table 4). Granulosa cell tumors are prone to hemorrhage and may present with hemoperitoneum. Due to their hyperestrogenic state, 25% of these tumors will be associated with endometrial hyperplasia, and 5% with endometrial cancer.[37,38] Inhibin is the most useful marker for granulosa cell tumors. Inhibin is secreted by the ovary in response to FSH and LH and should be low in menopausal women. Theca cells can be found in 75% of these cases. While thecomas, fibromas, and sclerosing stromal tumors are benign ovarian neoplasms, they may contribute to morbidity through secondary effects, such as

Table 4. Serum tumor marker elevations in sex cord-stromal tumors.

| | Inhibin | E2 | Testost | Andro | DHEA |
|---|---|---|---|---|---|
| Granulosa cell | YES | Possible | NO | NO | NO |
| Thecoma-fibroma | Possible | Possible | Possible | Possible | NO |
| Sertoli-Leydig | Possible | NO | YES | YES | NO |

*Notes*: E2: estradiol; testost: testosterone; andro: androstenedione; DHEA: dehydroepiandrostenedione.

unopposed estrogen secretion by thecomas on the endometrium, leading to hyperplasia or carcinoma, or with signs and symptoms mimicking malignancy such as Meigs syndrome and fibromas.

## Histology

Granulosa cell tumors are usually large and unilateral. They are often multicystic and filled with serous fluid or clotted blood. Tumors and tumor implants may appear yellow due to the accumulation of lipids. Adult-type granulosa cell tumors, which make up 95% of granulosa cell tumors and occur mostly in middle-aged and older women, classically have coffee bean nuclei seen on microscopy. There are few mitoses. Cells are arranged in rosettes around a central cavity in Call-Exner bodies. Juvenile-type granulosa cell tumors, which comprise the remaining 5%, occur more commonly in children and young women, do not have coffee bean nuclei or Call-Exner bodies. These cells possess a macro-follicular pattern with immature cells containing many mitoses. Immunohistochemical staining for inhibin appears to be the most sensitive and specific for granulosa cell tumors, but is not absolutely specific for a sex cord-stromal tumor of the ovary.[39,40]

Sertoli-Leydig tumors have a smooth surface and are firm, solid, lobulated masses. Poorly differentiated tumors may have areas of hemorrhage and necrosis. The presence of a retiform pattern may indicate hepatocellular differentiation and the elevation of serum alpha-fetoprotein levels.[41] Microscopically, cells are organized in tubules, with Sertoli cells lining the tubules and Leydig cells in the stroma. Most tumors are low-grade. Heterologous elements may also be present.

Gynandroblastomas are extremely rare tumors with only 17 cases authenticated in the literature.[42] These tumors contain both granulosa cells and Sertoli cells with their corresponding stromal cells. Sex cord-stromal tumors with annular tubules represent a histologically intermediate form between granulosa cells and Sertoli cells. Up to a third of these tumors are associated with Peutz-Jeghers syndrome.[43] Unclassified sex cord-stromal tumors encompass the majority of steroid cell tumors. The majority of these tumors lead to androgen excess, 10–15% to estrogen excess, and a very small percentage to cortisol excess.

## Treatment

### *Surgery*

The initial management of patients with sex cord-stromal tumors is surgical, with the combined goals of obtaining definitive tissue diagnosis, establishing surgical stage, and tumor debulking. Conservative surgery to preserve fertility in apparent early-stage disease may be considered. Women who underwent conservative surgery for stage I–II sex cord-stromal tumors have been shown to have comparable survival to women who underwent standard surgery including hysterectomy.[44] If childbearing is completed or there is bilateral or advanced disease then a hysterectomy, bilateral salpingo-oophorectomy with staging biopsies is appropriate; however, given the low incidence of lymph node metastases, complete pelvic and para-aortic lymphadenectomy may be unnecessary.[45] If conservative surgery is elected with preservation of the uterus, then a thorough sampling of the endometrial lining should be performed to exclude pathology related to elevated estrogen states.[35]

Due to the rarity of these tumors, even expert gynecologic pathologists may not be able to definitively diagnose these tumors on frozen section. Therefore it is important for preoperative discussions and informed consent to address the possibility of benign, malignant, or indeterminate intraoperative findings and that desires for fertility preservation and potential incomplete staging be documented. While the value of optimal tumor debulking has not been established for these tumors as it has been with epithelial ovarian cancers, maximum effort at tumor cytoreduction should be attempted in the presence of metastatic disease.[35] The surgical effort should be weighed with the additional evidence that age less than 50, size of tumor, and the presence of residual disease have been shown to hold prognostic significance.[46]

## *Chemotherapy*

Beyond primary surgery, there is no standard therapy for patients with sex cord-stromal tumors. Since the 1980s postoperative chemotherapy most often consisted of various platinum-based regimens. Bleomycin, etoposide, with cisplatin emerged as the regimen of choice, with reports of high response rates in patients with poor-prognosis sex cord-stromal tumors of the ovary.[47] The GOG also found BEP to be effective in treating incompletely resected stage II to stage IV, or recurrent sex cord-stromal tumors.[48] For patients with stage II to stage IV sex cord-stromal tumors, the NCCN guidelines recommend adjuvant chemotherapy using BEP, the regimen used for germ cell tumors. Chemotherapy should also be considered for patients with high-risk stage I tumors such as ruptured stage IC tumors. Typically, three or four cycles are given after primary surgery in these cases.

Of patients with poor-prognosis sex cord-stromal tumors, even though the majority will respond to BEP, only 14% attain a durable remission.[47] Use of BEP in advanced stages in the GOG trial was only able to achieve a sustained remission in one of seven cases and nearly half of the patients with recurrent disease had disease progression in spite of high response rates.[48] Furthermore, BEP has a number of significant toxicities that were also reported in these trials, including two deaths due to bleomycin-related pulmonary fibrosis.[47,48] Consequently, recent studies have focused on the efficacy of regimens with more favorable side effect profiles.

Taxanes have been recently studied as an alternative regimen to address these issues.[49] Data from MD Anderson Cancer Center has shown that when 11 patients who received BEP for primary therapy were compared to 11 who received taxane with platinum, there was no significant difference in response rate, progression-free survival, or overall survival. Of 21 patients treated with BEP, 5 were reported to have toxicity greater than grade 2 attributed to their therapy, compared to 7 of 44 patients treated with taxanes, though this did not reach statistical significance.[50] Other regimens that have been proposed include etoposide plus cisplatin (EP), cyclophosphamide, doxorubicin, and cisplatin (CAP); or a platinum agent alone. However, attempts to eliminate bleomycin from the BEP regimen have resulted in loss of therapeutic activity in testicular germ cell tumors.

## Outcome

While the majority of sex cord-stromal tumors are early-stage at the time of diagnosis and have a good prognosis, the prognosis for recurrent disease remains poor. Recurrence patterns for sex cord-stromal tumor are associated with initial surgical stage and histology. Granulosa cell tumors are known to be indolent and recur late, with a median time to relapse of five years.[51,52] In contrast, more than 90% of Sertoli-Leydig tumors recur within five years. Patients with poor-prognosis or advanced-stage disease rarely achieve a lasting remission with surgery and current chemotherapy regimens. There is no consensus approach to recurrent disease.[34,53] Treatment for recurrent disease has included secondary debulking surgery, salvage chemotherapy regimens, hormonal therapy, and radiation therapy.

Given the absence of consensus in treatment for recurrent disease, treatment must be individualized. Although secondary cytoreductive surgery for recurrent disease is controversial, it is a valid approach in patients with indolent tumor types and can have palliative benefits.[35,54] Chemotherapy regimens in the setting of recurrent disease have primarily included platinum-based regimens. When BEP was used for recurrent disease in the GOG experience, 21 of 41 patients were progression-free with a mean follow-up interval of three years; however, severe toxicities were found to be associated with it.[48] In the MD Anderson series, BEP showed improved response rates compared to taxane regimens, but no statistically significant difference in median progression-free survival. Taxanes used in recurrent disease in combination with platinum had better toxicity profiles.[50]

Radiation therapy presents another therapeutic option for patients with local or metastatic tumor that cannot be treated surgically. In a report from MD Anderson Cancer Center, 6 of 14 patients with clinically measurable disease achieved a complete clinical response, of whom three remained alive 10 to 21 years after treatment. The other three patients relapsed between four and five years later.[55] Given the functional nature of many of these tumors, there is also a rationale for hormonal therapy, although there is limited data in this area. The successful use of medroxyprogesterone acetate, megestrol, tamoxifen, and gonadotropin-releasing hormone agonists has been described in case reports yielding complete responses lasting as long as five years.[56–58]

## REFERENCES


1. Gershenson DM, Copeland LJ, Kavanagh JJ, *et al.* Treatment of malignant nondysgerminomatous germ cell tumors of the ovary with vincristine, dactinomycin, and cyclophosphamide. *Cancer* 1985;56(12):2756–2761.
2. Gershenson DM. Management of ovarian germ cell tumors. *J Clin Oncol* 2007;25(20):2938–2943.
3. Sekiya S, Seki K, Nagai Y. Rise of serum CA 125 in patients with pure ovarian yolk sac tumors. *Int J Gynaecol Obstet* 1997;58(3):323–324.
4. Tavassoli FA, Devilee P. Pathology and Genetics of Tumours of the Breast and Female Genital Organs. Lyon, France: *International Agency for Research on Cancer,* 2003.
5. Lai CH, Chang TC, Hsueh S, *et al.* Outcome and prognostic factors in ovarian germ cell malignancies. *Gynecol Oncol* 2005;96(3):784–791.
6. Billmire D, Vinocur C, Rescorla F, *et al.* Outcome and staging evaluation in malignant germ cell tumors of the ovary in children and adolescents: an intergroup study. *J Pediatr Surg* 2004;39(3):424–429; discussion 424–429.
7. Bafna UD, Umadevi K, Kumaran C, *et al.* Germ cell tumors of the ovary: is there a role for aggressive cytoreductive surgery for nondysgerminomatous tumors? *Int J Gynecol Cancer* 2001;11(4):300–304.
8. Slayton RE, Park RC, Silverberg SG, *et al.* Vincristine, dactinomycin, and cyclophosphamide in the treatment of malignant germ cell tumors of the ovary. A Gynecologic Oncology Group Study (a final report). *Cancer* 1985; 56(2):243–248.
9. Williams SD, Blessing JA, Moore DH, Homesley HD, Adcock L. Cisplatin, vinblastine, and bleomycin in advanced and recurrent ovarian germ-cell

tumors. A trial of the Gynecologic Oncology Group. *Ann Intern Med* 1989;111(1):22–27.
10. Gershenson DM, Copeland LJ, Kavanagh JJ, *et al.* Treatment of malignant nondysgerminomatous germ cell tumors of the ovary with vinblastine, bleomycin, and cisplatin. *Cancer* 1986;**57**(9):1731–1737.
11. Williams SD, Blessing JA, DiSaia PJ, Major FJ, Ball HG 3rd, Liao SY. Second-look laparotomy in ovarian germ cell tumors: the gynecologic oncology group experience. *Gynecol Oncol* 1994;52(3):287–291.
12. Williams SD, Birch R, Einhorn LH, Irwin L, Greco FA, Loehrer PJ. Treatment of disseminated germ-cell tumors with cisplatin, bleomycin, and either vinblastine or etoposide. *N Engl J Med* 1987;316(23):1435–1440.
13. Gershenson DM, Morris M, Cangir A, *et al.* Treatment of malignant germ cell tumors of the ovary with bleomycin, etoposide, and cisplatin. *J Clin Oncol* 1990;8(4):715–720.
14. Williams S, Blessing JA, Liao SY, Ball H, Hanjani P. Adjuvant therapy of ovarian germ cell tumors with cisplatin, etoposide, and bleomycin: a trial of the Gynecologic Oncology Group. *J Clin Oncol* 1994;12(4):701–706.
15. Dimopoulos MA, Papadopoulou M, Andreopoulou E, *et al.* Favorable outcome of ovarian germ cell malignancies treated with cisplatin or carboplatin-based chemotherapy: a Hellenic Cooperative Oncology Group study. *Gynecol Oncol* 1998;70(1):70–74.
16. Mann JR, Raafat F, Robinson K, *et al.* The United Kingdom Children's Cancer Study Group's second germ cell tumor study: carboplatin, etoposide, and bleomycin are effective treatment for children with malignant extracranial germ cell tumors, with acceptable toxicity. *J Clin Oncol* 2000;18(22):3809–3818.
17. Stern JW, Bunin N. Prospective study of carboplatin-based chemotherapy for pediatric germ cell tumors. *Med Pediatr Oncol* 2002;39(3):163–167.
18. Brewer M, Gershenson DM, Herzog CE, Mitchell MF, Silva EG, Wharton JT. Outcome and reproductive function after chemotherapy for ovarian dysgerminoma. *J Clin Oncol* 1999;17(9):2670–2675.
19. Culine S, Lhomme C, Kattan J, Michel G, Duvillard P, Droz JP. Cisplatin-based chemotherapy in the management of germ cell tumors of the ovary: The Institut Gustave Roussy Experience. *Gynecol Oncol* 1997;64(1): 160–165.
20. Williams SD, Blessing JA, Hatch KD, Homesley HD. Chemotherapy of advanced dysgerminoma: trials of the Gynecologic Oncology Group. *J Clin Oncol* 1991;9(11):1950–1955.

21. Williams SD, Kanderer J, Burnett AF, Lentz SS, Aghajanian C, Amstrong DK. Adjuvant therapy of completely resected dysgerminoma with carboplatin and etoposide: a trial of the Gynecologic Oncology Group. *Gynecol Oncol* 2004;95(3):496–499.
22. Dark GG, Bower M, Newlands ES, Paradinas F, Rustin GJ. Surveillance policy for stage I ovarian germ cell tumors. *J Clin Oncol* 1997;15(2):620–624.
23. Bonazzi C, Peccatori F, Colombo N, Lucchini V, Cantic MG, Mangioni C. Pure ovarian immature teratoma, a unique and curable disease: 10 years' experience of 32 prospectively treated patients. *Obstet Gynecol* 1994;84(4): 598–604.
24. Murugaesu N, Schmid P, Dancey G, *et al.* Malignant ovarian germ cell tumors: identification of novel prognostic markers and long-term outcome after multimodality treatment. *J Clin Oncol* 2006;24(30):4862–4866.
25. Sklar CA, Mertens AC, Mitby P, *et al.* Premature menopause in survivors of childhood cancer: a report from the childhood cancer survivor study. *J Natl Cancer Inst* 2006;98(13):890–896.
26. Tangir J, Zelterman D, Ma W, Schwartz PE. Reproductive function after conservative surgery and chemotherapy for malignant germ cell tumors of the ovary. *Obstet Gynecol* 2003;101(2):251–257.
27. Zanetta G, Bonazzi C, Cantù M, *et al.* Survival and reproductive function after treatment of malignant germ cell ovarian tumors. *J Clin Oncol* 2001; 19(4):1015–1020.
28. Nichols CR, Breeden ES, Lochrer PJ, Williams SD, Einhorn LH. Secondary leukemia associated with a conventional dose of etoposide: review of serial germ cell tumor protocols. *J Natl Cancer Inst* 1993;85(1):36–40.
29. Kondagunta GV, Bacik J, Donadio A, *et al.* Combination of paclitaxel, ifosfamide, and cisplatin is an effective second-line therapy for patients with relapsed testicular germ cell tumors. *J Clin Oncol* 2005;23(27): 6549–6555.
30. McCaffrey JA, Mazumdar M, Bajorin DF, Bosl GJ, Vlamis V, Motzer RJ. Ifosfamide- and cisplatin-containing chemotherapy as first-line salvage therapy in germ cell tumors: response and survival. *J Clin Oncol* 1997; 15(7):2559–2563.
31. Motzer RJ, Nichols CJ, Margolin KA, *et al.* Phase III randomized trial of conventional-dose chemotherapy with or without high-dose chemotherapy and autologous hematopoietic stem-cell rescue as first-line treatment for

patients with poor-prognosis metastatic germ cell tumors. *J Clin Oncol* 2007;25(3):247–256.

32. Koonings PP, Campbell K, Mishell DR Jr, Grimes DA. Relative frequency of primary ovarian neoplasms: a 10-year review. *Obstet Gynecol* 1989;74(6):921–926.
33. Werness BA, Ramus SJ, Whittemore AS, *et al.* Histopathology of familial ovarian tumors in women from families with and without germline BRCA1 mutations. *Hum Pathol* 2000;31(11):1420–1424.
34. Colombo N, Parma G, Zanagnolo V, Insinga A. Management of ovarian stromal cell tumors. *J Clin Oncol* 2007;25(20):2944–2951.
35. Gershenson DM, Hartmann LC, Young RH. Ovarian sex cord-stromal tumors. Barakat RR, ed., *Principles and Practice of Gynecologic Oncology*, 5th ed. Philadelphia: Lippincott, 2009.
36. Chen VW, Ruiz B, Killeen JL, Coté TR, Wu XC, Correa CN. Pathology and classification of ovarian tumors. *Cancer* 2003;97(10 Suppl):2631–2642.
37. Hildebrandt RH, Rouse RV, Longacre TA. Value of inhibin in the identification of granulosa cell tumors of the ovary. *Hum Pathol* 1997;28(12):1387–1395.
38. Lappohn RE, Burger HG, Bouma J, Bangah M, Krans M, de Bruijn HW. Inhibin as a marker for granulosa-cell tumors. *N Engl J Med* 1989;321(12):790–793.
39. McCluggage WG. Recent advances in immunohistochemistry in the diagnosis of ovarian neoplasms. *J Clin Pathol* 2000;53(5):327–334.
40. Movahedi-Lankarani S, Kurman RJ. Calretinin, a more sensitive but less specific marker than alpha-inhibin for ovarian sex cord-stromal neoplasms: an immunohistochemical study of 215 cases. *Am J Surg Pathol* 2002;26(11):1477–1483.
41. Mooney EE, Nogales FF, Tavassoli FA. Hepatocytic differentiation in retiform Sertoli-Leydig cell tumors: distinguishing a heterologous element from Leydig cells. *Hum Pathol* 1999;30(6):611–617.
42. Martin-Jimenez A, Condom-Munró E, Valls-Porcel M, Giné-Martin L, Del Amo E, Balagneró-Lladó L. [Gynandroblastoma of the ovary. Review of the literature]. *J Gynecol Obstet Biol Reprod (Paris)* 1994;23(4):391–394.
43. Young RH, Welch WR, Dickersin GR, Scully RE. Ovarian sex cord tumor with annular tubules: review of 74 cases including 27 with Peutz-Jeghers syndrome and four with adenoma malignum of the cervix. *Cancer* 1982;50(7):1384–1402.

44. Zhang M, Cheung MK, Shin JY, *et al*. Prognostic factors responsible for survival in sex cord-stromal tumors of the ovary — an analysis of 376 women. *Gynecol Oncol* 2007;104(2):396–400.
45. Abu-Rustum NR, Restivo A, Ivy J, *et al*. Retroperitoneal nodal metastasis in primary and recurrent granulosa cell tumors of the ovary. *Gynecol Oncol* 2006;103(1):31–34.
46. Chan JK, Zhang M, Kaleb V, *et al*. Prognostic factors responsible for survival in sex cord stromal tumors of the ovary — a multivariate analysis. *Gynecol Oncol* 2005;96(1):204–209.
47. Gershenson DM, Morris M, Burke TW, Levenback C, Matthews CM, Wharton JT. Treatment of poor-prognosis sex cord-stromal tumors of the ovary with the combination of bleomycin, etoposide, and cisplatin. *Obstet Gynecol* 1996;87(4):527–531.
48. Homesley HD, Bundy BN, Hurtedu JA, Roth LM. Bleomycin, etoposide, and cisplatin combination therapy of ovarian granulosa cell tumors and other stromal malignancies: A Gynecologic Oncology Group study. *Gynecol Oncol* 1999;72(2):131–137.
49. Brown J, Shvartsman HS, Deavers MT, Burke TW, Munsell MF, Gershenson DM. The activity of taxanes in the treatment of sex cord-stromal ovarian tumors. *J Clin Oncol* 2004;22(17):3517–3523.
50. Brown J, Shvartsman HS, Deavers MT, *et al*. The activity of taxanes compared with bleomycin, etoposide, and cisplatin in the treatment of sex cord-stromal ovarian tumors. *Gynecol Oncol* 2005;97(2):489–496.
51. Bjorkholm E, Silfversward C. Prognostic factors in granulosa-cell tumors. *Gynecol Oncol* 1981;11(3):261–274.
52. Evans AT, 3rd Gaffey TA, Malkasian GD Jr, Annegers JF. Clinicopathologic review of 118 granulosa and 82 theca cell tumors. *Obstet Gynecol* 1980; 55(2):231–238.
53. Schumer ST, Cannistra SA. Granulosa cell tumor of the ovary. *J Clin Oncol* 2003;21(6):1180–1189.
54. Pectasides D, Pectasides E, Psyrri A. Granulosa cell tumor of the ovary. *Cancer Treat Rev* 2008;34(1):1–12.
55. Wolf JK, Mullen J, Eifel PJ, Burke TW, Levenback C, Gershenson DM. Radiation treatment of advanced or recurrent granulosa cell tumor of the ovary. *Gynecol Oncol* 1999;73(1):35–41.
56. Briasoulis E, Karavasilis V, Pavlidis N. Megestrol activity in recurrent adult type granulosa cell tumour of the ovary. *Ann Oncol* 1997;8(8):811–812.

57. Fishman A, Kudelka AP, Tresukosol D, *et al*. Leuprolide acetate for treating refractory or persistent ovarian granulosa cell tumor. *J Reprod Med* 1996; 41(6):393–396.
58. Hardy RD, Bell JG, Nicely CJ, Reid GC. Hormonal treatment of a recurrent granulosa cell tumor of the ovary: case report and review of the literature. *Gynecol Oncol* 2005;96(3):865–869.

# 11

# GESTATIONAL TROPHOBLASTIC DISEASE AND MOLAR PREGNANCY

*Janos L. Tanyi*

## INTRODUCTION

Gestational trophoblastic neoplasia (GTN) and molar pregnancy comprise a spectrum of diseases which derive from the placenta, and include complete (CHM) and partial hydatidiform molar pregnancy (PHM), invasive mole, placental site trophoblastic tumor (PSTT), and choriocarcinoma (CCA). These diseases have different characteristics but all are capable of local invasion and metastasis. GTN can develop after molar or even normal pregnancies and is one of the rarest human malignancies, though highly treatable with chemotherapy and surgery.[1] This chapter reviews the immunobiology, diagnosis, and basic principles in the management of patients with molar pregnancies and GTN.

## HYDATIDIFORM MOLE

### Epidemiology

Molar pregnancies have been known since antiquity with the first written description of the disease recorded by Hippocrates, who called it "dropsy of the uterus". The name "hydatid mole" was first used by William Smellie in the 1700s. There are significant differences in the reported incidence of molar pregnancy all over the world.[2–4] The incidence of all molar pregnancies was found to be 1 per 1,500 live births in the United States.[3] The highest incidence of CHM has been reported in Asia, with 1 per

125 live births, which is 8–10 times higher than the known North American incidence rate.[2,3] It is well known that advanced maternal age increases the incidence of CHM.[3] Women older than 40 years have a five- to ten-fold increased incidence, while as many as 1 in 3 pregnancies in those over 50 years of age are reported to be molar.[3,5] An Italian epidemiologic study found an increased risk associated with both increasing paternal and maternal age for CHM, though no similar association between reproductive age and PHM was seen.[6] A patient's reproductive history also influences the risk of molar pregnancies. Women with a history of previous molar pregnancy generally have a ten-fold increased risk for another molar pregnancy. Bagshawe reported that the risk for a second and third molar pregnancy is 1 in 76 and 1 in 6.5 pregnancies, respectively.[7] Other factors of reproductive history such as prior infertility and spontaneous abortions were found also to increase the incidence of both CHM and PHM.[8] Nutritional factors such as low dietary carotene (vitamin A precursor) and animal fat consumption were associated with an increased incidence of CHM in both Asia and Italy.[9,10] Epidemiologic studies suggest that the prevalence of PHM is increased when there is an abnormal reproductive history, while the prevalence of CHM is more dependent upon age and nutritional factors.[11,12] There are molecular pathogenetic abnormalities linked with CHM. Increased expression of p53, p21, Rb, c-fms and MdM2 have been observed in CHM and CCA.[13,14] Increased expression of EGFR and c-erbB3 in the extravillous trophoblast has been noted to be associated with the development of postmolar tumors.[15] cDNA microarray studies were applied to analyze the different gene expression profiles between normal placenta and molar tissues, and identified 91 up-regulated and 122 down-regulated genes in CHM.[15]

## Complete Mole

Molar pregnancies present as two distinct entities, complete or partial hydatidiform mole, with assignment based on different karyotype, morphology, and histological characteristics (Table 1). Complete moles lack identifiable embryologic or fetal tissues because the fetus is reabsorbed before the development of the circulatory system. The chorionic villi display generalized swelling with hyperplasia and atypia, and fetal

Table 1. Features of complete and partial hydatidiform moles.

| | Complete mole | Partial mole |
|---|---|---|
| **Clinical symptoms** | | |
| Usual diagnosis | Molar gestation | Missed abortion |
| Uterine size | Large for dates | Small for dates |
| Theca lutein cysts | 25–30% | Rare |
| Medical complications | 10–25% | Rare |
| Postmolar GTN | 6.8–20% | 2.5–7.5% |
| **Pathologic characteristics** | | |
| Hydatidiform swelling with chorionic villi | Diffuse | Focal |
| Scalloping of chorionic villi | Absent | Present |
| Trophoblastic hyperplasia | Diffuse | Focal |
| Implantation-site trophoblast | Marked atypia | Mild atypia |
| Trophoblastic stromal inclusions | Absent | Present |
| Fetal or embryonic tissue | Absent | Present |
| **Karyotype** | 46,XX, 46,XY | 69,XXY, 69,XYY |

*Sources*:

1. Berkowitz RS, Goldstein DP. Molar pregnancy and gestational trophoblastic neoplasm. In: Barakat RR, Markman M, Randall ME, eds., *Principles and Practice of Gynecologic Oncology*, 5th edition. New York: Wolters Kluwer, 2009, pp. 875–895.
2. Soper J and Creasman WT. Gestational Trophoblastic Disease. In: DiSaia PJ, Creasman WT, eds., *Clinical Gynecologic Oncology*, 7th edition. Philadelphia: Elsevier, 2007, pp. 201–233.

red blood cells are not observed.[16,17] CHM has a diploid karyotype where all the chromosomes are derived from paternal sources: in 90% of cases, an empty ovum has been fertilized by a single haploid (23,X) sperm which then duplicates, rendering a 46,XX karyotype.[18] Approximately 5–10% of CHMs have a 46,XY chromosomal pattern, indicating that dispermic fertilization accounts for some complete moles.[18,19] There is a rare, recently reported form of CHM, called familial recurrent hydatidiform mole (FRHM). FRHM is the repeated appearance of CHM in subsequent pregnancies of a patient and accumulates in families. The responsible gene is located on chromosome 19q13.4 and its mutation creates dysregulation of imprinting in the female germline, resulting in a biparental, rather than androgenetic origin of these CHMs.[20]

The clinical presentation has changed over the last decades, as better diagnostic modalities are available. Patients are aware that they are pregnant, but vaginal bleeding usually occurs in the first trimester and is still the most frequent presenting symptom of CHM. Vaginal bleeding varies from spotting to heavy bleeding and occurs in 84–97% of the patients as molar tissues separate from the decidua and disrupt maternal vessels.[21,22] Sometimes the passage of molar vesicles accompanies the bleeding. Prolonged bleeding results in maternal anemia in over 50% of patients and creates the liquefied and oxidized character of discharge which is called "prune juice" bleeding.[21]

Excessive uterine size is another of the classic signs but is seen in only half of the patients (38–51%). Excessive hCG production stimulates the proliferation of trophoblastic tissue, causing its overgrowth; retained blood also stretches the uterine wall.[22,23] Theca lutein cysts are typically over 6 cm in size; they are commonly multicystic, bilateral, contain serosanguineous fluid, and are seen in 15–46% of CHM cases. They sometimes reach over 20 cm in size. Formation is caused by hyperstimulation of the ovaries due to increased serum levels of beta-hCG and prolactin.[24] They regress spontaneously after evacuation of the CHM within 2–4 months. Surgical intervention is necessary only rarely, when torsion, bleeding, or necrosis occur.

The incidence of pre-eclampsia in the first trimester is pathognomonic and is seen in 12–27% of CHM cases. It is believed to be caused by elevated beta-hCG levels and increased uterine size. Clinical evaluation for CHM should be initiated if pre-eclampsia presents before 20 weeks of gestation, although convulsions rarely occur.[25,26]

Hyperemesis gravidarum requiring antiemetic treatment develops in 8–26% of patients but sometimes may be confused with the usual nausea associated with normal pregnancies. Similar to pre-eclampsia, hyperemesis is associated with elevated beta-hCG levels, increased uterine size, and elevated circulating estrogen levels.[23,27]

Hyperthyroidism is observed in approximately 7% of CHM and is almost always associated with high hCG levels. Laboratory evidence of hyperthyroidism is frequently detected in asymptomatic patients with CHM but thyroid function test values rapidly return to normal after evacuation of the molar pregnancy.[28] There is still controversy over the exact mechanism of hyperthyroidism in molar pregnancies. hCG was found to be the likely thyroid stimulator, as it binds to the TSH receptor site causing thyroid hyperfunction. Those patients who have new-onset or uncontrolled hyperthyroidism before surgical evacuation of the molar pregnancy require extra precautions in order to avoid thyroid storm. It is important to administer beta-adrenergic blocking agents even before the induction of anesthesia. The signs and symptoms of thyroid storm are convulsion, atrial fibrillation, hyperthermia, delirium, heart failure, and occasional cardiovascular collapse. Clinical symptoms of hyperthyroidism quickly disappear when CHM is evacuated.

Respiratory distress caused by trophoblastic embolization is very rare but presents with dramatic clinical manifestations. It develops in less than 2% of all patients with CHM.[26] Interestingly, respiratory complications were observed in 27% of those patients whose uterus reached 16-weeks size.[29,30] The typical symptoms are tachypnea, tachycardia, anxiety, and confusion, which frequently resolve immediately after the surgical evacuation. The symptoms of respiratory distress usually respond within 72 hours if appropriate pulmonary support is provided. The reason for respiratory distress is multifactorial, including direct embolization of the trophoblast into the pulmonary vasculature, co-existing pre-eclampsia, thyroid storm, and aggressive fluid replacement.

## Partial Mole

Partial hydatidiform moles have different characteristics from CHM: their chorionic villi vary in size and show only focal swelling and cavitations. Focal trophoblastic proliferation is more subtle compared to CHM. They present with focal trophoblastic hyperplasia and atypia at the implantation site. Marked villous scalloping and prominent stromal trophoblastic inclusions are seen on histology.[31,32] Fetal red blood cells are observed in the vessels of the villi and fetus, and fetal tissue can be identified. These fetuses rarely survive beyond 20 weeks. Most of the PHMs (90–93%) have a triploid karyotype (Table 1) containing 69 chromosomes, where the extra haploid set is derived from the father as the normal egg is fertilized by two sperm.[33–35] The identified fetal tissues usually have the stigmata of triploidy, including growth retardation and congenital anomalies.[36] The main symptom among 81 patients with partial mole evaluated at the

New England Trophoblastic Disease Center (NETDC) was vaginal bleeding (72.8%), while absence of fetal heartbeat (14.8%), excessive uterine enlargement (3.7%), and pre-eclampsia (2.5%) were observed in a much lower percentage of the patients.[37] No hyperthyroidism, hyperemesis gravidarum, or the presence of theca lutein cysts were found in this series.[37]

## Diagnosis

In the 1960s and 1970s, CHM was usually diagnosed in the second trimester when the characteristic clinical symptoms manifested, but recently ultrasonography and serum qualitative beta-hCG measurement have made first-trimester diagnosis much more common.[38] Ultrasonography itself is a very sensitive method to detect CHM as the complete mole has a characteristic vesicular "snowstorm" sonographic pattern.[38] In the case of PHM, ultrasonography is less sensitive, though two characteristic findings of focal cystic changes in the placenta and a ratio above 1.5 between the transverse and anteroposterior dimension of the gestational sac have been described.[39]

The measurement of pre-evacuation serum hCG levels shows marked elevations above 100,000 mIU/ml in 41–46% of patients with CHM.[40,41] A single measurement of hCG however is not diagnostic, as high values can be seen with multiple gestations, bleeding, or in cases of placental abruption. Therefore, hCG determination and ultrasound should be used together in the diagnosis of molar pregnancy.[22,42] The hCG measurements in partial moles are not as helpful. In one series, only 2 of 30 patients with PHM had values higher than 100,000 mIU/ml.[37]

## Treatment

### *Surgical treatment*

When the diagnosis of molar pregnancy is established, the patient should first be carefully evaluated for co-existing conditions such as anemia, hyperthyroidism, pre-eclampsia, and electrolyte imbalance. Beta-adrenergic blocking agents should be given to patients with hyperthyroidism, and treatment with Rh-negative immune globulin should be provided to Rh-negative patients as the RhD factor is expressed on trophoblast.

Suction curettage is the most preferred method to evacuate the molar pregnancy of those patients who desire to preserve fertility. Oxytocin infusion is suggested even before cervical dilatation. After initiating dilatation, heavy bleeding frequently occurs secondary to retained blood products, but it should not deter the completion of the dilatation and suction curettage. Gentle manual massage of the uterus during suction may be employed if the uterus size is over 14 weeks in order to stimulate contractions. When suction evacuation is completed, a gentle sharp curettage is used to remove any residual molar tissue.[43,44]

If the patient does not wish to preserve her fertility, hysterectomy may be performed. Larger theca lutein cysts causing pressure symptoms may be aspirated to facilitate their resolution. The patient must be counseled that though hysterectomy eliminates the risk of local invasion, it does not prevent distant metastases.

### *Prophylactic chemotherapy*

Several studies have been published implying that chemoprophylaxis significantly reduces the risk of postmolar GTN;[45] others, however, found that exposing patients to toxic treatment is controversial when the risk of the development of postmolar GTN is only 20%.[46] One of the earliest studies, applying a single dose of actinomycin D at the time of evacuation of high-risk CHM, found that only 10 of 247 patients (4%) had persistent invasive mole, but no metastasis, and all resolved after one further dose of chemotherapy.[47] Another study using a single dose of actinomycin D as chemoprophylaxis found that only 11% of the patients developed postmolar tumor from high-risk CHM.[46] Similar results were published in two other prospective randomized trials using prophylactic chemotherapy in patients with high-risk CHM, reducing the occurrence of postmolar tumor from 47% to 14% and from 50% to 13.8%, respectively.[48,49]

## Follow-up

After treatment, all patients should be followed with weekly determination of the $\beta$-subunit of hCG until normal for three consecutive weeks; patients should then be followed monthly until achieving six consecutive normal values. After reaching normal serum hCG levels, the risk of developing postmolar GTN is almost zero.[50,51] Patients should be encouraged to start effective contraception during the follow-up period. Hormonal oral contraceptive pills (OCPs) or barrier methods are preferred as intrauterine devices can cause perforation, infection, or bleeding if residual disease is present. Although one study found increased incidence of postmolar GTN with OCPs, the Gynecologic Oncology Group (GOG)[52] and NETDC data[53] suggest that the use of OCPs does not increase the risk of postmolar GTN. Oral contraceptive pills are safe to use over the follow-up period.

## GESTATIONAL TROPHOBLASTIC NEOPLASIA

Gestational trophoblastic neoplasia (GTN) is a group of diseases comprising invasive, persistent, metastatic, or nonmetastatic molar pregnancy; placental-site trophoblastic tumor (PSTT); and choriocarcinoma (CCA). The rapid recognition of malignant GTN is very important because any delay in the diagnosis may increase the patient's risk and have an unfavorable impact on the response to therapeutic efforts. Invasive moles are defined as the presence of edematous chorionic villi with proliferation invading the myometrium. CCA is an epithelial tumor containing both neoplastic syncytiotrophoblast and cytotrophoblast but no formed chorionic villi. PSTT is a rare tumor characterized by a proliferation of intermediate trophoblast cells with the absence of villi. There are no syncytiotrophoblast cells in PSTT and the tumors secrete very low levels of hCG. PSTT tends to metastasize late while CCA has a tendency for early metastasis.

### Epidemiology

The incidence of postmolar GTN is reported to be 18–29% in the United States compared to a rate of 8–10% in Europe.[54,55] Although there are different definitions of postmolar GTN in the US, the most accepted definition is the re-elevation or persistent plateau of hCG for at least three consecutive weeks after completion of therapy. Locally invasive GTN or metastasis can develop in 15% and 4% of the patients with CHM after evacuation, respectively.[56,57] Berkowitz and Goldstein reviewed 858 patients with CHM in order to identify predictors for the development of GTN. They found that at the time of presentation, 41% of patients had the following three signs of trophoblastic proliferation: (1) enlarged uterine size, (2) hCG level >100,000 mIU/ml, and (3) theca lutein cysts >6 cm in diameter. After treatment, 31% of these patients developed invasion and 8.8% had metastasis. Of those patients who did not have marked trophoblastic growth, only 3.4% developed invasion.[56] Other studies reported postmolar GTN in 57%[25] and 55%[58] of patients who had excessive uterine size and theca lutein cysts, respectively. Tow reported that GTN develops in 37% of patients who are older than 40 years of age.[59] In women over 50 years with a previous history of PHM, postmolar GTN was found in only 2–4%.[60]

## Diagnosis

The current International Federation of Gynecology and Obstetrics (FIGO) requirements for the diagnosis of postmolar GTN are the following:

1. Four or more values of plateaued hCG (+/–) over at least three weeks: days 1, 7, 14, and 21.
2. Elevation of hCG of 10% or greater for three values or more over at least two weeks: days 1, 7, and 14.
3. Persistence of hCG beyond six months after mole evacuation.
4. Histological diagnosis of choriocarcinoma.

The pretherapy evaluation of patients with GTN starts with an assessment of history for clinical risk factors and a thorough physical examination. Laboratory surveys should include baseline hCG level, thyroid, hepatic, and liver function tests. Radiology survey starts with a chest X-ray but if the X-ray is negative, a computed tomographic (CT) scan of the chest may be performed. When physical examination does not detect vaginal metastases and chest imaging studies are negative, the likelihood of liver or brain metastases is minimal. However, in all patients with symptoms, vaginal or lung metastasis, or pathologic diagnosis of choriocarcinoma, CT scan or magnetic resonance imaging (MRI) should be obtained to identify any possible brain or liver involvement. Ectopic location of a molar pregnancy is rare, and was diagnosed only in 0.8% of all GTN in a series published by the New England Trophoblastic Disease Center.[61] Usually, the classic symptoms of ectopic pregnancy, such as pain, bleeding, or shock due to tubal rupture, occur before the diagnosis of molar pregnancy is made. False positive serum hCG levels, or "phantom" hCG may present a diagnostic dilemma. These elevations are caused by heterophilic antibodies, which are not secreted into the urine based on their large size, resulting in negative urine testing. They create a low-level serum hCG elevation, usually only up to 300 mIU/ml. These heterophilic antibodies will not be affected by serial dilution of the patients' sera.

## Classification

Both nonmetastatic and metastatic GTN exist, although nonmetastatic GTN has a uniformly good outcome. Metastatic GTN is divided into good and poor prognostic groups. All metastatic GTN diagnosed less than four months after any type of gestation, with pretherapy hCG levels $<40,000$ mIU/ml, no brain or liver metastases, no antecedent term pregnancy, and no prior chemotherapy, are deemed good-prognosis metastatic GTN. Patients with the following risk factors are considered to have poor-prognosis metastatic GTN: disease diagnosed over four months following any form of gestation, pretherapy hCG level above 40,000 mIU/ml, presence of brain or liver metastasis, antecedent term pregnancy, and prior chemotherapy.

### *Nonmetastatic disease*

Invasive but nonmetastatic GTN occurs in about 15% of cases after CHM, but is very rarely seen after normal pregnancies.[57] Nonmetastatic GTN usually presents clinically with irregular vaginal bleeding, uterine subinvolution or enlargement, persistent or increasing serum hCG levels, and persistent theca lutein cysts. Intra-abdominal bleeding, pain, and sepsis are seen rarely in advanced GTN when the tumor invades and perforates the uterine wall to the abdominal cavity.

## *Metastatic disease and choriocarcinoma*

Choriocarcinoma is the most frequently metastasizing GTN. Metastatic GTN develops in 4% of cases after CHM.[56] Choriocarcinoma gives rise to early hematologic metastasis and reaches widespread dissemination. Berkowitz and Goldstein evaluated the most common sites of metastases: lungs (80%), followed by the vagina (30%), pelvis (20%), brain (10%), and liver (10%), with bowel, kidney, and spleen usually less than 5%.[26] Characteristic clinical symptoms and signs are pain and heavy bleeding at metastatic sites, as well as rising hCG levels.

Hemoptysis, chest pain, and dyspnea are typically the earliest symptoms of pulmonary metastases. Characteristic lung involvement can be seen on chest radiograph in both symptomatic and asymptomatic patients. Pulmonary hypertension can develop rapidly when trophoblastic emboli create pulmonary artery occlusion. Sometimes, pulmonary symptoms are the first manifestation of metastatic GTN, so this disease should be on the differential diagnosis for every woman of reproductive age who experiences sudden pulmonary symptoms.

## Staging

FIGO created a staging system for GTN (Table 2). Stage I includes all the diseases with elevated hCG levels and the tumor confined to the uterus.

Table 2. The FIGO anatomic staging of trophoblastic neoplasia.

| | |
|---|---|
| Stage I | Disease confined to the uterus |
| Stage II | The disease extends outside the uterus but is confined to the genital structures such as vagina, adnexa and broad ligament |
| Stage III | The disease extends into the lung with or without known genital disease |
| Stage IV | Metastatic to all other site/distant metastasis |

*Source*: Kohorn EI. The new FIGO 2000 staging and risk factor scoring system for gestational trophoblastic disease: description and critical assessment. *Int J Gynecol Cancer* 2000;11:73.

Stage II includes all patients whose tumor extends outside the uterus, but remains localized to the vagina and the pelvic organs such as internal genital structures, adnexa, and broad ligament. Stage III disease is diagnosed in those patients who have lung involvement with or without known genital tract disease. Stage IV comprises all patients with involvement of the liver, kidneys, gastrointestinal tract, and the brain.

## Prognostic Indicators

Although the anatomic staging system provides a good structure for comparable reporting in the literature, it does not predict the outcome for patients after treatment. The World Health Organization (WHO) recommended a prognostic scoring system based on the work of Bagshawe,[7] which predicts the likelihood of the drug resistance and disease outcome (Table 3). According to the new FIGO system, establishing the patient's disease status will include both the anatomic stage and FIGO risk score.

Table 3. Scoring system based on prognostic factors as adapted by FIGO.

| | **Scores** | | | |
|---|---|---|---|---|
| | **0** | **1** | **2** | **4** |
| Age (years) | <40 | ≥40 | | |
| Antecedent pregnancy | Mole | Abortion | Full-term | |
| Interval months from previous pregnancy | <4 | 4–6 | 7–<13 | ≥13 |
| Largest tumor size | $<10^3$ | $10^3$–$<10^4$ | $10^4$–$<10^5$ | $\geq 10^5$ |
| Site of metastases | Lung | Spleen/Kidney | Liver/GI | Brain |
| Number of metastases | — | 1–4 | 5–8 | >8 |
| Previous failed chemotherapy | — | — | Single drug | 2 or more drugs |

*Notes*: Format for reporting to FIGO Annual Report: The stage is represented by a Roman numeral: I, II, III, and IV. The arabic number shows the actual risk score of the patient, e.g., stage II:5, stage IV:8. GI: gastrointestinal.

*Source*: Kohorn EI. The new FIGO 2000 staging and risk factor scoring system for gestational trophoblastic disease: description and critical assessment. *Int J Gynecol Cancer* 2000;11:73.

The factors used in this scoring system are age, the form of antecedent pregnancy, the duration of the disease, history of prior chemotherapy, and the hCG level. Further anatomic variables included in this system are the tumor size, and the number and location of the metastases. The score can range between 0 and 26 and it is suggested by FIGO that when the score is 7 or greater the patient is considered to be "high-risk" and will require combination chemotherapy. In general, all patients with stage IV disease are considered high-risk and all those with stage I disease are low-risk. This scoring system is of most benefit to cases of stage II and III disease.

## Treatment

The treatment of GTN is determined by the risk score and stage of the disease. Options include chemotherapy as well as surgical methods. Depending on risk, chemotherapy may consist of single-agent or combination treatments. Surgical modalities include a wide variety of options starting with dilatation and curettage and hysterectomy, but may also include thoracotomy or craniotomy depending on the location of the metastasis.

### *Treatment of patients with stage I disease*

When disease is confined to the uterus, the treatment is in part determined by the patient's reproductive desires, although in this early stage, almost all patients can be treated without the need for hysterectomy (Table 4). If the patient wishes to retain fertility, single-agent chemotherapy is the suggested first-line treatment. Single-agent therapy can be sequential methotrexate (MTX) or actinomycin D (ACT D). Berkowitz *et al.* found that a single course of MTX and folinic acid (FA) achieved complete remission in 90.2% of patients with stage I GTN.[62] MTX is usually administered in a five-day course, 0.4 mg/kg daily intravenously or intramuscularly with CBC and platelet count checked daily (see Table 5). If no response is observed, the dose can be elevated to 0.6 mg/kg, or the treatment may be switched over to actinomycin D. Alternatively, MTX may be administered as "pulse treatment" at a dose of 40 mg/m$^2$ given intramuscularly weekly. An eight-day regimen with folinic acid may also be

Table 4. Summary of treatment protocols of gestational trophoblastic diseases.

| Stage | Risk score | Status | Therapy |
|---|---|---|---|
| I | | Initial | Single-agent chemotherapy ± hysterectomy |
| | | Resistant | Combination chemotherapy ± hysterectomy or local uterine resection |
| | | Follow-up | Weekly until 3 normal, then monthly for 12 months |
| | | Contraception | 12 months with normal hCG values |
| II–III | Low-risk | Initial | Single-agent chemotherapy |
| | | Resistant | Combination chemotherapy if resistant to both single agents |
| | High-risk | Initial | Combination chemotherapy |
| | | Resistant | Second-line combination therapy |
| | | Follow-up | Weekly until 3 normal, then monthly for 12 months |
| | | Contraception | 12 months with normal hCG values |
| IV | | Initial | Combination chemotherapy ± surgery and whole-head irradiation (3000 cGy) |
| | | Resistant | Second-line combination chemotherapy |
| | | Follow-up | Weekly until 3 normal, then monthly for 24 months |
| | | Contraception | 24 months with normal hCG values |

*Note*: hCG: human chorionic gonadotropin.

*Source*: Berkowitz RS, Goldstein DP. Molar pregnancy and gestational trophoblastic neoplasm. In: Barakat RR, Markman M, Randall ME, eds., *Principles and Practice of Gynecologic Oncology*, 5th edition. New York: Wolters Kluwer, 2009, pp. 875–895.

administered. The usual adverse events include thrombocytopenia (1.6%), granulocytopenia (5.9%), and hepatotoxicity (14.1%)[62] though mucositis, serositis, gastrointestinal toxicity, and alopecia are also reported. Before using methotrexate, liver function should be checked as the drug undergoes hepatic metabolism. Hematologic, renal, and hepatic indices should be monitored before each chemotherapy cycle and hCG should be checked weekly. Actinomycin D is also given in a five-day protocol at 12 $\mu$g/kg administered daily intravenously. If there is no response, the dose can be increased further by 2 $\mu$g/kg or the treatment should be switched to

MTX. If ACT D is administered in a pulse fashion, 1.25 mg/m$^2$ should be given every other week.

The serum hCG level should be measured weekly following each course of treatment. If the hCG level falls progressively, no further treatment is needed. However, if the hCG level plateaus or starts to increase over three consecutive weeks, a second course of chemotherapy should be administered. If the hCG values do not decline by one log after repeated treatment, the patient should be considered resistant and another single-agent treatment should be considered. Hammond *et al.* using single-agent methotrexate, noted disease resistance in only 4 of 58 (7%) patients who were then successfully salvaged with single-agent actinomycin D.[63] In a more detailed analysis from Lurain *et al.* only 10.7% of the 253 patients initially treated with single-agent methotrexate required treatment with a second single agent, 1.2% of the patients needed multiple-agent therapy, and 0.8% of them underwent hysterectomy.[64] If the patient's disease is resistant to all single agents, then combination therapy should be started. Usually MAC (methotrexate, actinomycin D, and cyclophosphamide or chlorambucil) is the most frequently used combination chemotherapy (Table 5). If MAC fails, EMA/CO (etoposide, methotrexate, actinomycin D, cyclophosphamide, and vincristine) is used. In rare situations, when the patient is resistant to both single and combined treatment, a local uterine resection can be an option to preserve fertility.[65] Careful evaluation of the localization of the residual tumor with MRI, ultrasound, or arteriogram is needed before performing the operation.

If the patient does not wish to retain fertility, hysterectomy with adjuvant single-agent chemotherapy is the generally accepted first-line treatment. Early hysterectomy also reduces the duration and the amount of chemotherapy needed to produce remission. Adjuvant chemotherapy is safe and beneficial for the following three reasons: (1) it reduces the possibility of the tumor cells disseminating during surgery, (2) chemotherapy may maintain a sufficiently cytotoxic level to treat cells that have already spread into the blood stream, and (3) it treats occult metastases which already exist at the time of surgery. Most centers in the United States will start treatment with weekly IM methotrexate or bolus actinomycin D, with hysterectomy performed during the first cycle of chemotherapy. Chemotherapy is continued until hCG levels normalize, with at least one

### *Treatment of patients with stage IV disease*

These patients have the greatest risk of developing chemotherapy-resistant disease with rapid progression. All patients with stage IV disease must be treated with primary combination chemotherapy (EMA/CO). Combined modality therapy with radiation or surgery may be considered. Radiation combined with multiagent chemotherapy yielded 75% cure rates in those patients who initially presented with brain metastases.[68,69] Brain metastases usually respond well to whole-brain (3,000 cGy in ten fractions) radiation combined with multiagent chemotherapy. Concurrent use of chemotherapy and radiation therapy has been suggested by Yordan *et al.* in order to reduce the occurrence of spontaneous cerebral hemorrhage.[70] Craniotomy may be necessary for acute decompression or control of life-threatening hemorrhage as well as resection of resistant tumor nodules. Further therapy of patients with high-risk GTN who have chemoresistant tumor is very difficult and is influenced by previous chemotherapy exposure. The combination of etoposide and cisplatin with or without bleomycin or doxorubicin and vinblastine-bleomycin-cisplatin achieved a 50–86% remission rate in the salvage setting.[71] Chemotherapy should be continued until hCG values are normalized. After initial remission, 13% of patients with high-risk disease will develop recurrence.[71] The follow-up of patients with stage IV disease is extended for a two-year period with contraception prescribed over the interval.

## FUTURE FERTILITY

Patients with any form of hydatidiform mole can expect normal reproductive capacities in the future.[72,73] A patient with one prior CHM has a 1–2% risk of subsequent molar pregnancy.[74] It is reasonable to suggest that if the patient becomes pregnant following prior CHM, she should undergo comprehensive ultrasound evaluation to verify normal fetal anatomy and growth as well as an hCG measurement six weeks postpartum to rule out GTN. Garner *et al.* evaluated the outcome of subsequent pregnancies in those patients with a history of prior molar pregnancies and reported 68.6% full-term live births, 7.4% preterm deliveries, 0.9% ectopic pregnancies, 0.5% stillbirths, and 1.5% repeat molar pregnancies.[74] These outcomes, as well as the frequency of congenital malformation, were similar to that of the general population.[74] Subsequent pregnancy outcomes appear similar regardless of whether the mole was complete or partial. The recently used standard chemotherapy protocols in the treatment of malignant GTN do not significantly influence patients' ability to reproduce. The largest study which evaluated post-treatment reproductive outcomes found that 83% of women had at least one subsequent live birth.[75] No differences were found in the rate of subsequent pregnancy outcomes between patients treated with single-agent methotrexate versus multiagent chemotherapy.[75]

## REFERENCES


1. Lurain JR. Advances in management of high-risk gestational trophoblastic tumors. *J Reprod Med* 2002;47(6):451–459.
2. Palmer JR. Advances in the epidemiology of gestational trophoblastic disease. *J Reprod Med* 1994;39(3):155–162.
3. Bracken MB. Incidence and aetiology of hydatidiform mole: an epidemiological review. *Br J Obstet Gynaecol* 1987;94(12):1123–1135.
4. Jeffers MD, O'Dwyer P, Curran B, Leader M, Gillan JE. Partial hydatidiform mole: a common but underdiagnosed condition. A 3-year retrospective clinicopathological and DNA flow cytometric analysis. *Int J Gynecol Pathol* 1993;12(4):315–323.
5. Di Cintio E, Parazzini F, Rosa C, Chatenoud L, Benzi G. The epidemiology of gestational trophoblastic disease. *Gen Diagn Pathol* 1997;143(2–3):103–108.
6. Mazzanti P, La Vecchia C, Parazzini F, Bolis G. Frequency of hydatidiform mole in Lombardy, Northern Italy. *Gynecol Oncol* 1986;24(3):337–342.
7. Bagshawe KD. Risk and prognostic factors in trophoblastic neoplasia. *Cancer* 1976;38(3):1373–1385.
8. Fulop V, Mok SC, Berkowitz RS. Molecular biology of gestational trophoblastic neoplasia: a review. *J Reprod Med* 2004;49(6):415–422.
9. Berkowitz RS, Cramer DW, Bevnstein MR, Cassells S, Driscoll SG, Goldstein DP. Risk factors for complete molar pregnancy from a case-control study. *Am J Obstet Gynecol* 1985;152(8):1016–1020.
10. Parazzini F, La Vecchia C, Mangili G, *et al.* Dietary factors and risk of trophoblastic disease. *Am J Obstet Gynecol* 1988;158(1):93–99.

11. Parazzini F, Mangili G, La Vecchia C, Negri E, Bocciolone L, Faśoli M. Risk factors for gestational trophoblastic disease: a separate analysis of complete and partial hydatidiform moles. *Obstet Gynecol* 1991;78(6):1039–1045.
12. Berkowitz RS, Bernstein MR, Harlow BL, *et al.* Case-control study of risk factors for partial molar pregnancy. *Am J Obstet Gynecol* 1995;173(3 Pt 1): 788–794.
13. Cheung AN, Srivastava G, Pittaluga S, Man TK, Ngan H, Collins RJ. Expression of *c*-myc and *c*-fms oncogenes in trophoblastic cells in hydatidiform mole and normal human placenta. *J Clin Pathol* 1993;46(3):204–207.
14. Cheung AN, Srivastava G, Chung LP, *et al.* Expression of the p53 gene in trophoblastic cells in hydatidiform moles and normal human placentas. *J Reprod Med* 1994;39(3):223–227.
15. Tuncer ZS, Vegh GL, Fulop V, Genest DR, Mok SC, Berkowitz RS. Expression of epidermal growth factor receptor-related family products in gestational trophoblastic diseases and normal placenta and its relationship with development of postmolar tumor. *Gynecol Oncol* 2000;77(3):389–393.
16. Vassilakos P, Riotton G, Kajii T. Hydatidiform mole: two entities. A morphologic and cytogenetic study with some clinical consideration. *Am J Obstet Gynecol* 1977;127(2):167–170.
17. Montes M, Roberts D, Berkowitz RS, Genest DR. Prevalence and significance of implantation site trophoblastic atypia in hydatidiform moles and spontaneous abortions. *Am J Clin Pathol* 1996;105(4):411–416.
18. Kajii T, Ohama K. Androgenetic origin of hydatidiform mole. *Nature* 1977; 268(5621):633–634.
19. Pattillo RA, Sasaki S, Katayama KP, Roesler M, Mattingly RF. Genesis of 46,XY hydatidiform mole. *Am J Obstet Gynecol* 1981;141(1):104–105.
20. Fisher RA, Hodges MD, Newlands ES. Familial recurrent hydatidiform mole: a review. *J Reprod Med* 2004;49(8):595–601.
21. Goldstein DP, Berkowitz RS. Current management of complete and partial molar pregnancy. *J Reprod Med* 1994;39(3):139–146.
22. Kohorn EI. Molar pregnancy: presentation and diagnosis. *Clin Obstet Gynecol* 1984;27(1):181–191.
23. Berkowitz RS, Goldstein DP, Bernstein MR. Evolving concepts of molar pregnancy. *J Reprod Med* 1991;36(1):40–44.
24. Osathanondh R, Berkowitz RS, de Cholnoky C, Smith BS, Goldstein DP, Tyson JE. Hormonal measurements in patients with theca lutein cysts and gestational trophoblastic disease. *J Reprod Med* 1986;31(3):179–183.

25. Curry SL, Hammond CB, Tyrey L, Creasman WT, Parker RT. Hydatidiform mole: diagnosis, management, and long-term followup of 347 patients. *Obstet Gynecol* 1975;45(1):1–8.
26. Berkowitz RS, Goldstein DP. Pathogenesis of gestational trophoblastic neoplasms. *Pathobiol Annu* 1981;11:391–411.
27. Depue RH, Bernstein L, Ross RK, Judd HL, Henderson BE. Hyperemesis gravidarum in relation to estradiol levels, pregnancy outcome, and other maternal factors: a seroepidemiologic study. *Am J Obstet Gynecol* 1987; 156(5):1137–1141.
28. Galton VA, Ingbar SH, Jiminez-Fonseca J, Hershman JM. Alterations in thyroid hormone economy in patients with hydatidiform mole. *J Clin Invest* 1971;50(6):1345–1354.
29. Twiggs LB, Morrow CP, Schlaerth JB. Acute pulmonary complications of molar pregnancy. *Am J Obstet Gynecol* 1979;135(2):189–194.
30. Garner EI, Chang-Lee WY, Lu KH, Goldstein DP, Berkowitz RS. Trophoblastic pulmonary embolization after hysterectomy for invasive complete mole. A case report. *J Reprod Med* 1999;44(10):908–912.
31. Wells M. The pathology of gestational trophoblastic disease: recent advances. *Pathology* 2007;39(1):88–96.
32. Szulman AE, Surti U. The syndromes of hydatidiform mole. I. Cytogenetic and morphologic correlations. *Am J Obstet Gynecol* 1978;131(6):665–671.
33. Niemann I, Petersen LK, Hansen ES, Sunde L. Differences in current clinical features of diploid and triploid hydatidiform mole. *BJOG* 2007;114(10): 1273–1277.
34. Lawler SD, Fisher RA, Dent J. A prospective genetic study of complete and partial hydatidiform moles. *Am J Obstet Gynecol* 1991;164(5 Pt 1): 1270–1277.
35. Lai CY, Chan KY, Khoo US, *et al.* Analysis of gestational trophoblastic disease by genotyping and chromosome *in situ* hybridization. *Mod Pathol* 2004;17(1):40–48.
36. Philipp T, Grillenberger K, Separovic ER, Philipp K, Kalousek DK. Effects of triploidy on early human development. *Prenat Diagn* 2004;24(4):276–281.
37. Berkowitz RS, Goldstein DP, Bernstein MR. Natural history of partial molar pregnancy. *Obstet Gynecol* 1985;66(5):677–681.
38. Lazarus E, Hulka C, Siewert B, Levine D. Sonographic appearance of early complete molar pregnancies. *J Ultrasound Med* 1999;18(9):589–594; quiz 595–596.

39. Fine C, Bundy AL, Berkowitz RS, Boswell SB, Berezin AF, Doubilet PM. Sonographic diagnosis of partial hydatidiform mole. *Obstet Gynecol* 1989; 73(3 Pt 1):414–418.
40. Savage P, Seckl M, Short D. Practical issues in the management of low-risk gestational trophoblast tumors. *J Reprod Med* 2008;53(10):774–780.
41. Genest DR, Laborde O, Berkowitz RS, Goldstein DP, Bernstein MR, Lage J. A clinicopathologic study of 153 cases of complete hydatidiform mole (1980–1990): histologic grade lacks prognostic significance. *Obstet Gynecol* 1991;78(3 Pt 1):402–409.
42. Soper JT, Mutch DG, Schink JC. Diagnosis and treatment of gestational trophoblastic disease: ACOG Practice Bulletin No. 53. *Gynecol Oncol* 2004; 93(3):575–585.
43. Berkowitz RS, Goldstein DP. Current management of gestational trophoblastic diseases. *Gynecol Oncol* 2009;112(3):654–662.
44. Sebire NJ, Seckl MJ. Gestational trophoblastic disease: current management of hydatidiform mole. *BMJ* 2008;337:a1193.
45. Uberti EM, Fajardo Mdo C, da Cunha AG, *et al.* Prevention of postmolar gestational trophoblastic neoplasia using prophylactic single bolus dose of actinomycin D in high-risk hydatidiform mole: a simple, effective, secure and low-cost approach without adverse effects on compliance to general follow-up or subsequent treatment. *Gynecol Oncol* 2009;114(2):299–305.
46. Goldstein DP, Berkowitz RS. Prophylactic chemotherapy of complete molar pregnancy. *Semin Oncol* 1995;22(2):157–160.
47. Goldstein DP, Berkowitz RS, Bernstein MR. Management of molar pregnancy. *J Reprod Med* 1981;26(4):208–212.
48. Kim DS, Moon H, Kim KT, Moon YJ, Hwang YY. Effects of prophylactic chemotherapy for persistent trophoblastic disease in patients with complete hydatidiform mole. *Obstet Gynecol* 1986;67(5):690–694.
49. Limpongsanurak S. Prophylactic actinomycin D for high-risk complete hydatidiform mole. *J Reprod Med* 2001;46(2):110–116.
50. Wolfberg AJ, Growdon WB, Feltmate CM, *et al.* Low risk of relapse after achieving undetectable HCG levels in women with partial molar pregnancy. *Obstet Gynecol* 2006;108(2):393–396.
51. Lavie I, Rao CC, Castrillon DH, Miller DS, Schorge J. Duration of human chorionic gonadotropin surveillance for partial hydatidiform moles. *Am J Obstet Gynecol* 2005;192(5):1362–1364.

52. Curry SL, Schlaerth JB, Kohorn EI, *et al.* Hormonal contraception and trophoblastic sequelae after hydatidiform mole (a Gynecologic Oncology Group Study). *Am J Obstet Gynecol* 1989;160(4):805–809; discussion 809–811.
53. Berkowitz RS, Goldstein DP, Marean AR, Bernstein M. Oral contraceptives and postmolar trophoblastic disease. *Obstet Gynecol* 1981;58(4):474–477.
54. Bagshawe KD. Throphoblastic neoplasia In: Holland JF, Frei E, III, Bast R Jr, eds. *Cancer Medicine*. Baltimore: Williams & Wilkins, 1993, pp. 1691–1703.
55. Kohorn EI. Evaluation of the criteria used to make the diagnosis of nonmetastatic gestational trophoblastic neoplasia. *Gynecol Oncol* 1993;48(2): 139–147.
56. Berkowitz RS, Goldstein DP. Presentation and management of molar pregnancy. In: Hancock BW, Newlands ES, Berkowitz RS, eds., *Gestational Trophoblastic Disease*. London: Chapman and Hall, 1997, pp. 127–142.
57. Berkowitz RS, Goldstein DP. Management of molar pregnancy and gestational trophoblastic tumors. In: Knapp RC, Berkowitz R, eds., *Gynecologic Oncology*. New York: McGraw-Hill, 1993, pp. 328–350.
58. Morrow CP. Postmolar trophoblastic disease: diagnosis, management, and prognosis. *Clin Obstet Gynecol* 1984;27(1):211–220.
59. Tow WS. The influence of the primary treatment of hydatidiform mole on its subsequent course. *J Obstet Gynaecol Br Commonw* 1966;73(4):544–552.
60. Berkowitz RS, Goldstein DP. Chorionic tumors. *N Engl J Med* 1996;335(23):1740–1748.
61. Muto MG, Lage JM, Berkowitz RS, Goldstein DP, Bernstein MR. Gestational trophoblastic disease of the fallopian tube. *J Reprod Med* 1991;36(1):57–60.
62. Berkowitz RS, Goldstein DP, Bernstein MR. Ten year's experience with methotrexate and folinic acid as primary therapy for gestational trophoblastic disease. *Gynecol Oncol* 1986;23(1):111–118.
63. Hammond CB, Borchert LG, Tyrey L, Creasman WT, Parker RT. Treatment of metastatic trophoblastic disease: good and poor prognosis. *Am J Obstet Gynecol* 1973;115(4):451–457.
64. Lurain JR, Brewer JI, Torok EE, Halpern B. Gestational trophoblastic disease: treatment results at the brewer trophoblastic disease center. *Obstet Gynecol* 1982;60(3):354–360.
65. Berek JS, Hacker NF, Berkowitz RS, Goldstein DP. eds., Gestational trophoblastic neoplasia. In: *Practical Gynecologic Oncology*, 4th ed. Philadelphia: Lippincott Williams & Wilkins, 2005, pp. 603–623.

66. Bower M, Newlands ES, Holden L, *et al.* EMA/CO for high-risk gestational trophoblastic tumors: results from a cohort of 272 patients. *J Clin Oncol* 1997; 15(7):2636–2643.
67. Surwit EA, Childers JM. High-risk metastatic gestational trophoblastic disease. A new dose-intensive, multiagent chemotherapeutic regimen. *J Reprod Med* 1991;36(1):45–48.
68. Soper JT. Role of surgery and radiation therapy in the management of gestational trophoblastic disease. *Best Pract Res Clin Obstet Gynaecol* 2003; 17(6):943–957.
69. Small W Jr, Lurain JR, Shetty RM, Huang CF, Applegate GL, Brand WN. Gestational trophoblastic disease metastatic to the brain. *Radiology* 1996; 200(1):277–280.
70. Yordan EL, Jr, Schlaerth J, Gaddis O, Morrow CP. Radiation therapy in the management of gestational choriocarcinoma metastatic to the central nervous system. *Obstet Gynecol* 1987;69(4):627–630.
71. Lurain JR. Management of high-risk gestational trophoblastic disease. *J Reprod Med* 1998;43(1):44–52.
72. Uberti EM, Fajardo Mdo C, Ferreira SV, *et al.* Reproductive outcome after discharge of patients with high-risk hydatidiform mole with or without use of one bolus dose of actinomycin D, as prophylactic chemotherapy, during the uterine evacuation of molar pregnancy. *Gynecol Oncol* 2009;115(3):476–481.
73. Garrett LA, Garner EI, Feltmate CM, Goldstein DP, Berkowitz RS. Subsequent pregnancy outcomes in patients with molar pregnancy and persistent gestational trophoblastic neoplasia. *J Reprod Med* 2008;53(7):481–486.
74. Garner EI, Lipson E, Bernstein MR, Goldstein DP, Berkowitz RS. Subsequent pregnancy experience in patients with molar pregnancy and gestational trophoblastic tumor. *J Reprod Med* 2002;47(5):380–386.
75. Woolas RP, Bower M, Newlands ES, Secki M, Short D, Holden L. Influence of chemotherapy for gestational trophoblastic disease on subsequent pregnancy outcome. *Br J Obstet Gynaecol* 1998;105(9):1032–1035.

# 12

# ONCOLOGIC EMERGENCIES

*Sarah Adams*

## INTRODUCTION

Some women learn that they have a gynecologic cancer when visiting an emergency department with symptoms such as vaginal bleeding, pain, or intestinal obstruction. Women diagnosed with cancer may also require emergent medical care due to operative complications or symptoms resulting from chemotherapy, radiotherapy, or recurrent disease. Diagnosis of acute complications of therapy can be difficult in women with cancer who have multiple symptoms resulting from tumor burden, treatment toxicity, or other medical comorbidities. This chapter will review the presentation and management of clinical scenarios that require urgent care of women with gynecologic cancer, including hemorrhage, gastrointestinal obstruction, or perforation, thromboembolism, and sepsis. The common theme in managing all of these is the importance of early recognition and diagnosis, and the need to maintain a high index of suspicion in directing the care of women with gynecologic cancer.

## HEMORRHAGE

Vaginal bleeding may be the presenting symptom for women with gynecologic malignancies, but only rarely is severe enough to require emergency medical attention. Cervical cancer, endometrial cancer, and less common malignancies, such as sarcomas, gestational trophoblastic disease, and advanced vulvar cancer, may initially present with vaginal bleeding.[1]

## Cervical Cancer

Vaginal bleeding caused by cervical cancer is usually painless and typically occurs between menses or postcoitally.[1,2] Large tumors or advanced disease involving ulceration of the cervix or upper vagina, however, may present emergently with heavy vaginal bleeding.

After ensuring that the patient is stable, careful speculum exam is advised prior to bimanual exam in any woman presenting with bleeding. If the bleeding is confirmed to be cervical, it may be controlled directly with application of silver nitrite or Monsel's solution for discrete areas, or with vaginal packing for diffuse or heavy bleeding. Women who require vaginal packing will likely also require urinary catheterization and admission for observation and management.

Some cervical bleeding may resolve after packing. In patients who are not managed surgically, persistent or recurrent bleeding from a cervical tumor may require palliative radiation or arterial embolization for definitive control.[3] In a case series of six patients, four of whom had cervical cancer and bleeding persisting longer than four days, Mihmanli *et al.* reported 100% success in eliminating recurrent vaginal bleeding with bilateral uterine artery occlusion, without any complications.[4] In a larger series of patients with pelvic cancers, Pisco *et al.* reported cessation of bleeding in 70% of patients, with a decrease in bleeding severity in an additional 21%.[5] Only 11 patients continued to require transfusion following the procedure, and of these, six were unable to undergo bilateral arterial occlusion due to anatomic distortion or tumor effects.[5] Decisions about employing these procedures will depend on the extent of the patient's disease and plans for further management.

## Uterine Cancer

Although vaginal bleeding is the most common presenting complaint for women with endometrial cancer, it is seldom of sufficient magnitude to warrant an emergent evaluation. Women with recurrent disease in the vagina may also present with vaginal bleeding, but this too is seldom heavy and usually can be managed on an outpatient basis. An exception may be women with uterine sarcomas, which can cause vaginal hemorrhage in a subset of cases. In women who are not surgical candidates, or who cannot be resuscitated with transfusions, uterine artery embolization may be a temporizing option to reduce the severity of vaginal bleeding.[3] This may be done in preparation for surgery or in patients who decline transfusion for cultural or other reasons prior to initiating definitive therapy. Arterial embolization should be used with caution in these situations, however, as case reports of women treated with uterine artery embolization for fibroids who were later diagnosed with leiomyosarcomas demonstrated poor response to the procedure due to tumor vascularization from parasitic sources.[6,7] Severe complications from arterial embolization are rare, but include sepsis and pulmonary embolism.[6]

Women with gestational trophoblastic neoplasia most commonly present with vaginal bleeding.[8] Bleeding will be seen from the cervical os on speculum exam, and occasionally vesicular material also may be seen extruding through the os.[1] The definitive diagnosis is made by ultrasonography, which shows a distinctive multiechogenic pattern. A patient with gestational trophoblastic neoplasia should be admitted for further management.

## Vulvar Cancer

Severe bleeding caused by vulvar cancer is rare,[9] and women presenting with bleeding usually have an advanced vulvar lesion. Patients with advanced disease and bleeding should be admitted to initiate treatment. Options include surgical management or palliative radiation therapy.

## Intraoperative Bleeding

The primary treatment for most gynecologic malignancies includes surgical staging, which carries with it the risk of intraoperative bleeding complications. Patients with malignancies may be at a higher risk of bleeding due to tumor vascularity or impingement on major vessels. In addition, complications of anemia may be more severe in women with advanced or recurrent cancers who are malnourished or who have hepatic or cardiac disease, or pre-existing anemia due to prior radiation or chemotherapy.[10]

Surgical procedures which are most commonly associated with severe hemorrhagic complications during cancer staging include entry trocar

Table 1. Strategies to reduce risk of intraoperative hemorrhage.

| |
|---|
| Preoperative notation of any history of bleeding disorders or hepatic disease |
| Preoperative evaluation of coagulation factors and bleeding time |
| Careful patient selection for minimally invasive procedures |
| Preoperative investigation of cardiac function and reserve |
| Evaluation of imaging studies to determine the location and size of metastatic tumor implants |
| Insertion of peripheral large-bore IV lines or central access |
| Consideration of a vertical midline incision to improve access and visualization of the upper abdomen |
| Utilization of meticulous surgical technique |

injuries during laparoscopic or robotic procedures, lacerations of the great vessels during pelvic or para-aortic lymphadenectomy, splenic injury during debulking or total omentectomy, and bleeding from vascular tumors. Strategies to reduce the risk of intraoperative hemorrhage are detailed in Table 1.[11]

Despite these measures, intraoperative hemorrhage can occur as a result of distorted anatomy, tumor encroachment on large vessels, or the extent of resection necessary to achieve optimal debulking. Management of hemorrhage intraoperatively will be case-dependent but common strategies include suture ligation of vascular defects, the application of hemostatic clips, or vascular ligation proximal to the site of injury. Applying pressure to the site of bleeding to control blood loss until the patient can be stabilized may be necessary before proceeding with definitive measures.[11]

Venous bleeding can be more difficult to control than arterial bleeding due to the thin walls of veins and the less predictable course of venous structures. In many cases prolonged pressure may be sufficient to allow clotting, but larger venous injuries will require repair. Fine 5.0 suture can be used to directly repair venous lacerations after applying pressure with the hand or with a clamp. Presacral bleeding may require bone wax or compression with a sterile thumbtack if the injured vessel retracts into the sacral foramina.[11] If these measures fail, the patient's pelvis can be packed and re-explored at a second surgery following hematologic resuscitation. Alternately, a pack can be designed for removal at the bedside once the patient is stabilized in an intensive care setting.[11]

Compared with venous injuries, arterial lacerations are less frequent and can be easier to repair because of their thicker vessel walls and more predictable course. Strategies to control arterial bleeding include cautery of small vessels, suture ligation, or proximal ligation of select pelvic vessels.[11] After bleeding is controlled with a vascular clamp, 5.0 monofilament suture can be used to directly repair arterial vessels. More severe injuries may require a vein graft or patch, and postoperative anticoagulation is recommended to avoid having the site of repair become a nidus for clot formation.[11] Hypogastric artery ligation can be used to control bleeding from the uterus, the vaginal cuff, the broad ligament, or from pelvic tumor implants fed by this vessel.[3,5] Prophylactic ligation of the hypogastric artery has been described as a strategy to reduce the risk of intraoperative hemorrhage during radical hysterectomy to resect large pelvic tumors.[3] Typically a hypogastric artery ligation involves isolating the anterior division of the vessel for occlusion to reduce the risk of injury to the underlying internal iliac vein under the main arterial trunk; however, ligation of the main trunk may be performed to control bleeding from pudendal arteries of the pelvic floor.[11] Finally, any injury to mesenteric vessels requires evaluation of the bowel for any signs of ischemia. Devascularized bowel should be resected to avoid the risk of necrosis postoperatively.

## Postoperative Bleeding

Signs of significant postoperative bleeding are noted in Table 2.[2,10,11] Immediate management of the patient is facilitated by placing her in the

Table 2. Signs of postoperative hemorrhage.

| |
|---|
| Orthostatic hypotension |
| Pallor |
| Tachycardia |
| Tachypnea |
| Oliguria |
| Vaginal bleeding |
| Increased surgical drain output |
| Abdominal distention |
| Abdominal tenderness |

early to avoid severe sequelae. Management of these situations is focused on identifying the cause and rapidly initiating appropriate resuscitation or transfusion. Transfusion reactions, including anaphylaxis, underscore the importance of adopting a systematic and detail-oriented approach to managing patients with gynecologic cancers who develop bleeding complications.

## GASTROINTESTINAL COMPLICATIONS

Because of their location, most gynecologic malignancies affect bowel function, either directly through local spread, or indirectly with pressure from pelvic tumors or changes in bowel motility resulting from treatment regimens. As a result, gastrointestinal complications are common among women with these cancers, and are responsible for a large proportion of morbidity and mortality due to gynecologic tumors.

### Bowel Obstruction

Bowel obstruction is present at initial diagnosis in approximately 8–30% of patients with ovarian cancer,[12] and may be present in up to 51% of women with recurrent disease.[13,14] Women with bowel obstruction at the time of diagnosis of ovarian cancer have a diminished progression-free (19 vs. 21 months, $p = 0.001$) and overall survival (22 vs. 35 months, $p = 0.0008$).[12] In women with obstruction that results from disease recurrence and carcinomatosis, median survival is as low as one to three months,[14] and among women with ovarian cancer, bowel obstruction is the most common cause of death.[13]

Bowel obstruction in the setting of gynecologic malignancies may result from external compression by pelvic or abdominal tumors, direct infiltration of the bowel wall by metastatic disease, ileus due to intestinal muscle paralysis, postoperative adhesion formation, or radiation-induced bowel stricture.[2] Women with bowel obstruction typically present with persistent nausea and vomiting or anorexia, often have abdominal pain and distention, and may report an absence of flatus or bowel movements.[11,15] They may also be dehydrated, with resulting tachycardia or hypotension. Tympany, distention, and tenderness may be evident on abdominal exam, and radiographic studies will show air-fluid levels and bowel distention. It is critical to note overdistention of the large bowel, as a diameter greater than 10 cm is associated with a high risk of perforation and requires prompt decompression.[11] Women with bowel obstruction usually require admission for rehydration and management.

Medical management of bowel obstruction involves placement of a nasogastric tube to drain the stomach, decompress the bowel, and partially alleviate symptoms, as well as administration of intravenous fluid and close observation.[2] Relief of the obstruction is marked by the return of bowel activity with flatus, reduced nasogastric tube output, and the ability to tolerate liquids orally.[11] For these women the nasogastric tube can be removed and they can slowly resume a normal diet. Patients who do not respond rapidly to bowel rest will require parenteral nutritional supplementation. Women who develop progressive distention, fever, and leukocytosis associated with constant pain may have bowel necrosis from strangulation or perforation, and require immediate surgical evaluation.[11]

The decision to perform surgery for the managment of bowel obstruction can be difficult. Obstruction occuring acutely in the postoperative period generally should be managed surgically to evaluate for reversible causes, including torsion, ischemia, or mechanical obstruction with adhesions, which can be repaired.[11,16] Obstruction occurring as a result of recurrent cancer or an increasing tumor burden may also respond to surgical debulking, but the poor prognosis associated with this diagnosis suggests that the primary indication for surgery is palliation of symptoms.[13,14,16,17] The poor quality of life associated with bowel obstruction, however, supports palliative surgical intervention: a survey of patients with malignant bowel obstruction catalogued symptoms that included anorexia, fatigue, and poor overall well-being, with a deterioration in psychological functioning one month after diagnosis that continued to worsen after three months.[14]

A third option for the managment of a large bowel obstruction is the placement of a colonic stent to avoid the morbidity of surgery. These wire mesh stents can be placed endoscopically and expanded either directly or following balloon dilation of the colon.[14] Successful stent placement in women with gynecologic cancers was demonstrated in a series of 35 patients treated in 2001–2006 with a median length of obstruction of 6.5 cm.[18] Stent placement was performed in 27 women (77%), and one third of those women went on to have additional surgery to definitively manage their obstruction.[19] Failure of stent placement was due to bowel stricture or anatomic distortion. There were no complications reported for women who were successfully treated, although other series have reported a rate of bowel perforation of up to 5%.[18] Median survival among women who were successfully stented was 7.7 months compared with 1.9 months in cases when stenting failed, but these results did not reach statistical significance.[18]

## Bowel Perforation

Fortunately, bowel perforation is a rare event, but it can be catastrophic in women with recurrent gynecologic cancers. Bowel perforation can develop following obstruction and overdistention of the bowel or as a result of tumor infiltration of the intestinal wall.[11,20] Additional risk factors for perforation or fistula formation include massive dilation of the bowel (>12 cm), a history of prior obstruction, and treatment with anti-angiogenic chemotherapies such as bevacizumab.[20–22] In some cases the symptoms may be unexpectedly subtle, but most patients with bowel injury will have severe abdominal pain, possibly accompanied by fever, tachycardia, and abdominal rigidity resulting from acute peritonitis. A CT scan with Gastrografin may be helpful to confirm the diagnosis.[20]

With the success of bevacizumab, a humanized IgG1 antibody to the VEGF receptor, for primary or secondary treatment of women with gynecologic malignancies, more women may be at risk for bowel perforation.[21,22] Although bevacizumab is generally well-tolerated, toxicity from this drug can be severe, particularly in instances of bowel perforation.[20] The rate of bowel perforation associated with bevacizumab treatment is reported to be higher in women with ovarian cancer (0–15.4%, mean 5.4%) than in patients with other solid tumors (1.5–2.4%).[22] Risk factors for bowel perforation associated with bevacizumab are similar to general risk factors, and include a recent history of surgery, tumor involving the bowel, and prior radiation.[20] The mechanism of bowel disruption resulting from bevacizumab therapy is unknown but has been postulated to be related to necrosis of tumor involving the bowel wall, poor wound healing after bowel injury, or thrombosis of mesenteric vessels with resulting bowel ischemia.[21] The higher rates among women with ovarian cancer may result from the common development of peritoneal carcinomatosis with bowel obstruction, distention, and higher likelihood of prior bowel surgery.[21] More recently, an immunologic explanation was proposed when patients with ovarian cancer who developed bowel perforations were noted to have higher incidences of tumor-infiltrating T cells, leading investigators to speculate that immune-mediated tumor lysis results in a bystander effect with inflammation and weakening of the bowel wall.[23]

The development of bowel perforation in women with gynecologic cancers is associated with a high mortality rate.[11] Successful management depends on early diagnosis which requires a high index of suspicion. Imaging studies may confirm bowel perforation with signs such as free intraperitoneal air, extra-luminal contrast, and abscess formation.[20] If detected early, perforations can be treated with antibiotics and percutaneous drainage of abscess cavities, followed by intestinal diversion, but the decision to operate will depend on the anatomic location of the perforation and on the patient's overall performance status.[2,11] Management of bowel perforations occuring during bevacizumab treatment is particularly difficult due to impaired wound healing attributed to VEGF blockade. In a cohort of patients with colon cancer, Scappaticci *et al.* documented higher rates of postoperative complications, including wound dehiscence, bowel perforation, anastomotic leaks, fistula development, abscess, or hemorrhage, in patients treated with bevacizumab regimens, compared with patients receiving chemotherapy regimens that did not include bevacizumab (13% vs. 3%).[24] The half-life of bevacizumab is 20 days, and as a result, any elective surgical procedure should be delayed by at least 6–8 weeks after bevacizumab treatment if possible.

## Gastrointestinal Fistulas

Women with gynecologic malignancies may develop gastrointestinal fistulas as a consequence of tumor infiltration of the bowel, or as a complication of surgery or treatment with radiation or chemotherapy.[2,11] Fistulas developing in the postoperative period can result from an unrecognized enterotomy at the time of surgery, from erosion of a foreign body such as an intraperitoneal drain, or from infection and wound breakdown.[2] In patients treated with radiation or antiangiogenic chemotherapy, fistulas result from devascularization and breakdown of the affected tissue.[22] Patients with enterocutaneous fistulas may present with discharge from a prior incision site from surgery or a percutaneous drain site. Subcutaneous fluid collections may yield feculent material, and local necrosis or overlying cellulitis with erythema, warmth, or tenderness may be evident. Enterovaginal, or rectovaginal communications cause persistent vaginal discharge which may consist of caustic small bowel contents or feculent material if the distal intestinal tract is involved. It is often difficult to localize a fistulous tract due to patient discomfort, especially in patients who have vaginal stenosis from prior irradiation, but a gentle speculum exam may be helpful to confirm the diagnosis. CT fistulograms can also be performed to document the location of a tract for treatment planning. Women with a new fistula, or with evidence of infection from a chronic fistula, should be admitted and managed with broad-spectrum antibiotics and bowel rest, with surgical diversion or repair once any acute infection has resolved.

Overall, injury to the gastrointestinal tract resulting from tumor burden or treatment regimens results in a large proportion of morbidity experienced by women with gynecologic cancers. Attention to symptoms such as bloating, abdominal pain, nausea, or fever can alert the clinician to these conditions, and prompt earlier diagnosis and management. Complications due to advanced or recurrent disease are more difficult to manage, and careful consideration of the goals of care should be reviewed with patients before proceeding with surgical management.

## THROMBOEMBOLISM

Women with gynecologic cancers have an approximately threefold risk of thromboembolic events compared to women without a cancer diagnosis,[25] and deep vein thrombosis (DVT) or pulmonary embolus (PE) may be the presenting symptom that leads to a cancer diagnosis in some patients.

Studies of women with gynecologic cancer have demonstrated increased plasma viscosity and red cell aggregation, which impair blood flow and induce thrombosis and hypoxia, which in turn promotes resistance to therapy.[25] High levels of vascular endothelial growth factor (VEGF) produced by ovarian cancers can lead to fibrin clotting and leakage of fibrinogen into extravascular spaces, and cross-linked fibrin stranding and D-dimers have been documented in the plasma, ascites and cystic fluid of patients with ovarian cancer.[26] Studies of the peritoneum of women with ovarian cancer also documented high levels of multiple coagulation factors.[26] In addition to an acquired coagulopathy associated with malignancies, women with large pelvic tumors often also have vascular compression and venous stasis, which contributes to clot formation.[25]

The development of a venous thrombus in women with gynecologic cancers is associated with a poor prognosis. Among 95 patients with ovarian, endometrial, or cervical cancers, the median survival from the time of thrombus diagnosis was 7.8 months, with a five-year survival of only 20%, and a twofold increased risk of death.[25] Any patient presenting with a new venous thrombus should undergo evaluation for malignancy as a possible etiology of their coagulopathy: the incidence of cancer has been reported to be as high as 16.5% among patients with an idiopathic venous thromboembolism, including 5.6% who were diagnosed with ovarian and 2% with uterine cancer.[25] Finally, particular histologic subtypes of gynecologic cancers may confer higher susceptibility to thrombus formation: in a cohort of women with clear cell ovarian cancer, a thromboembolic event was documented in 42% of patients (relative risk 2.5).[27]

This risk of thrombotic events is increased in the postoperative period, and thromboembolism has been reported in up to 38% of women undergoing surgery for gynecologic cancers. Pulmonary embolus accounts for 3–4% of perioperative mortality in this group, and represents the leading cause of postoperative death in high-risk gynecologic cancer cases.[25] A proposed mechanism for this association implicates the physical disruption of the vascular endothelium following surgical trauma, which leads to release of tissue factor and exposure to pro-coagulant cytokines. In addition, immobility in the postoperative period favors clot formation.

The risk for thromboembolic events extends well past the typical postoperative hospital stay, with a rate of 7–17% within 42 days of

Classically, infected subcutaneous tissue does not bleed when incised, but the underlying muscle is spared. Identification of tissue which bleeds normally can be used to determine appropriate surgical margins but patients often require repeated debridement operations in addition to broad-spectrum antibiotics to completely treat the affected area. Patients subjected to extensive debridement will need intensive care, possibly in a burn unit.

### *Evisceration or vaginal cuff dehiscence*

Evisceration, with fascial separation, may present as an incisional mass or bulge with valsalva, and patients may report pain or nausea which can be sudden in onset or related to exertion or coughing. Risk factors for evisceration include a history of prior hernia, steroid use, immunosuppression, poorly controlled diabetes, obesity, infection, chronic cough, and tobacco use.[11] Evaluation of the wound will reveal a fascial defect and sometimes bowel herniation. If the bowel is exposed, the wound should be covered with sterile, moist towels, and arrangements made for the patient to be taken to the operating room for fascial closure.

Vaginal cuff dehiscence is a rare complication following hysterectomy that requires prompt medical attention. Risk factors include early resumption of intercourse postoperatively, increased intra-abdominal pressure, smoking, history of prior surgery or radiation, connective tissue disease, and steroid use.[31] Patients may present with vaginal pain or pressure or with protrusion of bowel into the vaginal vault.[31,32] The diagnosis can be confirmed with a sterile speculum exam and requires immediate surgical management.

## Indwelling Catheters or Drains

The placement of Foley catheters or surgical drains introduces a route for bacterial infection in the surgical patient. Correct sterile technique at the time of insertion of bladder catheters will prevent most infections, but the rate of urinary tract infection increases with the duration of use, and some practitioners will administer prophylactic antibiotics to women who require urinary catheterization for a prolonged period.[33] Surgical drains similarly should be used sparingly and removed as soon as possible. Removal of any indwelling drains or foreign bodies should be strongly considered in patients who present with fever or signs of infection.[10]

Vascular catheters, particularly central lines, can also place patients at risk for infection. These may be placed at the time of surgery, or later for chemotherapy administration. Peripherally inserted central catheters (PICC) do not appear to reduce the risk of infection associated with central venous lines.[2] Symptoms of a line infection include local inflammation and erythema at the site of insertion, which may be associated with purulence or tenderness, and may extend deep into the tract of the catheter line. If the bacteria contaminates the catheter lumen, patients may present with symptoms of bacteremia, including high fever and rigors.[2,10] Diagnosis of a line infection is made clinically based on signs and symptoms, but a culture of the line site may help to direct therapy. Blood cultures will reveal bacteremia resulting from luminal contamination. Treatment for line infections typically requires intravenous antibiotics, and is accelerated by removal of the infected line if possible. If the central line cannot be removed, it is preferable to initiate antibiotic therapy peripherally through a separate line. Choice of antibiotic therapy will be guided by culture results but empiric therapy should be started immediately with vancomycin alone in the case of superficial infection, and broad-spectrum combination therapy for patients with bacteremia or sepsis. Serial blood cultures should be monitored during treatment, and antibiotics should be continued for at least one week after documenting negative culture results.

Intraperitoneal catheters placed for chemotherapy administration are another potential nidus for infection in women with ovarian or other gynecologic cancers.[2] Like intravenous catheters, intraperitoneal lines may become superficially infected at the entry site, or they may be a conduit for bacteria resulting in peritonitis. Symptoms include tenderness, erythema, and fluctuance at the port site. The development of peritonitis may result in abdominal pain and fever, with rebound on examination. As with intravenous line infections, the diagnosis of an intraperitoneal catheter infection is made clinically, with cultures used to guide treatment. In patients who do not respond to intravenous antibiotics, the catheter should be removed. Intraperitoneal antibiotic therapy may speed resolution of the infection but requires careful dose calculation to avoid systemic toxicity from vascular absorption.

## Urosepsis

The most common source of infection in women with gynecologic cancers is the urinary tract, accounting for as many as 50% of hospital admissions for infection among women with pelvic tumors.[2,33] In addition to postoperative patients or patients requiring long-term bladder catheterization, women at risk for urinary tract infection include those undergoing pelvic radiation, and women with large tumors causing ureteral obstruction. Women with ureteral obstruction often present with nonspecific flank pain, occasionally radiating to the pelvis and groin. Urinary infection is associated with dysuria, fever, flank pain or suprapubic tenderness. Elevated leukocytosis and an abnormal urinalysis will confirm the diagnosis and culture will guide antibiotic choice. Patients in whom urosepsis is suspected, or patients who are debilitated or have been hospitalized for prolonged periods, should be treated with broad-spectrum antibiotics empirically until culture results are available. In the case of obstruction, definitive management will depend on the severity and etiology of the obstruction, but may require percutaneous nephrostomy tubes or urinary diversion to prevent recurrent infection.[34]

## Gastrointestinal Infections

Infections resulting from contamination by bowel flora may occur as a result of tumor erosion into the bowel, intraoperative injury, radiation-induced necrosis or fistula, or, rarely, bowel perforation.[2] The diagnosis and management of bowel perforation were reviewed in the discussion of gastrointestinal perforation earlier in this chapter. General principles guiding the management of infections from the intestinal tract include the early initiation of broad-spectrum antibiotics, drainage of any abscesses, and consideration of surgical repair of bowel injury in patients who are healthy enough to undergo an operation.[11]

A more common source of gastrointestinal infection affecting women with gynecologic cancers is the development of *Clostridium difficile* colitis. Women who are hospitalized, or who are treated with antibiotics or chemotherapy are at risk for *C. difficile* colitis, and may present with abdominal pain, fever, and frequent watery diarrhea.[2] Patients may require hospitalization for hydration and supportive care, and should be treated with oral metronidazole, or oral vancomycin in patients who do not respond to metronidazole.

## Neutropenic Fever

Women receiving chemotherapy for gynecologic malignancies may experience bone marrow suppression and neutropenia, leaving them particularly vulnerable to infection.[2,35] Most chemotherapeutic drugs cause some degree of myelosuppression, with neutropenic toxicity particularly associated with carboplatin and taxanes, common first-line agents for gynecologic tumors. Women with recurrent disease may have cumulative effects of multiple drug regimens, and be more prone to myelosuppressive toxicity. Neutropenia is defined as a neutrophil count of less than 1,000 cells/mm$^3$ (grade 3 toxicity), or 500 cells/mm$^3$ in cases of severe (grade 4) toxicity. Depressed neutrophil counts increase the risk of infection with skin flora such as *Staphylococcus* species, or gut flora, including *Escherichia coli* or *Klebsiella pneumoniae* as well as fungal and viral pathogens. Despite their immunosuppression, neutropenic patients may still mount a fever, even with counts as low as 100 cells/mm$^3$, which may be the only clinical sign of infection.

Neutropenia is typically diagnosed on routine blood tests scheduled during the anticipated nadir period following chemotherapy. Neutrophil counts should also be evaluated in patients undergoing chemotherapy who develop a fever higher than 100.5°F.[35] Women with neutrophil counts below 1,000 cells/mm$^3$ with fever should undergo a comprehensive evaluation and be admitted for empiric antibiotic therapy. Any evidence of hypotension or cardiovascular compromise which might suggest sepsis should direct admission of the patient to an intensive care unit. Cultures of blood, urine, and any fluid collections or abscesses should be collected, and radiographic imaging should be obtained. The current standard of care for initial antibiotic treatment of neutropenic patients is single-agent therapy with third- or fourth-generation cephalosporins or carbapenems, although culture results will direct the final choice of therapy. Treatment with antibiotics should continue until the neutrophil count returns to a level above 500–1000 cells/mm$^3$ and the patient is afebrile.

## Tumor Fever

Complicating the diagnosis of infection or sepsis in women with gynecologic cancers are the multiple symptoms attributable directly to tumor burden, including fevers.[2] Women with advanced or recurrent gynecologic cancers may have abdominal pain, distention, bowel obstruction, dehydration, tachycardia, hypotension, shortness of breath, and a myriad of other symptoms that can mimic the presentation of serious infections. Conversely, women undergoing chemotherapy, or women with advanced disease who are debilitated, may be unable to mount an inflammatory response to infection, making the diagnosis of septic complications difficult. Finally, the tumor itself may cause fever, although this is usually a diagnosis of exclusion. Tumor fever is typically associated with hepatic or pulmonary metastasis. Patients may feel relatively well with intermittent flares of high fever with rigors that do not respond to broad-spectrum antibiotics. If tumor fever is suspected after excluding infectious causes, women can be treated with anti-inflammatory agents for symptom relief.

Thus, the diagnosis of infections in women with gynecologic malignancies can be complicated by unusual or delayed symptoms, concomitant toxicity from chemotherapy or radiation, and by symptoms attributable to disease burden. Despite this, infectious complications of cancer treatment are often preventable through the use of prophylactic antibiotics and careful sterile technique.

## SUMMARY

Women with gynecologic cancers are susceptible to medical complications from their tumor burden as well as from surgery, chemotherapy, or radiation therapy that may require emergent medical attention. It is important to consider the effects and toxicities of these interventions when evaluating patients with a history of malignancy in the emergency setting, and to have a high index of suspicion to support early diagnosis and minimize morbidity and mortality in this vulnerable patient population.

## REFERENCES


1. DiSaia PJ, Creasman WT. *Clinical Gynecologic Oncology*, 6th ed. St. Louis: Mosby, 2002.
2. Hoskins WJ. *Principles and Practice of Gynecologic Oncology*, 4th ed. Philadelphia, PA: Lippincott Williams & Wilkins, 2005.
3. Dehaeck CM. Transcatheter embolization of pelvic vessels to stop intractable hemorrhage. *Gynecol Oncol* 1986;24(1):9–16.
4. Mihmanli I, Cantasdemir M, Kantarci F, Halif Yilmaz M, Numan F, Mihmanli V. Percutaneous embolization in the management of intractable vaginal bleeding. *Arch Gynecol Obstet* 2001;264(4):211–214.
5. Pisco JM, Martins JM, Correia MG. Internal iliac artery: embolization to control hemorrhage from pelvic neoplasms. *Radiology* 1989;172(2):337–339.
6. Common AA, Mocarski EJ, Kolin A, Pron G, Soucie J. Therapeutic failure of uterine fibroid embolization caused by underlying leiomyosarcoma. *J Vasc Interv Radiol* 2001;12(12):1449–1452.
7. Goldberg J, Burd I, Price FV, Worthington-Kirsch R. Leiomyosarcoma in a premenopausal patient after uterine artery embolization. *Am J Obstet Gynecol* 2004;191(5):1733–1735.
8. Kohorn EI. What we know about low-level hCG: definition, classification and management. *J Reprod Med* 2004;49(6):433–437.
9. Morley GW. Cancer of the vulva: a review. *Cancer* 1981;48(Suppl. 2): 597–601.
10. Marino PL, Sutin KM. *The ICU Book*, 3rd ed. Philadelphia, PA: Lippincott Williams & Wilkins, 2007.
11. Webb MJ, Kelly DG, Mayo Clinic. Division of Gynecologic Surgery. *Manual of Pelvic Surgery*, 2nd ed. Berlin; New York: Springer-Verlag, 1994.
12. Rauh-Hain JA, del Carmen M, Horowitz WS, *et al.* Impact of bowel obstruction at the time of initial presentation in women with ovarian cancer. *BJOG* 2010;117(1):32–38.
13. Ripamonti C, Bruera E. Palliative management of malignant bowel obstruction. *Int J Gynecol Cancer* 2002;12(2):135–143.

14. Selby D, Wright F, Stilos K, *et al.* Room for improvement? A quality-of-life assessment in patients with malignant bowel obstruction. *Palliat Med* 2010; 24(1):38–45.
15. Chase DM, Lopez S, Nguyen C, Pugmire GA, Monk BJ. A clinical pathway for postoperative management and early patient discharge: does it work in gynecologic oncology? *Am J Obstet Gynecol* 2008;199(5):541 e1–e7.
16. Rauh-Hain JA, Olawaiye AB, Munro EG, *et al.* Role of computed tomography in the surgical management of patients with bowel obstruction secondary to recurrent ovarian carcinoma. *Ann Surg Oncol* 2010; 17(3): 853–860.
17. Gwilliam B, Bailey C. The nature of terminal malignant bowel obstruction and its impact on patients with advanced cancer. *Int J Palliat Nurs* 2001;7(10):474–481.
18. Caceres A, Zhou Q, Iasonos A, Gerdes H, Chi OS, Barakat RR. Colorectal stents for palliation of large-bowel obstructions in recurrent gynecologic cancer: an updated series. *Gynecol Oncol* 2008;108(3):482–485.
19. Baraza W, Lee F, Brown S, Hurlstone DP. Combination endo-radiological colorectal stenting: a prospective 5-year clinical evaluation. *Colorectal Dis* 2008;10(9):901–906.
20. Badgwell BD, Camp ER, Feig B, *et al.* Management of bevacizumab-associated bowel perforation: a case series and review of the literature. *Ann Oncol* 2008;19(3):577–582.
21. Wright JD, Secord AA, Numnum TM, *et al.* A multi-institutional evaluation of factors predictive of toxicity and efficacy of bevacizumab for recurrent ovarian cancer. *Int J Gynecol Cancer* 2008;18(3):400–406.
22. Shord SS, Bressler LR, Tierney LA, Cuellar S, George A. Understanding and managing the possible adverse effects associated with bevacizumab. *Am J Health Syst Pharm* 2009;66(11):999–1013.
23. Tanyi J, *et al.* Clinical predictors of bevacizumab-associated gastrointestinal perforation. *Gyn. Oncol.* 2011;120(3):464–469.
24. Scappaticci FA, Fehrenbacher L, Cartwright T, *et al.* Surgical wound healing complications in metastatic colorectal cancer patients treated with bevacizumab. *J Surg Oncol* 2005;91(3):173–180.
25. Wang X, Fu S, Freedman RS, Kavanagh JJ. Venous thromboembolism syndrome in gynecological cancer. *Int J Gynecol Cancer* 2006;16 (Suppl. 1): 458–471.

26. Freedman RS, Deavers M, Liu J, Wang E. Peritoneal inflammation — A microenvironment for Epithelial Ovarian Cancer (EOC). *J Transl Med* 2004; 2(1):23.
27. Duska LR, Garrett L, Henretta M, Ferriss JS, Lee L, Horowitz N. When 'never-events' occur despite adherence to clinical guidelines: the case of venous thromboembolism in clear cell cancer of the ovary compared with other epithelial histologic subtypes. *Gynecol Oncol* 2010;116(3):374–377.
28. Einstein MH, Kushner DM, Connor JP, *et al.* A protocol of dual prophylaxis for venous thromboembolism prevention in gynecologic cancer patients. *Obstet Gynecol* 2008;112(5):1091–1097.
29. Leonardi MJ, McGory ML, Ko CY. A systematic review of deep venous thrombosis prophylaxis in cancer patients: implications for improving quality. *Ann Surg Oncol* 2007;14(2):929–936.
30. Wechter ME, Pearlman MD, Hartmann KE. Reclosure of the disrupted laparotomy wound: a systematic review. *Obstet Gynecol* 2005;106(2): 376–383.
31. Croak AJ, Gebhart JB, Klingele CJ, Schroeder G, Lee RA, Podratz KC. Characteristics of patients with vaginal rupture and evisceration. *Obstet Gynecol* 2004;103(3):572–576.
32. Robinson BL, Liao JB, Adams SF, Randall TC. Vaginal cuff dehiscence after robotic total laparoscopic hysterectomy. *Obstet Gynecol* 2009;114(2 Pt 1): 369–371.
33. Chamberlain DH, Hopkins MP, Roberts JA, McGuire EJ, Morely GW, Wang CC. The effects of early removal of indwelling urinary catheter after radical hysterectomy. *Gynecol Oncol* 1991;43(2):98–102.
34. Dudley BS, Gershenson DM, Karanagh JJ, Copeland LJ, Carrasco CH, Rutledge FN. Percutaneous nephrostomy catheter use in gynecologic malignancy: M.D. Anderson Hospital experience. *Gynecol Oncol* 1986;24(3): 273–278.
35. Rubin SC. *Chemotherapy of Gynecologic Malignancies*, 2nd ed. Philadelphia, PA: Society of Gynecologic Oncologists.

# 13

# SUPPORTIVE CARE

*Yevgeniya J. Ioffe and Premal H. Thaker*

## INTRODUCTION

During the second half of the 20th century the field of gynecologic oncology witnessed several therapeutic breakthroughs. As a result, the life expectancy of the patients afflicted with cancer was slowly but steadily rising. However, despite the increasing number of therapeutic options, a large number of patients were surviving for longer increments of time but were living with advanced disease. Due to this phenomenon, the issue of quality of life began to gain more attention. Several organizations and interest groups, such as the Multinational Association of Supportive Care in Cancer (MASCC), emerged over the last several decades. Some of the main goals of MASCC are as follows: (1) alleviating symptoms and complications of cancer, (2) reduction and prevention of toxicities of treatment, and (3) easing the emotional burden of patients and caregivers.

Palliative care is any form of medical treatment that concentrates on reducing the severity of disease symptoms and improving the patient's quality of life, rather than striving to provide a cure. Non-hospice palliative care is not dependent on prognosis and is offered in conjunction with curative approaches. The modern hospice is a relatively recent concept that originated in the United Kingdom after the founding of St. Christopher's Hospice in 1967; Dame Cicely Saunders is considered the founder of the modern hospice movement.[1,2]

Hospice in the United States began as a volunteer-based movement striving to care for people dying alone or isolated; over the last several decades hospice care became a full-fledged, and compensated healthcare component. Hospice is the only Medicare benefit that includes pharmaceuticals, medical equipment, 24-hour seven days a week access to care, and support for loved ones following a death.[3] Most hospice care is delivered at home. The first United States hospital-based palliative care programs began in the late 1980s at institutions such as the Cleveland Clinic and Medical College of Wisconsin. In the present day these programs are numbering over 1,200.[2]

Similar to palliative care, supportive care focuses on improving the quality of life of cancer patients suffering from tumor-related effects such as ascites, pleural effusion, pain, and bowel obstruction and treatment-related effects such as nausea and vomiting, peripheral neuropathy, and mucositis. The objective of this chapter is to review some of the common strategies and practices of supportive and palliative care in patients with advanced gynecologic malignancies.

## MANAGEMENT OF COMMON SYMPTOMS

### Nausea and Vomiting

Nausea and vomiting are common symptoms in patients with advanced cancer, occurring in approximately 21% to 68% of these patients. The physiologic center responsible for processing the input leading to nausea and emesis, i.e. the vomiting center, is located in the reticular formation of the medulla. This area receives input from the chemoreceptor trigger zone, the upper gastrointestinal tract and pharynx, the vestibular apparatus, and the higher cortical centers. In a patient with an advanced gynecologic malignancy, nausea and vomiting can stem from a large number of mechanical, metabolic, pharmacological, treatment-induced, and psychological stimuli.[4]

The mechanical causes of nausea usually are attributable to obstruction or occlusion of small or large bowel, as well as paralytic dysfunction of the bowels. The management of bowel obstruction is discussed in another section of this manual. Paralytic dysfunction of the bowels that leads to chronic nausea is managed somewhat differently from acute nausea, usually with a prokinetic agent such as metoclopramide.[5] Metoclopramide can be administered orally or parenterally at doses of 10 mg four times a day, or if needed every four hours. A continuous parenteral infusion of metoclopramide, at doses of 60 to 120 mg/day, may be helpful for patients with refractory chronic nausea. An infrequent complication of this antidopaminergic agent is extrapyramidal symptoms.[5,6] The addition of dexamethasone to metoclopramide may be useful in select cases, although one study has suggested that dexamethasone was not better than placebo in patients who were not controlled with metoclopramide. The exact mechanism of action and the optimal dose of corticosteroids for this indication are not known, and the duration of use of a corticosteroid is short-term.[7]

The metabolic and pharmacologic causes of nausea are common etiologies in the setting of advanced malignancy. A number of pharmacologic agents such as nonsteroidal anti-inflammatory agents (NSAIDs), opioids, and agents used for management of depression, such as selective serotonin re-uptake inhibitors (SSRIs), may also exacerbate the nausea. In a patient undergoing treatment with opioids, nausea frequently occurs with the initiation of treatment, but frequently resolves within several days.[6] However, nausea resulting from the accumulation of morphine-6-glucuronide, a morphine metabolite, may persist especially in patients with impaired renal function who are at increased risk. Other metabolic causes of nausea may include uremia, dehydration, and hypercalcemia. The management of hypercalcemia often includes rehydration and the use of diuretics, steroids, and bisphosphonates. While correcting the hypercalcemia, 5-hydroxytryptamine-3 (5-$HT_3$) serotonin receptor antagonists, antihistamines, and steroids can be used to control nausea.[8,9]

## *Chemotherapy-induced nausea and emesis*

Historically, chemotherapy-induced nausea and vomiting (CINV) has been a common side effect and one of the most feared complications of the treatment of cancer. Guidelines for the management of chemotherapy-induced nausea and emesis have been published by the American Society of Clinical Oncology (ASCO) and the National Comprehensive Cancer Network (NCCN), as well as other organizations. Currently, the antineoplastic agents are divided into four groups based upon their emetogenicity potential: high (producing emesis in 90% of cases), moderate (producing emesis in 30–90% of cases), low (producing emesis in 10–30% of cases), and minimal (fewer than 10%).[10–13]

Furthermore, the patterns of CINV are subdivided based upon the timing of symptom onset: acute, delayed, breakthrough, refractory, and anticipatory CINV. Acute CINV begins within the first 24 hours after initiation of chemotherapy, with acute delayed nausea and vomiting occurring 12–24 hours from the onset of treatment. Delayed nausea and vomiting develops more than 24 hours after chemotherapy initiation and may last for six to seven days. Some of the agents commonly used in the management of gynecologic malignancies such as carboplatin, cisplatin, cyclophosphamide, and doxorubicin are often associated with delayed nausea and vomiting.[13,14] Modern classes of antiemetics include 5-$HT_3$ serotonin receptor antagonists, substance P antagonists, neurokinin 1 receptor antagonists, motility agents, antihistamines, phenothiazines, benzodiazepines, cannabinoids, and corticosteroids.[6,9,13,14]

Antiemetic regimens used in offsetting the effects of at least moderately emetogenic chemotherapies almost uniformly include 5-$HT_3$ serotonin receptor antagonists (Table 1). These agents are well-established in the management of acute emesis, but less so in the management of delayed emesis. Palonosetron, the newest 5-$HT_3$ serotonin receptor antagonist, is approved by the US Food and Drug Administration (FDA) for prevention of acute CINV associated with moderately and highly emetogenic chemotherapy and for the prevention of delayed CINV associated with moderately emetogenic chemotherapy. A randomized double-blind trial of palonosetron versus ondansetron showed higher efficacy rates for palonosetron in controlling both acute and delayed emesis. However, palonosetron is only available in IV preparations.[15]

Aprepitant is an oral agent that is commonly used in a three-day course for the prevention of acute and delayed nausea and vomiting. This agent works by binding to the protachykinin-1 receptor. Aprepitant may also be useful when used in combination with oral dexamethasone. The latter agent is recommended for prevention of acute CINV for low and moderately emetogenic chemotherapy.[14,16]

Notably, benzodiazepines can be useful to reduce anxiety and the risk of anticipatory CINV, but the antiemetic potential of benzodiazepines such as lorazepam and alprazolam is low. In addition, nonpharmacologic

Table 1. List of treatment agents for chemotherapy-induced nausea and vomiting.

| Agent | Class | Route | Dosage/Emetogenicity |
|---|---|---|---|
| Ondansetron | $5\text{-}HT_3$ receptor antagonist | Oral, IV | 24 mg/high; 16 mg/moderate; 8 mg (0.15 mg/kg) |
| Granisetron | $5\text{-}HT_3$ receptor antagonist | Oral, IV | 2 mg; 1 mg (0.01 mg/kg) |
| Tropisetron | $5\text{-}HT_3$ receptor antagonist | Oral, IV | 5 mg; 5 mg |
| Dolasetron | $5\text{-}HT_3$ receptor antagonist | Oral, IV | 100 mg; 100 mg (1.8 mg/kg) |
| Palonosetron | $5\text{-}HT_3$ receptor antagonist | IV | 0.25 mg |
| Aprepitant | $NK_1$-receptor antagonist | Oral | 125 mg on day 1, 80 mg on days 2 and 3 |
| Dexamethasone | Corticosteroid | Oral, IV | 12 mg/highly emetogenic with aprepitant, 20 mg without aprepitant; 8 mg/moderately emetogenic; 8 mg/high & moderate given on days 2 and 3 |
| Lorazepam | Benzodiazepine/GABA receptor inhibitor | Oral, IV | 2.5 mg orally × 2 night before and after chemotherapy for anticipatory nausea; 1.5 mg/m$^2$ 45 minutes before chemotherapy |

therapies such as acupressure, acupuncture-point stimulation, hypnosis, and massage may provide some relief of CINV.[6,8,13]

## Fatigue

With a prevalence rate of 60%, fatigue is the most common symptom experienced by patients with cancer. Cancer-related fatigue (CRF) is often experienced alongside sleep disturbances, depression, and pain syndromes. For many patients, CRF is more distressing than any other cancer-related symptoms since it ubiquitously affects the activities of daily living. In the early 2000s, the National Institutes of Health identified treatment of CRF as one of the priorities in improving cancer care.

Contributing to the etiology of CRF are a number of factors including the cancer itself, treatment-related effects, anemia, infection, and psychological conditions such as depression. Clinicians faced with the treatment of fatigue can address the correctable physiologic conditions such as anemia, infection, and metabolic disturbances first. However, if the symptoms persist, nonpharmacologic and pharmacologic interventions aimed at the treatment of fatigue can be then utilized.[6]

There are a number of pharmacologic modalities that may be given consideration. It is a rather frequent occurrence that the diagnosis of cancer coexists with depression. An atypical antidepressant such as bupropion that has also been used in the treatment of chronic fatigue syndrome may be useful in alleviating both conditions. A systemic review of the literature by Carroll and colleagues identified two case series in which treatment with bupropion SR (100–300 mg/day) was associated with improvements in fatigue scores within 2–4 weeks of the initiation of treatment.[17] Several studies demonstrated improvement of CRF with the use of modafinil, a CNS stimulant, and psychostimulants such as methylphenidate and dexmethylphenidate. However, the use of these agents should be carefully weighed against the potential side effects of irritability, anorexia, tachycardia, mood lability, as well as insomnia.

In addition, nonpharmacologic treatments should be utilized when initiating the treatment of CRF. These interventions include exercise, nutritional and dietary assessment, and improved sleep hygiene. A replacement of L-carnitine, a micronutrient important in energy production, may be beneficial in individuals who have received chemotherapy.[6–9]

## Constipation

In patients with an advanced gynecologic malignancy, constipation is a common problem. It may develop as an adverse effect of narcotic analgesics or large bowel dysmotility secondary to tumor burden. In individuals afflicted with this problem, daily assessment for signs and symptoms of constipation should be performed. Assessment is performed via history taking regarding the frequency, quantity, and quality of bowel movements, as well as a flat plate radiograph of the abdomen to assess the quantity of stool content in the bowel as well as a digital rectal examination if necessary. Treatment options include a number of pharmacological agents as well as behavioral changes. If possible, an increase in fluid intake and the addition of fiber to daily diet as well as regular exercise should be encouraged.[6]

All patients receiving opioids should be started on a prophylactic bowel regimen at the time of initiation of narcotic therapy, including a stool softener (e.g., docusate) and a stimulant laxative (e.g., senna tablets).[18] Other stimulant agents such as bisacodyl, cascara, castor oil, phenolphthalein, polyethylene glycol (Miralax®), and danthron may also be useful. Saline laxatives include magnesium sulfate, milk of magnesia, magnesium citrate, phospho-soda, and sodium phosphate. The above-mentioned agents lead to bowel movement by drawing fluid into the intestine, causing distention and reflex peristalsis. If saline laxatives are used, attention should be paid to the fluid and electrolyte balance, since those may become depleted with repetitive use.[8] Prolonged use of stimulant laxatives may ultimately contribute to a loss of normal bowel function and cause laxative dependence. This issue should be weighed against the long-term prognosis and goal of palliative care in each individual patient.

For patients in whom stool softeners and stimulant laxatives are inadequate, enemas and suppositories are helpful especially in the management of proximal rectal dysmotility. A variety of enema preparations are available, including warm normal saline or simply warm tap water, phosphate/biphosphate, soapsuds, milk and molasses, and mineral oil. The two main types of suppositories in use are bisacodyl and glycerin. Methylnaltrexone subcutaneously can be used for refractory opioid-induced constipation without affecting pain control.[19]

Clinicians should also be aware that fecal impaction is frequently underdiagnosed. This complication may be particularly dangerous in a patient with an advanced malignancy and can lead to bowel perforation.[6]

## MANAGEMENT OF COMPLICATIONS OF CHEMOTHERAPY

### Neutropenic Fever

Several components of the immune system are affected by chemotherapy, starting with the skin and mucosal membrane barriers as well components of cellular and humoral immunity including immunoglobulin function, T lymphocytes, and macrophages. The neutrophil is one of the main components affected, thus leading to the risk of neutropenic fever. Historically, bacteria have been the predominant pathogen for neutropenic fever. However, the most prevalent bacterial species isolated in patients with this condition have fluctuated through the decades, somewhat in a cyclic nature.[20–22] After the turn of the millennium, Gram-negative bacteria have emerged as the leading pathogen. Also, new bacterial species have emerged in addition to the increase in antibiotic resistance as well as the rise in invasive fungal infections (IFI).[23,24]

Current Infectious Diseases Society of America (IDSA) guidelines from 2002 stipulate that at the onset of fever in a neutropenic patient, a careful clinical exam of the perineal area and inspection of vascular access sites should be performed to exclude a focus for fever and infection. Blood cultures should then be obtained from vascular catheters and a peripheral vein as well as urine cultures and a chest X-ray. If no site of infection is identified, empiric broad-spectrum antibiotics should be started intravenously. This approach has resulted in a substantial reduction in bacteremia-associated mortality to $<5\%$ in neutropenic patients with fever. The antibiotic agents considered by IDSA as appropriate monotherapy are ceftazidime, imipenem, meropenem, and cefepime. The recommended combinations are that of broad-spectrum beta-lactams (piperacillin, ceftazidime, cefepime) or carbapenems plus an aminoglycoside (amikacin, gentamicin, tobramycin).[21]

If the patient continues to have an antibiotic-unresponsive neutropenic fever (AUNF) after 3–7 days of antibiotic therapy, there is a possibility that a fungal infection is emerging. At this point, an antimycotic agent should be started; however, there is some debate over which agent has the highest efficacy and the lowest toxicity. Liposomal amphotericin B (LAB) may be the agent of choice since it has the least toxicity while maintaining efficacy, but the data is limited.[25]

In terms of neutropenic fever prevention, the 2002 IDSA guidelines urge against prophylactic antibiotic usage. It remains to be seen whether the recommendation will change in the updated version of guidelines that is pending release in the near future.

## Growth Factors

Granulocyte (G-CSF) and granulocyte macrophage colony-stimulating factors (GM-CSF) are myeloid growth factors. G-CSF modulates the formation of granulocytes (mostly neutrophils), while GM-CSF also controls the formation of macrophages and eosinophils. The current ASCO guidelines also recommend against the general use of G-CSF as an adjunct to antibiotics, except in special, high-risk situations such as expected prolonged (>10 days) and marked ($<0.1 \times 10^9$/L) neutropenia, age >65 years, uncontrolled primary disease, multi-organ dysfunction, hypotension, pneumonia, invasive fungal infection, or being hospitalized at the time of development of a fever.[26]

A recent work by Perez Velasco conducted a literature review in order to ascertain the benefit of G-CSF in cancer patients with febrile neutropenia. The trials reviewed were heterogeneous, with a number of limitations. The majority of the studies did show a decrease in time to defervescence and an increase in absolute neutrophil count to $>0.5 \times 10^9$/L. The author of the review concluded, not dissimilarly to ASCO's recommendations, that the use of G-CSF should be reserved for use in high-risk patients.[27]

In 2007, ASCO issued a set of updated guidelines regarding the use of erythropoiesis stimulants in cancer patients with anemia.[28] Prior to initiating therapy with hematopoietic factors, it is prudent to conduct a thorough history and physical examination to rule out correctable sources of anemia that are not connected to the administration of chemotherapy. Subsequently, if all the other causes of anemia have been ruled out, and anemia indeed appears to be chemotherapy-induced, the initiation of epoetin or darbepoetin may be carried out in order to avoid a blood transfusion. ASCO considers both of the agents, i.e., epoetin and darbepoetin to be equally efficacious. The threshold hemoglobin (Hb) concentration for initiation of factor supplementation is near or below 10 g/dl. In patients with less severe anemia (i.e., Hb < 12 g/dl), clinicians should make decisions on an individual basis regarding supplementation with erythropoietic factors.

Prior to initiating administration of erythropoiesis-stimulating agents (ESAs), clinicians should carefully weigh the risk of thromboembolism against the benefits of administering an ESA. It should also be noted that the updated 2007 ASCO guidelines highlighted the black box warning issued in March of 2007: "Use of ESAs increased the risk of death when administered to a target Hb of 12 g/dl in patients with active malignant disease receiving neither chemotherapy nor radiation therapy. ESAs are not indicated in this population." Therefore, it can be concluded that the use of ESAs should be limited to patients with chemotherapy- or radiation-induced anemia.[28] In February of 2010, the FDA notified healthcare professionals that ESAs must be used under a risk evaluation and mitigation strategy (REMS) risk management program, given studies showing increased tumor growth and shortened survival in patients using these products (www.fda.gov/Safety/MedWatch/SafetyInformation/SafetyAlertsofHumanMedicalProducts/ucm200391.htm).

## Palmar-Plantar Erythrodysesthesia

Hand-foot syndrome (HFS), also known as palmar-plantar erythrodysesthesia, acral erythema, and Burgdorf reaction, is a potential adverse reaction of a number of chemotherapeutic agents. It was originally described by Zuehlke in 1974 and by Burgdorf *et al.* in 1982. The early reports associated HFS with 5-fluorouracil (5-FU), doxorubicin, and cytarabine. In the last decade, the syndrome was also described in patients taking various tyrosine kinase inhibitors.[29]

The affected areas of HFS include hands and feet, particularly the finger pads. Several clinical variants exist, and the form that presents with bullous edema is the most severe one. The timing of onset of the cutaneous manifestations is variable, ranging from 24 hours to 10 months after the beginning of treatment. Generally, the data support a correlation between a greater cumulative dose of the chemotherapeutic agent and the severity of HFS. The management of the syndrome hinges on treatment interruption. Generally, HFS resolves 2–4 weeks after discontinuation of chemotherapy. Therapy may be restarted once HFS symptoms decline to grade 0 or 1, but at a lower dose. If grade 2 toxicity recurs for the fourth time or grade 3 toxicity recurs for the third time, therapy will need to be stopped altogether.

In terms of pharmacologic agents, pyridoxine is the best studied intervention. A single randomized controlled trial by Von Gruenigen *et al.* of pyridoxine administration of 100 mg twice daily to patients receiving liposomal doxorubicin for recurrent ovarian, breast, or endometrial cancer demonstrated neither symptom improvement via the Functional Assessment of Cancer Therapy (FACT-G) nor decrease in HFS.[30] Another strategy that has been used is placement of ice packs on the extremities during the infusion of chemotherapy. A recent controlled prospective trial by Mangili *et al.*[31] of 53 patients receiving pegylated liposomal doxorubicin showed a significantly reduced rate of HFS occurrence.

## Neurotoxicity

Adverse neurotoxic events attributable to chemotherapy include both peripheral and central nervous system dysfunction. Although chemotherapy is not a common cause of encephalopathy and acute cognitive dysfunction, it nevertheless remains on the differential diagnosis.[32] Chemotherapy-related encephalopathy (transient, diffuse, delayed irreversible or posterior reversible leukoencephalopathy, PRES) has been described in patients receiving high-dose methotrexate. Also, PRES has been described in patients receiving cisplatin, 5-fluorouracil, and bevacizumab, among other agents. The clinical features of this syndrome include hypertension, headaches, seizures, altered mental status, and visual disturbances, and are coupled with MRI radiographic findings.

Further, occurrences of intracranial hemorrhages and ischemic strokes have been increasingly recognized in association with the use of angiogenic inhibitors, i.e., bevacizumab.[33]

A more commonly recognized adverse neurotoxic effect of chemotherapy is peripheral neuropathy that can be subdivided into sensory, motor, and hearing components. The most common variant of this syndrome is a length-dependent axonal sensorimotor neuropathy. The drugs causing this adverse effect are immunomodulatory agents (thalidomide, lenalidomide) or antimicrotubule agents (vinca alkaloids, epothilones, and taxanes). Grade 2–3 sensory neuropathy occurs in 25% of patients receiving platinum- and/or taxane-based regimens and is described by patients as numbness, burning, and shooting pain in the distal extremities.[32] It appears that almost a quarter of the patients afflicted with a sensorimotor neuropathy suffer from residual symptoms 48 months after the discontinuation of chemotherapy.[34,35]

Classically, the treatment for peripheral nervous system adverse effects is discontinuation of the offending drug.[32] Neuropathic pain responds poorly to opioids and is usually better managed by anticonvulsant or antidepressant agents such as gabapentin, lamotrigine, topiramate, and amitriptyline. Preventative agents such as amifostine and vitamin E have been reported by some studies to reduce the incidence of neurotoxicity. However, the data on the successful use of these agents is not robust.[36–38]

## Mucositis

It is not uncommon for high-dose chemotherapy to cause inflammation and ulcerations of the alimentary tract, otherwise known as mucositis. Certain regimens such as those containing antimetabolites and alkylating agents are associated with a higher incidence of mucositis. Oral mucositis initially presents as erythema of the oral mucosa that progresses to erosions and ulcerations. The ulcers are usually covered by a white fibrinous pseudomembrane and usually arise on the nonkeratinized surfaces (lateral and ventral tongue, buccal mucosa, and soft palate). The oral manifestations of the syndrome include erythema and ulcerations; if severe enough, this adverse reaction may necessitate dose reduction or interruption of chemotherapy. The lesions typically heal 2–4 weeks after the last dose of stomatotoxic chemotherapy.[39,40]

Over the last several years, there has been progress in understanding the pathways leading to preferential development of mucositis in certain patients who are undergoing various regimens of chemotherapy at certain sites. For example, the investigation by the German 5-FU Toxicity Study Group discovered a significant genetic association between a dihydropyrimidine dehydrogenase (DPD) splice site mutation (DPYD*2A) and onset of mucositis. The finding relates to the fact that DPD rapidly metabolizes 5-FU, and paucity of this gene product leads to increased levels of 5-FU and onset of mucositis.[41,42]

The Mucositis Study Group of the Multinational Association of Supportive Care in Cancer and the International Society of Oral Oncology (MASCC/ISOO) has isssued guidelines for the management of mucositis in 2007; the issues to be addressed include pain control, oral decontamination, and therapeutic interventions aimed to reduce severity or prevent mucositis. Pain control may require topical and systemic agents. Topical agents includes saline mouth rinses, ice chips, rinses such as Magic Mouthwash® with 2% viscous lidocaine, mixed with equal volumes of diphenhydramine and soothing agents such as aluminium hydroxide. However, more than likely, systemic opioids will be required to achieve adequate pain control.[40]

Oral decontamination and hygiene should include brushing with a soft toothbrush, flossing, and the use of saline or sodium bicarbonate rinses. There are a few biochemical and pharmacological agents and approaches that have been used to decrease or prevent mucositis. A few interventions that are pertinent to gynecologic malignancies include the use of cryotherapy, low-level laser therapy, and the use of a proprietary oral L-glutamine solution. Cryotherapy is administered by placement of ice chips in the patient's mouth five minutes before the administration of chemotherapy for a total of 30 minutes. This technique may be effective in reducing the severity of mucositis in patients receiving 5-FU, melphalan, and edatrexate. Saforis® (MGI Pharma), a solution that enhances the uptake of the amino acid L-glutamine, has been shown to reduce the incidence of oral mucositis when compared to a placebo in a phase III trial.[43] Also, the MASCC/ISOO guidelines recommend the use of low-level laser therapy if available to reduce the severity of oral mucositis. The therapeutic mechanism is not clearly understood, but may involve the reduction in the levels of reactive oxygen species and the pro-inflammatory cytokines that are involved in the progression of mucositis.[44]

## MANAGEMENT OF ASCITES AND PLEURAL EFFUSIONS

### Ascites

Malignant ascites results from widespread microscopic and macroscopic tumor infiltration of the peritoneal cavity and the peritoneum and interference with the peritoneal fluid efflux and influx. As a result, several liters of fluid accumulate in the peritoneal cavity, leading to the troublesome symptoms of pain, early satiety, nausea, fatigue, and shortness of breath. Chemotherapy may be used at the initial presentation of the patient with ascites. However, this modality is not efficacious in patients with recurrent ascites resistant to chemotherapy.[38,45,46] In such cases, paracentesis becomes the treatment of choice, but if repetitive paracentesis is required then placement of a semi-permanent drainage tube, Tenckhoff® catheter, has been FDA-approved for symptomatic relief in patients with recurrent ascites. Albumin depletion is likely to follow, but temporary comfort becomes a priority in the treatment of the terminally ill patient.[6,8,38,45,46]

Recent work by Markus M. Heiss *et al.* describes a phase II/III trial utilizing a trifunctional antibody, catumaxomab (anti-epithelial cell-adhesion molecule, EpCAM+), in the treatment of malignant ascites. The group conducted targeted immunotherapy via intraperitoneal treatment of EpCAM-positive malignant ascites secondary to epithelial cancers, including advanced ovarian cancer. The patients who received catumaxomab in conjunction with conventional paracentesis experienced longer intervals between the procedures (median of 44 versus 11 days). The most commonly reported catumaxomab-related adverse events were pyrexia, nausea, vomiting, and abdominal pain. These events were generally mild to moderate in intensity and reversible.[47] Further studies are needed in the United States to assess the utility of this compound in conjunction with paracentesis. VEGF may also be implicated in the accumulation and exacerbation of ascites as it increases vascular permeability. Therefore, VEGF antagonists can serve to reduce the accumulation of the fluid.[38]

### Pleural Effusions and Dyspnea

Especially in advanced or recurrent ovarian cancer, dyspnea may arise as a byproduct of several pathologic mechanisms acting in unison. First, pleural effusions may act as an obstruction to normal lung excursion; second, cancer cachexia, malnutrition, and weakness may contribute to decreased activity capacity; third, an increase in ventilation requirements secondary to metabolic acidosis or anemia may increase the sensation of shortness of breath.[6,8,38]

If the patient has a chemotherapy-responsive tumor, the treatment may resolve the pleural effusion. However, if a pleural effusion occurs in the setting where only palliative treatments are being utilized, the repertoire of options includes pleurodesis, thoracentesis, placement of a PleurX® catheter, and symptomatic control. Benzodiazepines and oxygen may aid with ameliorating the sensation of breathlessness. Unfortunately if the interventions listed above are not adequate, it may become necessary to alter daily activities in order to prevent the onset of dyspnea.[38,48]

## MANAGEMENT OF CHRONIC BOWEL OBSTRUCTION

Patients with advanced recurrent epithelial ovarian cancer often suffer from chronic, progressive bowel obstructions that evolve to become inoperable. Some of the classic data on disease outcomes in ovarian cancer demonstrates that intestinal obstruction occurs in 42% of the patients with terminal ovarian cancer. The disease processes contributing to this phenomenon are as follows: (1) pseudo-obstruction secondary to tumor infiltration of the muscularis and the nerve plexuses, (2) generalized carcinomatosis of the bowel and the mesentery by military tumor, (3) extrinsic occlusion of the lumen by larger recurrent tumor masses, (4) postoperative abdominal and pelvic adhesions, and (5) chronic obstruction due to prior chemotherapy or radiation. Other factors also contribute to the process, including bowel edema from inflammation, constipating

has mandated the standards of care requiring prompt assessment and management of pain for every patient.[58] The American Pain Society has put forth improvement guidelines for cancer pain management that were refined and expanded in 2005. The outline of the pain management goals centers around these key concepts: (1) involve patients and families in pain management plan; (2) improve treatment patterns; (3) reassess and adjust pain management plan as needed; and (4) monitor processes and outcomes of pain management.[59]

Cancer pain, similar to postsurgical pain, is expected to be present continuously with spikes of increased pain with movement, deep breathing and coughing, and ambulation. Successful pain management requires accurate assessment and diagnosis of the pain syndrome. Pain can generally be broken down into three main types: (1) nociceptive, i.e., aching or throbbing; (2) visceral, i.e., squeezing or cramping; and (3) neuropathic, i.e., burning, tingling, electrical sensations, or painfully numb.

Key components of pain history that need to be explored along with the customary questions regarding location(s), intensity, and aggravating and alleviating factors are as follows: the meaning of pain to the patient and the family including suffering or existential distress, cultural factors, and a detailed medication history. A history of substance abuse may alter the patient's response to pain management.[6]

A multi-dimensional, clinically useful tool that has been used extensively in patients with cancer is the Brief Pain Inventory (BPI). It includes a diagram to note the location of pain, questions regarding pain intensity, as well as tools to evaluate morbidity due to pain; the BPI is available in a number of languages.[60]

It is estimated that up to 90% of cancer pain can be adequately managed with analgesics using the World Health Organization (WHO) analgesic ladder.[59]

- Step 1: non-opioid analgesics
- Step 2: weak opioids
- Step 3: strong opioids

The staple of cancer pain management are narcotic analgesics that can be delivered via a number of routes. Equianalgesic and conversion charts should be used when switching between regimens and calculating a 24-hour narcotic requirement. In such cases, when a patient is being tried on a new regimen, it is important to decrease the dose of the novel narcotic agent by approximately 25% in order to account for non-cross-resistance. If breakthrough pain is present with the current narcotic regimen, a rescue dose may be necessary. When calculating a rescue dose, consider administering 10% of the total 24-hour narcotic requirement using a fast-acting opioid formulation, such as of oral morphine or hydromorphone (MS IR® or Hydromorph IR®) (see Table 2). Unfortunately, narcotics are almost uniformly associated with constipation, and a bowel regimen should be prescribed. In patients with significant side effects from the systemic opioids such as intolerable constipation, nausea and vomiting, and cognitive impairment, or refractory pain that is non-responsive to high-dose opioids, consideration may be given to intrathecal catheter placement in coordination with the pain management service.

Both neuropathic and bone pain syndromes often require agents other than opioids for successful management. Nonsteroidal anti-inflammatory drugs (NSAIDs) and certain antidepressant and antiepileptic medications can produce a synergistic effect when used in conjunction with narcotics. Some of the newer agents used for neuropathic and myofascial pain include duloxetine (Cymbalta®) and pregabalin (Lyrica®). Note that if pain can be linked to bone metastasis, a course of palliative radiation therapy may lead to pain relief.[59]

In terms of nonpharmacologic interventions, transcutaneous electrical nerve stimulation (TENS), massage therapy, and meditation or other biofeedback methods may be helpful adjuncts in the treatment of pain in a patient with advanced cancer.[6,9,38]

## PALLIATIVE CARE

When available curative treatment options become ineffective or futile, the goal of care changes from cure to palliation. Palliative care addresses the treatment of the patient and her entire family unit, i.e., the treatment unit. The treatment interval spans from the time that the diagnosis of advanced or incurable disease is made until the patient's death and

Table 2. Commonly used opioid analgesics.

| Brand name | Generic name | Oral dose | Parenteral dose | Oral to parenteral dose ratio | Transdermal | Duration of effect (hrs) |
|---|---|---|---|---|---|---|
| Morphine | morphine | 30 mg q3–4h | 5 mg q3–4h | 6:1 | | 4–7 |
| Roxanol® | morphine | 30 mg q4h | | | | |
| Morphine IR® | morphine | 30 mg q4h | | | | |
| Oramorph SR® | morphine | 100 mg q12h | | | | |
| MS Contin® | morphine | 100 mg q12h | | | | |
| Avinza® | morphine | 200 mg q24h | | | | |
| Kadian® | morphine | 200 mg q24h | | | | |
| Dilaudid® | hydromorphone | 5 mg q4–6h | 1 mg q4h | 5:1 | | 4–5 |
| Codeine | codeine | 30 mg q4–6h | 45 mg q4–6h | 1.5:1 | | 4–6 |
| Duragesic® | fentanyl | | | | 100 mcg q72h | 72 |
| Actiq® | fentanyl | start with 200 mcg PO × 1 prn | | | | |
| Oxycontin® | oxycodone | start with 10 mg PO q12h 60–80 mg q12h (in opiate tolerant patients) | | | | 12 |
| Dolophine® | methadone | 2.5–10 mg q8–q12h in opioid naïve patients | | | | 8–12 |

beyond. The palliative care team should be multi-faceted and include healthcare professionals with expertise from various fields such as a case manager, a home health nurse, a psychiatric nurse, a social worker, and a palliative care physician.

The success of palliative care hinges on the quality of communication between the members of the healthcare team, the patient, and the family. Optimally, the treating physician would establish a level of trust and comfort with the patient and the entire treatment unit prior to "breaking bad news", discussing poor prognosis, the issue of a living will, and other legal issues. The physician should also strive to remain up to date with the patient's prognosis and keep the directions for resuscitative measures current on the chart.

Aside from being utilized as a method for exchange of information, communication may also prove to be therapeutic and alleviate anxiety. In terms of addressing the patient's physical needs, pain control becomes a central issue accompanied by other end-of-life supportive care issues such as nutrition, fatigue, and control of secretions. Referral to a hospice service may be beneficial in order to address all of these issues with the benefit of doing so at a patient's home.[6,8,9,38]

## CACHEXIA AND MALNUTRITION

Several factors contribute to cancer-associated weight loss and malnutrition. Patients with advanced cancer syndrome often do experience decreased appetite due to depression and adverse reactions to cancer treatment. However, systemic effects of the disease, local tumor effects, alterations in nutrient metabolism, and resting energy expenditure (REE) may also contribute to nutritional status and cancer-associated malnutrition of the patient.[61] Cachexia is usually defined as weight loss of >5% of an individual's baseline body weight over 2–6 months in the setting of a chronic illness. The consequences of malnutrition include impairment of immune functions, performance status, muscle function, and quality of life. More importantly, responses to chemotherapy are decreased, chemotherapy-induced toxicity and complications are more frequent and severe, and even survival time may be compromised.[61]

Several strategies are employed by physicians in battling cancer-associated weight loss. Nutritional counseling in conjunction with a nutritional support team, the use of dietary supplements and shakes (e.g., Ensure®), and in some cases home parenteral nutrition may improve the patient's response to treatment and quality of life. Some oncologists also use appetite stimulants such as eicosapentaenoic acid (alpha omega-3 fatty acid), marijuana derivatives, or megestrol acetate (Megace®) to counteract cancer-related cachexia. Out of the three above-mentioned appetite stimulants, megestrol acetate may prove to be the most effective one. However, the practitioner should keep in mind that megestrol acetate is associated with an increased risk of venous thromboembolism.[62,63]

## SPIRITUALITY

As emphasis on quality of life has increased, the ideas of incorporating religiosity and spirituality into cancer care have grown, especially at the end of life. The National Cancer Institute defines religion as a set of beliefs and practices associated with a religion or denomination and defines spirituality as the search for ultimate meaning through other paths or religion.[64] The National Consensus Project for Quality Palliative Care has put in place national palliative care guidelines which include religion and spirituality as one of eight important clinical domains.[65] Between 50% and 90% of cancer patients view religion and spirituality as personally important and want physicians to address these needs. Balboni and associates explored quality of life, treatment preferences, and advance care planning in 230 advanced cancer patients of diverse racial and ethnic backgrounds. Interestingly, nearly half of the patients felt that their spiritual needs were minimally or not at all supported by the religious community, and 72% of patients felt that their spiritual needs were not supported by the medical community. More importantly, spiritual support was significantly associated with improved quality of life and not wanting aggressive measures to extend life.[66] Therefore, physicians should recognize the spiritual needs of patients and advocate attention to them in order for patients to better cope with their illness and improve their quality of life.

## CONCLUSION

As we learn more about the importance of quality of life components from ongoing randomized clinical trials in gynecologic oncology, oncologists are realizing the prognostic value of quality of life and the need to encourage patients to discuss supportive care issues. Thereby the oncologist can address these issues in order to improve the quality of life of patients during active treatment as well as at the end of life.

## REFERENCES

1. Center to Advance Palliative Care, www.capc.org, accessed August 1, 2010.
2. Lynn J. Sick to Death and Not Going to Take It Anymore! Reforming Health Care for the Last Years of Life. Berkeley: University of California Press, 2004, p. 72.
3. Hill RR. Clinical pharmacy services in a home-based palliative care program. *Am J Health Syst Pharm* 2007;64(8):806, 808, 810.
4. Pereira J, Bruera E. Chronic nausea. In: Bruera E, Higginson I, eds., *Cachexia-Anorexia in Cancer Patients*. New York, NY: Oxford University Press, 1996, pp. 23–37.
5. Bruera E, Seifert L, Watanabe S, *et al*. Chronic nausea in advanced cancer patients: a retrospective assessment of a metoclopramide-based antiemetic regimen. *J Pain Symptom Manage* 1996;11(3):147–153.
6. Strasser F, Bevers MW, Bruera E. Palliative care for gynecologic malignancies. In: Eifel PJ, Gershenson DM, Kavanagh JJ, Silva EG, eds., *MD Anderson Cancer Center Series: Gynecologic Cancer*. New York: Springer Science+Business Media, Inc., 2006, pp. 280–303.
7. Bruera E, Moyano JR, Sala R, *et al*. Dexamethasone in addition to metoclopramide for chronic nausea in patients with advanced cancer: a randomized controlled trial. *J Pain Symptom Manage* 2004;28(4):381–388.
8. Ramondetta LM, Fields MM, Fisch MJ. Supportive care. In: Markman M, Bast RC Jr, eds., *Ovarian Cancer*. London: Remedica Pub Ltd, 2009, pp. 185–227.
9. Rubatt JM, Boardman C, Segreti EM, *et al*. Palliative care of the patient with advanced gynecologic cancer, www.emedicine.com; updated Feb 4, 2010.
10. Schnell F. Chemotherapy-induced nausea and vomiting: the importance of acute antiemetic control. *Oncologist* 2003;8:187–198.

11. Aapro M. Optimizing antiemetic therapy: what are the problems and how can they be overcome? *Curr Med Res Opin* 2005;21:895–897.
12. Viale P. Update on the management of chemotherapy induced nausea and vomiting. *J Intraven Nurs* 2006;29:283–291.
13. Nevadunsky NS, Matulonis U. Chemotherapy-induced nausea and vomiting. *US Oncology* 5(1):10–15.
14. Poli-Bigelli S, Rodrigues-Pereira J, Carides A. Addition of the neurokinin 1 receptor antagonist aprepitant to standard antiemetic therapy improves control of chemotherapy induced nausea and vomiting. Results from a randomized, double-blind, placebo-controlled trial in patients receiving high-dose cisplatin — the Aprepitant Protocol 052 Study Group. *J Clin Oncol* 2003;21:4112–4119.
15. Gralla R, Lichinitser M, van der Vegt S, *et al.* Palonosetron improves prevention of chemotherapy-induced nausea and vomiting following moderately emetogenic chemotherapy: results of a double-blind randomized phase III trial comparing single doses of palonosetron with ondansetron. *Ann Oncol* 2003;14:1570–1577.
16. Hesketh P, Grunberg S, Gralla R. The oral neurokinin-1 antagonist aprepitant for the prevention of chemotherapy induced nausea and vomiting: A multinational, randomized, double-blind, placebo-controlled trial in patients receiving high-dose cisplatin — the Aprepitant Protocol 052 Study Group. *J Clin Oncol* 2003;97:3090–3098.
17. Caroll JK, Kohli S, Mustian KM, *et al.* Pharmacologic treatment of cancer-related fatigue. *Oncologist* 2007;12:43–51.
18. Gordon DB, Dahl J, Miaskowski C, *et al.* American pain society recommendations for improving the quality of acute and cancer pain management. *Arch Intern Med* 2005;165:1574–1580.
19. Thomas J, Karver S, Cooney GA, *et al.* Methylnaltrexone for opioid-induced constipation in advanced illness. *N Engl J Med* 2008;358:2332–2343.
20. Ellis M. Febrile neutropenia evolving strategies. *Ann NY Acad Sci* 2008;1138:329–350.
21. Hughes WT, Armstrong D, Bodey GP, *et al.* Guidelines for the use of antimicrobial agents in neutropenic patients with cancer. *Clin Infect Dis* 2002; 34:739–751.
22. Leibovici L, Paul M, Cullen M, *et al.* Antibiotic prophylaxis in neutropenic patients: new evidence, practical decisions. *Cancer* 2006;107:1743–1751.

23. de Bock R, Cometta A, Kern W, *et al.* Incidence of single agent Gram-negative bacteremias (SAGNB) in neutropenic cancer patients (NCP) in EORTC-IATG trial of empirical therapy for febrile neutropenia [abstract L-773]. In: *Program and Abstracts of the 41st Interscience Conference on Antimicrobial Agents and Chemotherapy (Chicago).* Washington DC: American Society for Microbiology, 2001.
24. Fridkin SK. The changing face of fungal infections in health care settings. *Clin Infect Dis* 2005;41:1455–1460.
25. Ostrosky-Zeichner L, Marr KA, Rex JH, Cohen SH. Amphotericin B: time for a new "gold standard". *Clin Infect Dis* 2003;37:415–425.
26. Smith TJ, Chatcheressian J, Lyman GH, *et al.* 2006 Update of recommendations for the use of white blood cell growth factors: an evidence-based clinical practice guideline. *J Clin Oncol* 2006;24(19):3187–3125.
27. Perez Velasco R. Review of granulocyte colony-stimulating factors in the treatment of established febrile neutropenia. *J Oncol Pharm Pract* 2010; doi: 10.1177/1078155210374129.
28. Rizzo JD, Somerfield MR, Hagerty KL, *et al.* Use of epoetin and darbepoetin in patients with cancer: 2007 American Society of Clinical Oncology/American Society of Hematology clinical practice guideline update. *J Clin Oncol* 2008;26(1):1–17.
29. Lipworth AD, Robert C, Zhu AX. Hand-foot syndrome (hand-foot skin reaction, palmar-plantar erythrodysesthesia): focus on sorafenib and sunitinib. *Oncology* 2009;77:257–271.
30. von Gruenigen V, Frasure H, Fusco N, *et al.* A double-blind, randomized trial of pyridoxine versus placebo for the prevention of pegylated liposomal doxorubicin-related hand-foot syndrome in gynecologic oncology patients. *Cancer* 2010;116:4735–4743.
31. Mangili G, Petrone M, Gentile C, *et al.* Prevention strategies in palmar-plantar erythrodysesthesia onset: the role of regional cooling. *Gynecol Oncol* 2008;108:332–335.
32. Chamberlain MC. Neurotoxicity of cancer treatment. *Curr Oncol Rep* 2010;12:60–67.
33. Vardy J, Wefel JS, Ahles T, *et al.* Cancer and cancer-therapy related cognitive dysfunction: an international perspective from the Venice cognitive workshop. *Ann Oncol* 2008;19:623–629.

34. Huang HQ, Brady MF, Cella D, *et al.* Validation and reduction of FACT/GOG-Ntx subscale for platinum/paclitaxel-induced neurologic symptoms: a gynecologic oncology group study. *Int J Gynecol Cancer* 2007;17(2):387–393.
35. Pignata S, de Placido S, Biamonte R, *et al.* Residual neurotoxicity in ovarian cancer patients in clinical remission after first-line chemotherapy with carboplatin and paclitaxel: the Multicenter Italian Trial in Ovarian cancer (MITO-4) retrospective study. *BMC Cancer* 2006;6:5.
36. Vielhaber A, Portenoy RK. Advances in cancer pain management. *Hematol Oncol Clin North Am* 2002;16(3):527–541.
37. Albers J, Chaudhry V, Cavaletti G, *et al.* Interventions for preventing neuropathy caused by cisplatin and related compounds. *Cochrane Database Syst Rev* 2007;(1):CD005228.
38. Chase DM, Monk BJ, Wenzel LB, Tewari KS. Supportive care for women with gynecologic cancers. *Expert Rev Anticancer Ther* 2008;8(2):227–241.
39. Lalla RV, Sonis ST, Peterson DE. Management of oral mucositis in patients who have cancer. *Dent Clin North Am* 2008;52(1):61–68.
40. Peterson DE, Lalla RV. Oral mucositis: the new paradigms. *Curr Opin Oncol* 2010;22:318–322.
41. Schwab M, Zanger UM, Marx C, *et al.* Role of genetic and nongenetic factors for fluorouracil treatment-related severe toxicity: a prospective clinical trial by the German 5-FU Toxicity Study Group. *J Clin Oncol* 2008;26:2131–2138.
42. van Kuilenburg AB, Menisma R, Zoetekouw L, *et al.* High prevalence of the IVS14 + G > A mutation in the dihydropyrimidine dehydrogenase gene of patients with severe 5-fluorouracil-associated toxicity. *Pharmacogenetics* 2002;12:555–558.
43. Peterson DE, Jones JB, Petit RG 2nd. Randomized, placebo-controlled trial of Saforis for prevention and treatment of oral mucositis in breast cancer patients receiving anthracycline-based chemotherapy. *Cancer* 2007;109(2):322–331.
44. Schubert MM, Eduardo FP, Guthrie KA, *et al.* A phase III randomized double-blind placebo controlled clinical trial to determine the efficacy of low level laser therapy for the prevention of oral mucositis in patients undergoing hematopoietic cell transplantation. *Support Care Cancer* 2007;15:1145–1154.
45. Ayhan A, Gultekin M, Taskiran C, *et al.* Ascites and epithelial ovarian cancers: a reappraisal with respect to different aspects. *Int J Gynecol Cancer* 2007;17:68–75.

46. Smith EM, Jayson GC. The current and future management of malignant ascites. *Clin Oncol (R Coll Radiol)* 2003;15:59–72.
47. Heiss MM, Murawa P, Koralewski P, *et al.* The trifunctional antibody catumaxomab for the treatment of malignant ascites due to epithelial cancer: results of a prospective randomized phase II/III trial. *Int J Cancer* 2010;127:2209–2221.
48. Ripamonti C. Management of dyspnea in advanced cancer patients. *Support Care Cancer* 1999;7(4):233–243.
49. Roeland E, von Guten CF. Current concepts in malignant bowel obstruction management. *Curr Oncol Rep* 2009;11(4):298–303.
50. Mercandante S, Ripamonti C, Casuccio A, *et al.* Comparison of octreotide and hyoscine butylbromide in controlling gastrointestinal symptoms due to malignant inoperable bowel obstruction. *Support Care Cancer* 2000; 8:188–191.
51. van Ooijen B, van der Burg ME, Planting AS, *et al.* Surgical treatment of gastric drainage only for intestinal obstruction in patients with carcinoma of the ovary or peritoneal carcinomatosis of other origin. *Surg Gynecol Obstet* 1993;176(5):469–474.
52. Caceres A, Zhou Q, Iasonos A, *et al.* Colorectal stents for palliation of large bowel obstructions in recurrent gynecologic cancer: an updated series. *Gynecol Oncol* 2008;108(3):482–485.
53. Clarke-Pearson DL. Surgical management of intestinal obstruction in ovarian cancer. I. Clinical features, postoperative complications, and survival. *Gynecol Oncol* 1987;26(1):11–18.
54. Redman CW. Survival following intestinal obstruction in ovarian cancer. *Eur J Surg Oncol* 1988;14(5):383–386.
55. Caprotti R. Palliative surgery for recurrent bowel obstruction due to advanced ovarian cancer. *Minerva Ginecol* 2006;58(3):239–244.
56. Kucukmetin A, Naik R, Galaal K, *et al.* Palliative surgery versus medical management for bowel obstruction in ovarian cancer (Review). *Cochrane Database Syst Rev* 2010;(7):CD007792.
57. Mangili G, Aletti G, Frigerio L, *et al.* Palliative care for intestinal obstruction in recurrent ovarian cancer: a multivariate analysis. *Int J Gynecol Cancer* 2005;15:830–835.
58. JCAHO. *Comprehensive Hospital Accreditation Manual.* Oakbrook Terrace, IL, 2001.

59. Mercadante S. Pain treatment and outcomes for patients with advanced cancer who receive follow-up care at home. *Cancer* 1999;85:1849–1858.
60. Cleeland CS, Ryan KM. Pain assessment: global use of the Brief Pain Inventory. *Ann Acad Med Singapore* 1994;23(2):129–138.
61. Cutsem EV, Arends J. The causes and consequences of cancer-associated malnutrition. *Eur J Oncol Nurs* 2005;9:S51–63.
62. Femia RA, Goyette RE. The science of megestrol acetate delivery: potential to improve outcomes in cachexia. *BioDrugs* 2005;19(3):179–187.
63. Bernstein EG, Ortiz Z. Megestrol acetate for the treatment of anorexia-cachexia syndrome. *Cochrane Database Syst Rev* 2005;2:CD004310.
64. National Cancer Institute. Spirituality in Cancer Care. http://www.cancer.gov/cancertopics/pdq/supportivecare/spirituality
65. National Consensus Project. The Development of Clinical Cancer Practice Guidelines for Quality Palliative Care. http://www.nationalconsensusproject.org/
66. Balboni TA, Vanderwerker LC, Block SD, *et al.* Religiousness and spiritual support among advanced cancer patients and associations with end-of-life treatment preferences and quality of life. *J Clin Oncol* 2007;25(5):555–560.

# INDEX